"With *The Adrenal Thyroid Revolution*, Dr. Romm guides readers on a profound journey of transformational healing. Not only do we realize that our fears are misguided but, further, Dr. Romm reveals a clear path to leaving our symptoms behind and living to our highest potential."

—Gabrielle Bernstein, #1 *New York Times* bestselling author

"It has never been more critical to develop insight into the vital importance of adrenal and thyroid health. Now, in the era of patient-directed healing, Dr. Aviva Romm brings you a powerful, easy-to-use guide to begin your journey toward your most empowered self."

—Kelly Brogan, M.D., holistic women's health psychiatrist and author of *A Mind of Your Own*

"Initially, before my Graves' diagnosis, I was brushed off by my doctor as just being stressed out. Dr. Romm is an outstanding physician and a voice of hope for all of us women who are not being heard by conventional medicine."

—Amy Myers, M.D., author of *The Thyroid Connection* and *The Autoimmune Solution*

"Prescription-based remedies for thyroid and adrenal issues focus on short-term, symptom-based fixes. Gratefully, Dr. Romm reveals how specific lifestyle choices incorporated into a cohesive and encompassing program can address what actually underlies these issues, paving the way for radical improvement and taking back your health."

—David Perlmutter, M.D., board-certified neurologist, fellow of the American College of Nutrition, and author of *Grain Brain* and *The Grain Brain Whole Life Plan*

"*The Adrenal Thyroid Revolution* is the beginning of a new era in women's health where women can finally stop accepting exhaustion, brain fog, extra weight, and emotional imbalance as the norm and take more control of their health and well-being."

—Frank Lipman, M.D., *New York Times* bestselling author of
The New Health Rules

"Aviva Romm has helped thousands of women silently suffering from 'medically unexplained symptoms' that dramatically decrease the quality of life. This empowering new book will give you a plan to uncover what is at the root of these confusing health problems and show you how to love your body again."

—Vani Hari, founder of Foodbabe.com and *New York Times*
bestselling author of *The Food Babe Way*

"Don't live one more day heading down an unhealthy and unnecessary path. Buy this book, and let Dr. Aviva Romm remind you how good you deserve to feel and teach you how to find the balance and health your body, mind, and spirit are craving."

—Danielle DuBoise and Whitney Tingle, founders of Sakara

THE
ADRENAL THYROID REVOLUTION

THE
ADRENAL THYROID REVOLUTION

A Proven 4-Week Program to Rescue Your
Metabolism, Hormones, Mind & Mood

AVIVA ROMM, M.D.

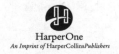

HarperOne
An Imprint of HarperCollinsPublishers

HarperOne

Image on page 65 by isaree | Shutterstock.

This book contains advice and information relating to health care. It should be used to supplement rather than replace the advice of your doctor or another trained health professional. If you know or suspect you have a health problem, it is recommended that you seek your physician's advice before embarking on any medical program or treatment. All efforts have been made to ensure the accuracy of the information contained in this book as of the date of publication. The publisher and the author disclaim liability for any medical outcomes that may occur as a result of applying the methods suggested in this book.

THE ADRENAL THYROID REVOLUTION. Copyright © 2017 by Aviva Romm, M.D. All rights reserved. Printed in the United States of America. No part of this book may be used or reproduced in any manner whatsoever without written permission except in the case of brief quotations embodied in critical articles and reviews. For information, address HarperCollins Publishers, 195 Broadway, New York, NY 10007.

HarperCollins books may be purchased for educational, business, or sales promotional use. For information, please email the Special Markets Department at SPsales@harpercollins.com.

FIRST HARPERCOLLINS PAPERBACK EDITION PUBLISHED IN 2019

Designed by Ad Librum

Library of Congress Cataloging-in-Publication Data is available upon request.

ISBN 978-0-06-247635-7

22 23 LSC(H) 10 9 8 7 6

To all women who have felt unseen and unheard,
you are not invisible and you are not alone.
To all who have been told "It's all in your head," it is not.
And to all who have felt like you've been
sleeping for too long, rise and shine.
Let's move mountains together.

When sleeping women wake, mountains move.

—Chinese proverb

Contents

THE
ADRENAL THYROID
REVOLUTION

INTRODUCTION
Feel Like Yourself Again

My mission in life is not merely to survive,
but to thrive, and to do so with some passion,
some compassion, some humor, and some style.
—MAYA ANGELOU

I DIDN'T GO INTO MEDICINE thinking I'd specialize in women's adrenal or thyroid function. I knew a great deal about the importance of these glands in women's health, but did not anticipate that they would play a central role in my medical practice. However, the unexplained symptoms my patients were experiencing, and the difficulties they'd experienced trying to get answers about their symptoms and conditions, brought the adrenals and thyroid to the center of my attention.

While I was seeing women with all of the concerns an integrative family doctor expects, from weight problems to headaches, high cholesterol to hormonal imbalances, I found that almost all of my patients had clusters of symptoms in common that weren't technically related—at least according to the way conventional medicine works. They were worrisome symptoms, too, not only to them, but also to me, because I knew that many of them were signs of chronic inflammation that heralded potentially more serious chronic disease in their future. Some had already progressed to those chronic diseases.

More than 80 percent were fatigued. Sometimes it was minor, causing them to rely on caffeine and sugar to get them through the day, but many were struggling with severe exhaustion, which affected their daily functioning and their ability to care for their families, perform at work, and enjoy their lives. The vast majority weren't sleeping well—some were unable to fall asleep, others were waking up in the night, and many woke in the morning wanting to pull the covers back over their heads because they were still exhausted. Most needed a coffee or two to get their day going. About a third were taking, or had recently been prescribed, a medication for depression, anxiety, or sleep—or all three.

Memory and concentration problems were common, even in women as young as their twenties, leading quite a few to express concerns about early dementia. Not only were weight and body image a problem, but so were signs of metabolic syndrome, a serious condition of prediabetes, high cholesterol, belly fat, and high blood pressure, even in women in their thirties and forties. Digestive troubles including constipation, reflux, bloating, and irritable bowel syndrome (IBS) were typical.

Most shocking was the number of women I was seeing with autoimmune conditions. Previously considered rare, at least one in eight of my patients came to me with at least one autoimmune condition, whether rheumatoid arthritis, Sjögren's syndrome, Crohn's disease, psoriasis, celiac disease, or, most commonly, Hashimoto's thyroiditis.

Almost all of my patients were perpetually overwhelmed, with a relentless sense of stress and dread over their never-ending to-do list of personal, professional, and family responsibilities, unable to carve out time for self-care, or even to prepare and eat regular meals. My patients were seeking my care for what is now increasingly called "the Western cluster"—a twenty-first-century set of chronic symptoms and frighteningly common medical conditions that in the past decade has become "the new normal." Overall, my patients felt sick, tired, frazzled, and foggy, and they didn't know why. Over and over I heard patients say, "Dr. Romm, I just want to feel like myself again."

Woman after woman came to me after having been seen by sometimes as many as five or more physicians and specialists who had no answers for them other than what could be written on a prescription pad—often a recommendation for an antidepressant—leaving them feeling alone, confused, unheard, and without solutions to the very real symptoms that were impacting the quality of their lives.

This book began in response to the needs of these women for a deeper understanding of what was going on with their health, and a much-needed way of preventing and reversing this Western cluster. *The Adrenal Thyroid Revolution* brings you the same plan that I developed for the women in my practice and that I use daily. I bring it to you because you also deserve to have the answers you need to feel at home in your body. This program is designed to reverse the symptoms that are keeping you from feeling your best, reversing the symptom overload that is keeping you from feeling your best and helping you get from depleted to replenished.

The Adrenal Thyroid Revolution focuses on two systems—the adrenal and thyroid glands—that are often the most overdriven and overwhelmed in a woman's body. The overwhelm of these important organs is the result of multiple influences on your health that you'll soon understand and learn to change.

Why a revolution? Because it's about time for a change in women's health care, and the medical profession needs to sit up and listen to what we're saying. Not only are women suffering needlessly, but too many are being dismissed, ignored, and disrespected. Women's lives are at stake, and it does not have to be this way. *It should not be this way.* This book offers a revolutionary new way to think about your health: it's that you can live energized and symptom-free, instead of feeling frustrated with, or even betrayed by, your body. And it puts the tools you need to take back your health right into your hands. That's revolutionary.

The solution you're about to discover will strengthen and balance multiple systems in your body by healing the root imbalances that are impacting you the most. It will show you how to make simple, powerful, and sustainable food and lifestyle changes that ease toxic multisystem overload and bring you into a symptom-free life with renewed energy. I've helped thousands of women transform their health and lives, and I'd love to help you, too.

WOMEN NOT SEEN, NOT HEARD

In medical school, I was taught to diagnose and treat an incredibly long list of diseases. I studied under some of the world's most brilliant and influential doctors at one of the most prestigious medical institutions. Yet somehow, the top concerns leading women to seek medical care—fatigue, chronic overwhelm, problems with memory and focus, hormonal imbalances, insomnia, depression, anxiety, and stubborn weight—were not being addressed in our medical education, beyond teaching us what drugs might relieve the symptoms. No connection was made between these various symptoms and their causes, other than to say it was genetic, or "all in the patient's head," and there was no discussion about why increasing numbers of women were suffering from these seemingly disparate symptoms. Like you perhaps are, my patients were among the tens of millions of women struggling with a complex array of confusing symptoms. Many had been dismissed with "medically unexplained symptoms" or treated as "difficult patients."

Let me introduce you to just a few of the women I've worked with whose symptoms had been dismissed or overlooked by their doctors, and for whom my program has made a world of difference.

Bethany: Running on Empty and Paying the Price

Bethany, at forty-seven, was so tired that she was pumping herself up with coffee and sugary snacks all day to keep going. By 4:00 P.M. she was already longing for the moment when she could get her kids into bed and crash for the night. Diagnosed with high cholesterol, high blood pressure, and prediabetes—which together are called metabolic syndrome—she was at high risk for heart disease, and her primary care doctor recommended that she start a cholesterol-lowering (statin) drug. She didn't want to, but she was worried because even after doing a restrictive detox program, and diligently going to a spin class five mornings a week, she hadn't been able to lose more than a few of the thirty-five extra pounds she'd put on after her fourth child was born five years before. Her TSH—an important thyroid lab—had doubled in the past year, indicating that she had hypothyroidism, but her doctor had assured her that her thyroid was normal. He'd chalked up her symptoms to fatigue from being a busy mom.

Using the program you'll find in part 2 of this book, Bethany was able to receive proper thyroid testing, which led to a proper diagnosis and treatment, and a complete turnaround in her energy. She was able to get off of the sugar and caffeine roller coaster, and over a few months, her cholesterol normalized and she returned to close to her prebaby weight.

Liz: Foggy, Groggy, and Hormonally Imbalanced

Liz, at thirty-nine, wanted to start a family, so was coming in for hormonal advice. Her hormone struggle began in her twenties and included severe PMS and endometriosis. Liz was now struggling to get pregnant. On top of that, she felt so exhausted that she needed to rest between seeing patients in her graduate nursing studies, and she couldn't seem to concentrate on her studies, describing a feeling of "brain fog." She was worried about whether she'd be too physically tired and mentally unfocused to be a good nurse, or mom, should she eventually have a baby.

After following my program for only a few months, Liz was able to become pregnant, and is now the mother of a lovely little girl, for whom she is able to provide the level of attention and care she'd hoped for due to her improved energy and focus.

Anna: Fatigued and Frustrated, and a Hidden Diagnosis

Anna, thirty-six, became so fatigued six months prior to coming to see me that she'd had to cut back to half of her work hours at a job she'd been at full-time with no problem for more than a decade. She'd gained twenty-eight pounds in that time, though she hadn't changed her diet at all. After meals she looked six months pregnant due to bloating. She was frustrated with her exhaustion and appearance, and had just been diagnosed with an autoimmune condition: Hashimoto's thyroiditis.

Once Anna began my program, she recognized gluten as a dietary trigger for many of her symptoms. We cut gluten from her diet and used the SOS Solution to further heal her gut and eventually reverse her Hashimoto's thyroiditis diagnosis. Anna dropped the weight that was a result of over-whelming inflammation and thyroid problems, and regained her energy.

Debra: Strain, Pain, and Feeling Older Than Her Age

Debra, in her late fifties, felt that she had suddenly gone from vibrant and energetic to exhausted, old, and flabby. She, too, had gained weight—twenty pounds over the past three months—and had trouble focusing on her work as an accountant. She wasn't sleeping well and suffered from a variety of unexplained aches, pains, and digestive symptoms, including constipation. When Debra came to me, she'd already seen several doctors who had given her a host of diagnoses and a list of medications to match. "I just want to feel like myself again, Dr. Romm," she said. "I feel like I'm eighty years old."

Shortly after starting the program, Debra was able to sleep and her joint pain improved. She experienced more mobility and more energy, and her old self began to return as she learned to eat in a way that prevented and reduced inflammation, especially by learning to avoid foods that had been hidden triggers for her.

It's hard to imagine that before trying the SOS Solution, Bethany, Liz, Anna, and Debra were told to accept their symptoms as facts of life. Yet dismissal by the medical system is nothing new for women. It's based on centuries-old biases that persist and pervade the institution and practice of medicine today. "Hysteria," which stems from the Greek word for uterus, *hystera*, was a medical *diagnosis* given to "unstable" women as recently as the early 1900s. "Hypochondriac" is another word historically ascribed to women with "complaints" that have no "diagnosable" physical basis. Women are far more likely than men to have a missed diagnosis or be undertreated. It can take five or more years for women dealing with chronic symptoms related to fatigue, memory and focus issues, aches and pains, hormonal problems, and more to even receive a proper diagnosis. Sadly, because so many women have experienced being rebuffed, made to feel small, like a complainer, "difficult"—or like a hypochondriac—in a doctor's office, we've also stopped seeking medical care, sometimes even when we need it for serious medical conditions.

You, too, may have seen several doctors attempting to understand why you feel the way you do, and what you can do to feel better. Like millions of women, you may have left your doctor's office without solutions. With an average doctor visit lasting fifteen minutes or less, this isn't surprising. I've had patients who were told their symptoms were the result of unlucky genes, just a normal part of life, the result of menopause or aging (I had a patient in her twenties whose doctor told her this!), and that they should just accept it. Perhaps, like so many of my patients, you were told that your symptoms result from your own habits; for example, if you would eat less and exercise more, you'd be able to lose weight. Chances are you were offered a prescription for an antidepressant, antianxiety medication, or another pharmaceutical. More than a few women have confided their fear that their symptoms were really in their heads since they'd heard that so many times from a practitioner, and nobody can find "anything wrong" with them.

The fact that you've picked up this book tells me that you still have hope for a natural solution and a different approach. I'm so glad, because that is why I've written it. I've worked with so many women who have transformed their health with the steps I share in this book, and it all starts with the first step you've already taken: being here! While your symptoms seem like a big, unrelated mess, I assure you, they are not. In the following chapters I'll show you exactly how they are connected by *Root Causes* that are preventable—and reversible—and I'll finally dispel the notion that this is all in your head.

Let me repeat that: *Your symptoms are not all in your head. You are not crazy.*

Recognizing, understanding, and treating your symptoms at their roots, as you will soon learn to do, will bring you a lasting solution and is the key to sustained energy and vitality.

SYSTEM OVERWHELM LEADS TO SYMPTOM OVERLOAD

Since you have picked up this book, chances are you're struggling with one or more of the following symptoms: fatigue, memory or focus issues, anxiety, depression, or your weight—unsure why you've been gaining it, or why you can't lose it regardless of how strictly you diet or how hard you exercise. Sleep may be evading you, worsening your mood and focus, yet you're still having to function during the day, driving you to coffee, sugar, or other "pick-me-ups" just to keep up your energy and attention.

On top of this you may be struggling with hormonal problems such as PMS, polycystic ovarian syndrome (PCOS), endometriosis, fertility problems, or acne. Perchance you're wrestling with one or more accompanying symptoms: digestive problems, chronic headaches and migraines, regular illness, cold sores, urinary infections, seasonal allergies, or food intolerances.

Further, irritable bowel syndrome, chronic fatigue syndrome, fibromyalgia, rheumatoid arthritis, or an autoimmune condition such as Hashimoto's thyroiditis may be putting a damper on your life. Perhaps you've already been diagnosed with high blood pressure, high cholesterol, insulin resistance, metabolic syndrome, or diabetes and want to reverse it.

You may have only a few of these symptoms, or like most of my patients, five or more. You, too, may have had to miss work or beg off from activities you wish you could do; or sometimes have been too exhausted to play with your kids, or go out with your partner or girlfriends. You, like so many of the women I've worked with, may be trying to look like you're coping, when you feel like you're hanging on by a thread.

From the perspective of conventional medicine, the disparate symptoms women are experiencing don't fit neatly into a diagnosis, but I knew there had to be an explanation. So I asked myself: What's really going on here? What's similarly affecting so many women from so many different backgrounds? Why are so many women experiencing symptom overload? What core or underlying imbalances could be at the root? It wasn't long before I connected the dots.

IT'S ALL CONNECTED

My thirty years of experience as a midwife and herbalist taught me to guide women in holistic lifestyle changes, not just reach for a prescription pad as the first and only way to help my patients. Midwifery and herbal medicine are predicated on the beliefs that the body possesses its own innate healing wisdom, that the human organism intrinsically wants to move toward repair and wellness, that there is no separation between mind and body, that the human body is an interconnected whole rather than separate systems, and that chronic disease doesn't begin at the time of a diagnosis but, with rare exception, is the result of a combination of cumulative factors that eventually tip the balance away from health and toward disease.

These ideas are not new (though my solutions are!), nor is the mind-body-health connection "woo-woo" philosophy. Twenty-five years of hard science has now emerged from the field of *psychoneuroimmunology* (PNI; the study of the interconnectedness of the immune, nervous, and endocrine systems) that unequivocally demonstrates the connections between stress and our emotions, immunity, mood, cognitive function, and hormones. As I began exploring this phenomenon more deeply, I found myself revisiting the first PNI book I ever read to help me connect the dots on what was really going on.

I'd first read *Why Zebras Don't Get Ulcers*, by MacArthur Genius Award winner and Stanford University neuroendocrinology professor Robert Sapolsky in 1998. Sapolsky draws vastly on science demonstrating not only the physiologic interconnectedness of what appear to be separate body systems and symptoms, but also the impact of a variety of forms of stress on the human body as a result of their triggering a primitive survival system, called the hypothalamic pituitary adrenal axis (HPA axis), which controls the *stress response*. This axis begins in your brain and extends throughout your body, connecting your nervous system, immune system, and digestive and circulatory systems, via cascades of chemical and hormonal messengers. Disruption in any area can and does lead to any—and all—of the symptoms and conditions my patients were struggling with.

I knew I'd hit on the heart of the problem, and over time it led to the development of the program I use in my practice—and that I bring to you in this book.

ARE YOU IN SOS?

The HPA axis controls a relatively short-lived stress response lasting minutes to hours. It's not supposed to be activated as often as it is for most of us today, which is repeatedly or chronically each day, due to the stress of modern living. When activated, this system puts us into "survival mode" to protect us from immediate threats to our safety—from infection to food scarcity to animal attacks, to name just a few. But the brain doesn't readily differentiate between perceived danger, or danger that isn't truly life-threatening—for example, bills that need to be paid, or phone calls, texts, and emails that must be answered—and real and immediate threats such as a tractor trailer veering into your lane, your company downsizing and you wondering if you'll still have a job in a few weeks, or the greater global stresses and concerns we're all facing. So this system remains in a persistent state of high alert, as if it's stuck in the ON position, and we become chronically triggered to remain in survival mode.

From the perspective of psychoneuroimmunology, what I saw in my patients suddenly made sense. When the HPA axis is activated, a complex set of responses ensues, allowing your body to survive the hazard. These include acutely heightened mental hyperawareness, ramped-up blood sugar and insulin release, and immune system stimulation. At the same time, energy is diverted away from important but less immediately pressing functions such as digestion and reproduction. It is these responses, and others that are related and that you'll soon learn about, that when chronically triggered are responsible for both the symptoms and the medical conditions so many women are facing and that this book is dedicated to helping you reverse.

Most of my patients easily related to the idea that they were living in chronic survival mode. In fact, quite a few of my patients had said just that to me. So I began to call the connection between chronic overwhelm and the downstream impacts on health *Survival Overdrive Syndrome*, or *SOS*.

But even after coining the term, I knew I was still missing an important connection. While many of my patients had gone through an obviously high-stress period of time before they started having symptoms, or had more than average stress in their lives, some did not. Yet, in spite of the lack of significant mental or emotional stress, they, too, had chronic symptoms and illnesses that smacked of SOS. So I investigated further. What was the dot I still needed to connect? Why were these women, too, showing the same SOS symptoms?

MORE THAN A FEELING

A deep dive into the science of the stress response led me to some intriguing discoveries. The most important was that it's not only chronic emotional and mental stress that can trigger SOS. It's any of a number of triggers that behave as stressors, overwhelming our naturally self-corrective internal healing systems. It was reversing these triggers in my patients that really began to produce big results consistently and that became part of the core of my SOS Solution. These triggers include chronic inflammation, exposure to environmental toxins and underfunctioning internal detoxification systems, lack of sleep, dietary triggers, blood sugar imbalances, disruptions in gut health, and even viral infections that my patients didn't realize they were harboring.

THE ROOTS OF IMBALANCE

What we call symptoms—and even diseases—are surface manifestations of what's going on at a deeper, less obvious level in the body, the hidden *roots*, or *Root Causes*, of health problems. There are five Root Causes that get your stress response into overdrive, leading to system overload and Survival Overdrive Syndrome:

1. **Chronic emotional and mental stress:** when the daily stuff of life never turns off or leaves you no time to hit the pause button and take care of yourself or to get proper sleep

2. **Food triggers:** foods that might be causing hidden inflammation, nutrients your body might be missing that you need for healing, and blood sugar ups and downs that get your stress response going

3. **Gut imbalances:** damage to your gut lining or your microbiome from food triggers, stress, and certain medications

4. **Toxic overload:** household, food, and environmental exposures as well as underfunctioning natural detoxification processes due to nutrient insufficiencies and poor elimination

5. **Stealth infections:** new infections or reactivation of prior infections, usually viral in origin, that activate your immune system chronically

When you address the Root Causes by removing the obstacles to your body's innate healing responses and adding in the important healing elements your body needs, your body begins to recalibrate naturally. Science is on our side: it has been shown that even simple lifestyle and dietary changes can prevent and reverse most of your symptoms and some very real diseases, including 93 percent of diabetes, 81 percent of heart attacks, 50 percent of strokes, and 36 percent of all cancers. These same changes will boost your energy, relieve brain fog, balance your hormones, help you lose weight, and do so much more.

OUT OF SURVIVAL MODE: THE SOS SOLUTION

I formulated the SOS Solution, which you'll discover in part 2 of this book, to remove the hidden influences that are keeping you sick and tired, preventing you from getting back to your best self, and to help you replace the important elements your body needs for wellness. My program is based on two core philosophies:

1. Your body is innately wise and wants to move toward balance and health.

2. We simply have to remove what is harming you, and supply the missing elements your body needs for healing.

Unlike so many programs that restrict practically everything, the SOS Solution gives you a life blueprint for nourishment and enjoyment. No deprivation here! You just have to *give your body what it needs*, including the right nutrients and lifestyle habits, and *remove the obstacles*—the Root Causes—that lead to SOS. I know that sounds crazily simple, but actually that's all it takes, along with a commitment to waking up your inner healer.

In as short as two weeks after starting the SOS Solution, I've watched my patients lose up to twelve pounds, lose inches around their waists, and drop clothing sizes. Brain fog clears up—as one patient said, "Dr. Romm, I feel like someone turned the windshield wipers on in my brain and I can think clearly again." Cravings for sugar and junk food disappear. Digestion improves. My patients sleep better, and they feel more calm and energized than they have sometimes in years. They look younger, too, because their cells are getting nourished, making their skin healthier and more vibrant. I've seen chronic, even long-standing joint aches and pains clear up in a matter of two weeks, diabetes reversed, and autoimmune conditions that are supposed to be "incurable" go into complete remission. All of this happens because my patients have begun to crack the code on what's keeping them sick and tired. And what's amazing is that because they see the benefits of the plan, they love and stick with it as a lifestyle.

In the SOS Solution I teach you how to take back your health with antidotes to the Root Causes—the five solutions that can have a major impact in as soon as two to four weeks. I like to think of this plan as the start of the best rest of your life.

Here's what you'll be doing:

Reboot: Upleveling your diet is the biggest needle mover toward health. In a 21-Day Reboot you'll learn which foods are SOS triggers for most women, and which are unique triggers for *you*, allowing you to personalize your program. You'll also have some fun doing a pantry, medicine cabinet, and body products detox to eliminate hidden exposures that can be causing havoc in your hormones, mind, immune system, thyroid, and more. You'll also learn to balance your blood sugar and replace the nutrients most women are missing and that your body can't heal without.

Reframe: It's not just our diets and homes that get a detox in the SOS Solution—you're going to learn to shift your mindset from one that's keeping you stressed out, anxious, and overwhelmed to one that gives you enough time and energy to live your life more sanely. Yes, that really is possible. You'll learn to let go of beliefs and behaviors that can be holding you back in a big way from a much easier life. Examples include Perfectionism, Good-Girl Syndrome, and FOMO (Fear of Missing Out). I'm also going to help you renew your relationship with one of your best friends—good sleep—and teach you how to get into the You Zone.

Repair: In chapter 6 we'll work, step-by-step, through healing the multiple systems involved in SOS—your digestive, immune, hormonal, and detoxification systems. Using the latest information on the safest and most effective nutritional and botanical supplements, you are going to revitalize these systems so they work for—not against—you, with the necessary steps for reversing SOS and healing your adrenals and thyroid.

Recharge: In chapter 7 you'll learn the secrets of directly recharging your adrenal and thyroid glands with the help of herbs, supplements, and natural energy boosts that really work. I'll also teach you which thyroid tests you need to uncover a hidden thyroid problem, the treatments that really make a difference, when thyroid hormone supplementation is necessary, how to work with your doctor to choose the right supplement at the right dose for *you*, and all the other adrenal-thyroid information you've been wanting to know but didn't have anyone to ask.

Replenish: Once you've finished Rebooting, Reframing, Repairing, and Recharging, you'll be well on your way to feeling Replenished. You'll use your personally tailored dietary information to move forward with a long-term sustainable plan for optimal vitality. The Replenish Lifestyle is a real-food, energy-boosting, fat-burning version of the Mediterranean diet, full of fantastic foods (including chocolate and guacamole!) that you (and your entire family) can enjoy. You'll learn how to keep your energy tank full, never letting yourself live on fumes again.

#TAKEBACKYOURHEALTH

Being plagued by a host of chronic symptoms is not inevitable and does not have to be your fate. You do not have to be relegated to a life of pills for every ill or a life of symptoms and disease. *Your body has the ability to heal beyond what you've ever been led to believe, and you have much more control over your health than you have ever been taught.* There is an explanation for why you feel sick and tired. It is not just normal aging or bad genes. But you have to give your body the ingredients it needs to mobilize its self-healing responses—daily.

That's why I've written this book. I've taken everything I've learned based on decades of research in natural medicine, and now more than ten years of research in psychoneuroimmunology, adrenal, and thyroid health, along with experience helping patients every day in my medical practice, and have put it into your hands, with easy explanations that will help you feel empowered and be successful. As one of the world's most sought-after experts on women's botanical medicine and nutrition, I am also uniquely qualified to provide you with this guidance. I'm going to give you a plan that will remove the trial and error you may be going through trying differ- ent supplements, herbs, and thyroid medications, and remove the dietary and nutritional guesswork and the challenge of identifying and reducing environmental triggers. This plan *is* the new medicine for women, and it's based on nourishment, self-care, and personal empowerment. It's about recharging your batteries—and keeping them recharged.

It's specifically meant to not overwhelm you or be "one more thing to do." It's meant to be an adventure—the best thing you can do for yourself starting right now. You're going to love how you feel.

Say what, Dr. Romm? I can do this in just four weeks?

Yes! If you let me join you for just twenty-eight days of your life, we'll work wonders together. My patients do, and you can, too. Getting healthy doesn't have to be hard. This is a gentle, achievable, supportive plan that is—at last—going to give you the results you've been looking for.

So let's get going on the four weeks that are the new start to the rest of your life!

The journey of a thousand miles begins with a single step.

Part 1

THE ROOTS OF SOS

YOUR BODY AND BRAIN ARE SENDING OUT AN SOS

*Viewed from the perspective of the evolution of the animal
kingdom, sustained psychological stress is a recent invention,
mostly limited to humans and other social primates.*

—ROBERT SAPOLSKY

BARBARA SAT DOWN with a heavy sigh. She looked defeated.

"Dr. Romm, I'm exhausted all the time, and these cravings are driving me nuts. Nuts and chocolate and chips, more accurately," she said with a wry smile. "I'm constantly fighting an inner battle over food. I've been dieting for years and haven't lost a pound. Honestly, I hate my body most of the time, and it's not just my weight. It feels like I'm always chasing off a cold or a yeast infection. And now I have arthritis in my knees. Life is so overwhelming, and just when I think I'm gaining control, something throws me off."

At forty-five, Barbara had metabolic syndrome, a prediabetic condition with high blood pressure, high cholesterol, and high blood sugar. Her conventional doctor had nothing more to offer her than drugs for these serious problems, and painkillers and surgery for her knee pain. She didn't like the idea of becoming dependent on medications. "I'm only forty-five and already have so many problems. You'd think I was an old lady!"

Barbara is not alone. Every day women visit my practice feeling defeated. They're overwhelmed and frazzled, not sleeping well, getting sick more often than they expect to, and even when they're not sick, feel they're operating at 50 percent of their best. They have trouble losing weight and can't stick to a diet or kick their sugar habit. They feel they have no willpower. They feel stuck in overdrive. They're in survival mode, and life feels out of control.

That day in my office, I asked Barbara a question: "How do you *want to feel?*"

"Nobody's ever asked me that before," she said with tears in her eyes. "I'm just so overwhelmed by everything in my life. I'm pretty sure my teenagers hate me. They just ignore me, and my daughter is struggling with anxiety. My husband, bless his heart. He's patient, but I'm pushing him away. I never want to be intimate with him because I don't feel sexy. I'm always overwhelmed and feel like my health is completely out of control."

"Yes. That's a lot," I said, leaning toward her. "So, how do you want to feel?" I asked her again, gently but firmly.

"I just want to feel like myself again, I want my life back, I want to remember what feeling good feels like. And," she added, "I don't want to go down this road of pills and surgery. I want to be healthy and really live my life."

Like Barbara, many of my patients arrive with symptoms mirroring a disturbing and growing trend in the health of women throughout the United States over the past couple of decades. Here are just a few of the troubling statistics:

Stress, poor sleep, and overwhelm: According to the Annual Stress Survey by the American Psychological Association, 75 percent of women experience moderate to severe stress, 49 percent report sleep problems, and more than 40 percent report physical symptoms as a direct result of stress. Recent studies show that most are also experiencing chronic overwhelm and exhaustion. Millions of women take a sleep medication nightly, and many more "on occasion." Frighteningly, stress, poor sleep, and chronic overwhelm can set the stage for future heart disease and cancer. Women—especially women who have to juggle multiple roles—feel the effects of it, sometimes in the form of a long list of symptoms and a variety of illnesses.

Obesity: Thirty-four percent of adults age twenty years or over are overweight, 34 percent are obese, and 6 percent are extremely obese. Between ages twenty and sixty, women are much more likely to be overweight than men. Terrifyingly, 50 percent of the entire adult population is expected to have diabetes by 2030, and this is one of the major predictors of heart disease and is also associated with dementia.

Depression and anxiety: One in four women experiences an extended time of major depression in her life, and as many women are on an antidepressant, an antianxiety medication, or often both, not living their lives with the joy and satisfaction we are meant to experience.

Autoimmune disease: Autoimmune disease is now the third most common category of disease in the United States, and one of the ten leading causes of death for women. Conservative estimates show that 78 percent of autoimmune disease sufferers are women. Hashimoto's thyroiditis is the most prevalent, and affects women almost exclusively.

Some of these conditions have become so common that many doctors are chalking them up to being normal facts of life or aging.

Women in the United States are also dangerously overmedicated, at a rate higher than men, for problems that generally require lifestyle—not pharmaceutical—solutions. Women are also more likely to experience adverse medication reactions. Statin drugs for cholesterol, for example, are some of the most commonly prescribed medications for women and have been found to *cause* diabetes in 50 percent of the people who use them, even when prescribed to otherwise healthy women for disease prevention. Considering that half of women over age fifty are on at least two medications, 10 percent of Americans take five medications in any thirty-day period, and the third leading cause of death in the United States, after heart disease and cancer, is prescription medications, this is no small matter. While some of these medications may resolve symptoms, none treats the underlying and reversible causes, and all can have unintended consequences.

WHY YOUR DOCTOR
DOESN'T KNOW THIS STUFF

Why doesn't modern medicine have a solution? Why doesn't your doctor have the answers you're looking for? The majority of M.D.s simply haven't been taught to connect the dots. In our training, we aren't taught to understand the complex array of nutritional, environmental, and lifestyle factors that contribute to disease. In my seven years of medical training, I had only one fifty-minute class on nutrition, and when I brought up the impact of endocrine disruptors—plastics and chemicals that mimic the estrogen in our bodies and can cause serious hormonal imbalances and even cancer—with a prominent endocrinology professor at my Ivy League medical institution, he looked at me as if I'd lost my senses and said: "You don't really believe in all that BPA crap, do you?" Yet research on endocrine disruptors had been in the scientific literature for years at that point, and the harms were well known. But here's the problem: a 2011 study found that it takes an estimated seventeen years for new scientific and medical information to reach most doctors and change the way they practice.

Doctors are also sorely unprepared to understand and treat the new chronic diseases Americans are facing. The serious infectious diseases doctors have long been trained to handle have largely been surpassed by diseases such as diabetes and obesity, and in younger and younger populations in overwhelming numbers. So too have stress-related conditions and mental health problems. When it comes to lesser-known diagnoses, doctors are even more lost. Less than ten years ago, neither fibromyalgia nor chronic fatigue syndrome, both of which primarily affect women, was recognized as a real condition by the medical establishment. Not long before that, neither was irritable bowel syndrome (IBS). All were considered "fringe" diagnoses. Women who told their physician, "I think I might have chronic fatigue syndrome," report having received eye rolls and dismissive responses—much like women today who say they think they have a thyroid or adrenal problem. These patients also might be labeled as "difficult," or "that kind" of patient—code for a psychological problem.

While fibromyalgia, chronic fatigue syndrome, and IBS are now recognized medical diagnoses, many health care providers remain ignorant or skeptical. Chronic fatigue syndrome, for example, is still commonly mistaken for a mental health condition, or "a figment of the patient's imagination." Misconceptions or dismissive attitudes by health care providers make the path to diagnosis long and frustrating for many patients, compounded by the fact that less than one-third of medical schools include information about this and other marginalized conditions in their curricula.

Further complicating the problem is that there were no diagnostic tests that could "prove" that you had one of these conditions, so you were simply told that you didn't. Medicine has black-and-white criteria for diagnoses. You either meet the criteria or you don't. But in reality, there are fifty shades of not okay, and lab tests should be interpreted in the context of a woman's symptoms and the trends in her labs, and in light of the fact that as medicine evolves, so do criteria for disease diagnosis. You'll learn more about this when we talk about thyroid testing later in the book.

SO WHAT'S REALLY GOING ON?

I had to ask myself that same question, What *is* going on? Why are so many women suffering with symptoms and medical conditions that have historically never before plagued us to even nearly this extent, or which were not ever previously seen?

What I discovered came not from the hallowed halls of medicine but from a fascinating branch of science called psychoneuroimmunology (PNI), as I shared in the introduction. I discovered that at their root, these common problems share the fact that women are living in chronic overload emotionally and physically. We are stuck in survival mode.

PNI has proven that there is interconnectedness among the nervous system, our immunity, hormones, mood, cognitive function, digestion, circulation, and the stress response. PNI illuminates what conventional medicine hasn't figured out: that a compartmentalized approach to disease misses the main point—it's all connected. What we do, eat, think, and are exposed to in the environment affect us tip to toe. Even if you're not a science geek like I am (admittedly textbooks are often my bedtime pleasure reading), I think you'll be amazed to learn that what drove you to pick up this book—whether an autoimmune problem, fatigue, creeping weight gain, lack of focus and concentration, out-of-whack hormones—can be traced to a common cause: overdrive of your body's stress response.

"But wait," you may be thinking, "I'm not feeling *that* stressed, so how could it be my stress response?" Great question. Here's the thing: it's not only stress in the way we think of it traditionally—the mental and emotional kinds—that gets your stress response working overtime. It's anything that overwhelms your body's capacity to respond effectively to the challenges you're exposed to.

As I detailed in the introduction, there are actually five Root Causes that get your stress response in overdrive: chronic emotional and mental stress, food triggers, gut disruption, environmental toxins, and stealth infections.

We're going to dive into all of these in the next chapter, and then you're going to turn them around with the SOS Solution. Right now, though, it's time to discover how a chronically triggered stress response is at the heart of your symptoms.

MEET THE STRESS RESPONSE

We've all had moments of heightened anxiety—a racing heartbeat, rapid breathing (or holding our breath), cold sweat, clenched hands, heightened awareness of our surroundings (for example, when you're alone in your house at night and hear an unexpected sound). These familiar responses are signs that what is commonly called the *fight-or-flight reaction*, and technically referred to as the *stress response*, has been activated.

The stress response is a cascade of hormones and neurotransmitters (the nervous system's chemical messengers) that connect your brain, numerous survival reactions that begin in your "lizard brain," and your body. Didn't know you had a lizard brain? You do! It's so nicknamed because it's such an ancient, primal response system that it can be tracked back to earliest evolution.

Your lizard brain contains two small almond-shaped structures on either side of your brain, called the *amygdala*, which serve as the brain's emotional interpretation center. It's where you process fear and danger-related images, sounds, and experiences, which your brain then catalogs for fast future reference to instantaneously warn you of related dangers. Within split seconds of perceiving a threat, your lizard brain mobilizes and sounds the alarm, sending a chemical distress signal to your brain's executive hormone director, the hypothalamus.

The hypothalamus, a tiny gland in the front center of your brain, serves as a rapid relay station, receiving, responding to, and regulating signals from all over your body, communicating through an elaborate network called your *autonomic nervous system* (ANS), using chemical and hormonal signals to get the information delivered to where it needs to go. This ANS controls your breathing and heartbeat, the constriction and relaxation of your blood vessels, blood pressure, immune system responsiveness, and your level of alertness. The stress response signals, once registered, get passed on to the pituitary gland, another major hormonal regulatory center in your brain, and from there, all the way down to your adrenal glands, where your body translates these signals into action.

Help Is on the Way: Your Adrenal Glands

Your adrenal glands are two small triangular-shaped glands (meaning they secrete chemicals and hormones), weighing barely a few ounces, that sit one atop each kidney. Tiny as they are, they're mighty, and central to your survival. The adrenal glands produce and secrete, among a number of hormones and chemicals, adrenaline and cortisol. Together, these regulate your body's ability to protect you from infection (immunity); regulate your blood sugar, fat storage, and mobilization to provide you with energy (metabolism); and drive your sexual desire, hormonal cycles and levels, and ability to get pregnant, carry, and nourish babies (reproduction). They also drive you into fast action when you're in danger and provide the fuel you need to sustain that action.

First Response: Adrenaline

The adrenal glands initially respond to a real, potential, or perceived threat by pumping out a chemical called *adrenaline*, which you've no doubt heard of. Under adrenaline's influence, your heart rate quickens to get more blood coursing to your muscles in case you need to run or fight, and your respiratory passages dilate, letting you take in as much oxygen as possible because oxygen provides the "gas" your brain and muscles need for extra focus and action. Your blood vessels constrict, causing your blood pressure to go up, infusing your brain and muscles with oxygen-rich blood. Your immune system mobilizes germ-fighting cells and inflammatory messenger chemicals called *cytokines* to protect you in the event of injury or infection. Your body directs energy away from any functions that aren't needed in the immediate face of danger, such as digestion and reproduction (those can always happen later!), temporarily affecting your gut and hormone balance. Your pupils dilate to take in more peripheral vision and help you see if it's dark, and your senses sharpen, leading to a state of hypervigilance, which means you are keenly aware of and sensitive to every possible threat or hint of danger in your environment. All the while the amygdala is imprinting every aspect of the possible threat so you remember in exquisite detail the sounds, sights, smells, and feelings associated with this hazard, as a protective mechanism against possible future threats. It's this same hypervigilance, also sometimes called *hyperarousal*, that keeps you on the edge of your seat and makes you jump at the slightest sound when you're watching a scary movie—which, if you're a sensitive type, your brain perceives as real danger even though it's just a film.

In the short run, some people actually love the feel of adrenaline. It gives you a rush. It's the same feeling we get when we're thrilled by something, experience something new and wonderful, or experience a feeling of positive stress, as with extreme sports or a roller coaster ride. But when this rush becomes chronic, as happens when activated too often by regular stress, it's not fun anymore. It can turn into anxiety, feeling wired and unable to find inner quiet; it keeps your blood pressure elevated and can cause dangerous heart rate variations, to name a few problems. Moreover, when stress becomes prolonged for days, weeks, months, or most of the time, as is the case for most of us these days, adrenaline isn't enough to keep you protected for the long game. Your body has to ramp up cortisol production for extra reinforcement.

Cortisol: Our Best "Frenemy"

Cortisol is a steroid hormone. Like the steroids doctors prescribe for inflammation, one of the main jobs of your body's naturally occurring cortisol is to keep inflammation from getting out of hand. Cortisol has received a bad reputation as "the stress hormone," and it's true that when it's too high or too low, problems abound, as you'll soon learn. But cortisol isn't a villain. It's an essential survival hormone, responsible for regulating major biological processes including metabolism of fats, carbohydrates, and protein, the responsiveness of your immune system to infection and inflammation, your hormonal balance, sex drive, and reproduction—as well as your thyroid hormone production.

Cortisol is meant to be secreted by your adrenal glands in a daily, rhythmic fashion, called a diurnal pattern, that looks like a ski slope on a graph (see page 28). It is highest in the morning, when it gives you a natural surge of energy called the *cortisol awakening response* (CAR—an easy way to remember that: it gives you drive, and when your CAR won't start in the morning, you don't have the energy you need to get going) to wake up and get your day going. As the day progresses, your cortisol level should taper. Then, at about midnight, when cortisol secretion, and thus the amount circulating in your body, reaches its nadir, you enter into a rest, detoxification, and repair phase while you sleep. Slowly, cortisol begins to climb again, until about 7:00 or 8:00 A.M., when it reaches its zenith and the cycle begins anew. We all have a natural energy drip that wears off as the day goes on and replenishes itself while we sleep.

In addition to this daily cortisol rhythm, cortisol production and release ramp up whenever the stress response gets activated due to stress, which could be due to a life issue, threatening situation, infection, or other overwhelming challenge to your resilience or reserves.

Cortisol gets you mobilized for protection: it tells your liver to convert stored energy into sugar, which is rapidly pumped into your bloodstream and then to your muscles, so you have an immediate burst of energy if you need to run or fight. Simultaneously, insulin is pumped out of your pancreas to perform its primary function of regulating this now extra circulating blood sugar. You don't want too much blood sugar hanging around for too long because it causes cellular damage, so insulin is ready, and when the crisis calms down, it quickly clears any sugar you haven't burned up. Your immune system is simultaneously mobilized to be ready to fight infection and control inflammation should you be injured in the possible fight or flight. Along with adrenaline, cortisol keeps your blood pressure

Examples of Abnormal Cortisol Rhythms

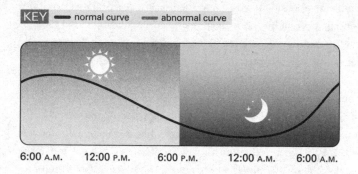

KEY — normal curve — abnormal curve

6:00 A.M.   12:00 P.M.   6:00 P.M.   12:00 A.M.   6:00 A.M.

1. This is an example of a normal cortisol curve.

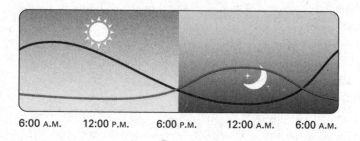

6:00 A.M.   12:00 P.M.   6:00 P.M.   12:00 A.M.   6:00 A.M.

2. This is an example of a flipped cortisol curve; it is low in the morning and high in the evening. In this case one might find it hard to wake in the morning, there's likely to be morning depression, you might actually have an evening burst of energy, but you might feel tired but wired before bed and have difficulty sleeping.

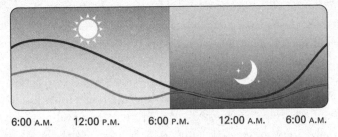

6:00 A.M.   12:00 P.M.   6:00 P.M.   12:00 A.M.   6:00 A.M.

3. Here the cortisol curve is a bit low in the morning, dips in the afternoon, which can often be associated with afternoon fatigue, poor concentration, and sugar or caffeine cravings, but it is generally normal in the evening.

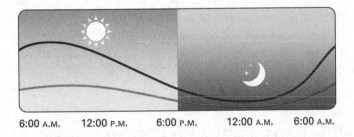

6:00 A.M.   12:00 P.M.   6:00 P.M.   12:00 A.M.   6:00 A.M.

4. Here the cortisol curve is generally low throughout the day and evening.

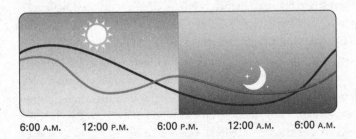

6:00 A.M.   12:00 P.M.   6:00 P.M.   12:00 A.M.   6:00 A.M.

5. Here the cortisol curve is normal in the early morning, with a late-morning dip that may be associated with fatigue, poor concentration, and sugar or caffeine craving, and a slight elevation in the evening that might be associated with sleep troubles.

elevated during the crisis, so should you be injured, you have the buffer you need to prevent you from going into shock. Higher blood pressure also means more blood flow—and thus more oxygen—to your brain to keep you vigilant and aware.

When responding to a temporary threat, this system works with perfect elegance. When the threat is over, your body quickly resets to its former calm, leaving no lasting consequences. This primitive survival response has kept us alive since the dawn of human existence on this planet. We're hardwired to withstand a significant amount of stress, from famines, to storms, to injuries, infections, and attacks from fanged and clawed animals, and even invading unfriendly tribes.

"But," you might be thinking, "if this system works so well to protect us, why has Dr. Romm implicated it pretty much in every health problem I'm having?" Well, Lovely, that's because it works perfectly—until it's triggered too often, or just doesn't turn off, meaning we barely ever get a rest from being in high alert. That's when all of these protective responses become liabilities.

WHEN STRESS BECOMES DISTRESS

At the heart of our twenty-first-century chronic health issues is, not surprisingly, a modern chronic problem. We rarely ever "turn off." And neither does our stress response, which is where all of the trouble begins. The stress response evolved to handle immediate and short-lived threats. All of the protective reactions I described above help us in emergencies and high-stress events, but they eventually cause us harm when they just don't stop. Then they can backfire, turning into chronic symptoms—or worse, medical problems. The havoc plays out in your hormones, digestion, immune system, metabolism, brain, mood—and pretty much everywhere else! Your brain and body get stuck in survival mode with all of the consequences thereof.

The effects of SOS on your mind and performance can actually be tracked on a graph, called the Yerkes-Dodson Curve, in psychoneuroimmunology often called the "inverted-U curve." I refer to it as the *You Curve*.

What you see in the image on page 32 is that stress itself is not inherently "bad"; a small amount of contained stress—what we might even call "good stress"—heightens our awareness and memory, mobilizes energy, increases stamina, and boosts immunity. This explains the phenomenon of why so many of us perform better under a deadline, or don't get sick until after a big stress is over.

It also shows that it's when stress crosses into stress overload that we experience problems.

It's not just mood, mind, and performance that can be tracked on this curve—so can a number of health parameters, such as immunity, which is stimulated by small amounts of stress, but when stuck in overactivation, can cause a big health hit. Here's a glimpse of the problems that result from stress overload:

Chronic anxiety, overwhelm, and sleep problems: While hyper-vigilance makes you more alert in the short run, in the long run it translates into feelings of oversensitivity, anxiety, feeling constantly stressed out or overwhelmed, "wired," and becoming sleep-deprived. Over time, resultant exhaustion can lead to depression, cognitive problems, sugar cravings, and weight gain, and increases your risk for heart disease and even cancer.

Brain fog: Sleep problems themselves can cause difficulty with memory and concentration, but as you'll soon learn, cortisol has some very special actions in the brain that sabotage your memory, focus, and even willpower.

Digestive problems: When your body mobilizes energy to run or fight, it does so by diverting energy away from other important functions, such as digestion. Over time, this can lead to digestive symptoms, irritable bowel syndrome, and even damage to your intestinal lining and microbiome.

Sugar, fat, and salt cravings and belly fat: Cortisol tells your body to store energy in case an emergency persists, so when cortisol is chronically elevated as a result of your chronically activated stress response, your body holds on to calories and turns them into fat. This fat is packed preferentially around your waist and around your organs, while excess fat gets stored as cholesterol, all setting you up for metabolic syndrome.

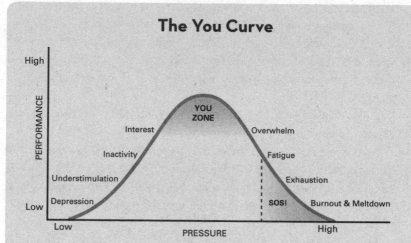

The You Curve

PERFORMANCE

High

Low

YOU ZONE

Interest

Inactivity

Understimulation

Depression

Overwhelm

Fatigue

Exhaustion

SOS!

Burnout & Meltdown

Low   PRESSURE   High

The You Curve is a visual reminder that stress can be beneficial, and interestingly, viewing stress in a positive light reduces its potential harmful impact on your health. One study looked at two groups of employees who were each shown a film—one was on all the positive aspects of the stress response, how it makes you more alert and responsive, while the other was about how stress sabotages you. Then they each were given the exact same public speaking challenge (studies have found public speaking is one of people's greatest anxiety triggers). The group who saw stress as a problem tanked on the test, while the ones who saw it as a challenge that made them stronger succeeded, which demonstrates that how we think about stress—as an intrinsic, manageable part of life, or as an enemy—makes a difference in how it affects us.

In fact, when you go into the stress response, a cascade of stress-balancing hormones is supposed to be released simultaneously, increasing stress resilience. Oxytocin, sometimes called "the cuddle hormone," is produced in the pituitary gland, and prompts us to bond with others, which helps us feel safe and meets our primitive survival need to "connect" and "belong," and also boosts our sense of courage and confidence. DHEA (dehydroepiandrosterone), produced by the adrenals, and upregulated in times of stress, plays a role in improving your resistance to viral, bacterial, and parasitic infections; builds muscle mass and healthy bone; promotes hormone production; keeps your body fat low; and lowers "bad" cholesterol, counteracting the harmful effects of prolonged cortisol exposure.

Unfortunately, being under chronic stress blunts production of oxytocin and DHEA. The good news is that getting out of SOS can improve your stress resilience.

You need more energy to keep up with the stress response reactions, so you end up with sugar and carbohydrate cravings, because they provide fast fuel, and you store the extra calories in the form of dangerous inflammatory fat around your waist.

Hormonal problems: When your stress response gets activated, your body diverts energy away from what evolutionary biologist Robert Sapolsky calls "optimistic activities" such as hormone production, preferentially making more cortisol from the shared building blocks of your sex hormones estrogen, progesterone, and testosterone and telling your pituitary gland to release a chemical called *prolactin,* which also suppresses your sex hormones. Sex drive and reproduction require an enormous amount of energy, so out goes your libido, and often fertility, too.

Metabolic syndrome and high blood pressure: When blood sugar and insulin are perpetually required in elevated amounts, over time the sugar can damage your blood vessels, and your pancreas can underfunction from the extra demand, resulting in insulin resistance, which down the road can lead to diabetes and heart disease. And that elevated blood pressure can stay elevated, turning into chronic hypertension.

Immune system problems and autoimmune disease: While immediate activation of your immune system can protect you from danger, long-term activation leads to all kinds of confusion in your immune system, resulting in a host of troublesome responses, from allergies, hives, and eczema, to getting sick too often, to major immune system backfiring in the form of autoimmune diseases.

Inflamm-aging: Persistent activation of the stress response leads to a tremendous amount of wear and tear on the body and brain that can ultimately lead to a phenomenon called *inflamm-aging*, premature aging with all of the wrinkles, sagging skin, and health problems that come with it. No. Thank. You.

Chronic overload, due to overactivation of the stress response, pushes you beyond your natural capacity to bounce back—a phenomenon known as *allostatic load* or, as I explain to my patients and explained to you in the introduction, Survival Overdrive Syndrome, which so vividly describes what's going on. The perfect shorthand for Survival Overdrive Syndrome is SOS. After all, symptoms—and even medical conditions—are a call from your body for rescue.

ARE YOU IN SOS?

Does being ON all the time sound familiar? Like most women, there's a good chance you start your day by checking email, maybe even before you've gotten out of bed. If you have time, you squeeze in a quick work-out. Probably, though, you're in a hurry to get out the door for work, leaving no time for exercise. If you have kids, you're juggling to get them out of the door, too, so you skip breakfast, having just a cup of coffee or tea, and maybe once in a while you've got time to make a smoothie. You might have to battle traffic on the way to work, with the feeling that you're perpetually running late.

Then your day really gears up. You have incessant deadlines, an unrelenting to-do list, an insane workload, and in the midst of it, your kid's birthday party to plan and that Pap smear you need to fit in. You're constantly on the go, reaching for coffee, energy bars, or sugary treats to keep you energized, and maybe, with any luck, grabbing a decent salad for lunch. Then there's traffic to deal with on the way home, groceries to pick up, dinner to make. The kids need help with homework; you have more work deadlines to meet after they're tucked in.

By 10:00 P.M., if you're lucky, it's finally "you time," which you take with your fave TV show and a glass (or three) of wine. You're way too tired for sex, and frankly, way too tired to care. If you're lucky, you hit the pillow and fall asleep, only to start over the next day. If you're like half of all women, though, you're more likely to be staring at the ceiling for quite some time, wishing sleep would come, waking up in the night, or struggling to wake the next morning. Life can make you feel that you're being chased by a hungry lion.

That's what your survival hardwiring thinks is happening, too.

Evolutionary biologists call the modern crisis we're experiencing an *evolutionary mismatch*. *Mismatch theory* states that humans have traits that have been passed down and preserved by natural selection because they helped us to survive in a given environment. However, because the environment we're living in now differs drastically from the environment in which we evolved, the traits that were once adaptive are now "mismatched" and do more harm than good. Here's an example: Our cavewoman grandmothers didn't get diabetes. But one in three of us does. Sugars and fats were uncommon in our ancestors' diets so our bodies processed them slowly, and evolved protective mechanisms to keep our blood sugar high enough for us to survive on. Modern life makes sugar easy to get, and stress makes us crave it. This mismatch is making us fat and giving us diabetes, and is just one of many examples of how evolutionary systems get overloaded and backfire.

Being ON all the time is exhausting, and so many of us are experiencing burnout and serious health symptoms as a result. You remain in overdrive, "all systems go." Your body tries to adapt, until it can't anymore. You end up feeling like you really do want to shout out "SOS!"

ARE YOU IN OVERDRIVE? EXHAUSTION? THE TWO FACES OF SOS

The stress response problems I am referring to can be differentiated into two main categories, what I call *SOS with Overdrive* (SOS-O), and its end result, *SOS with Exhaustion* (SOS-E). In SOS-O cortisol is chronically elevated, or elevated when it should be low. In SOS-E cortisol is chronically low, or depressed when it should be elevated. The latter is what is commonly called *adrenal fatigue*, though this is actually a misnomer; it's not that the adrenals get fatigued, it's usually that the adrenal glands' chemical stimulator in the brain, CRH (corticotropin-releasing hormone), stops driving the adrenals so hard to give you a break, and as a result, the production of stress response hormones declines, leaving you in a state of low cortisol and low adrenaline.

One can also have both SOS-O and SOS-E at varying points during the day; both patterns are flip sides of the same coin—the downstream impacts of the stress system impacting the normal cortisol rhythm. You can see the symptoms of each below.

Both patterns have also been associated with autoimmune conditions—for example, Hashimoto's thyroiditis, Graves' disease, Crohn's disease, rheumatoid arthritis, Sjögren's syndrome, psoriasis, celiac disease, fibromyalgia, and chronic fatigue syndrome, in addition to the symptoms I describe below.

Adrenal Overdrive: SOS-O

SOS-O is the amped-up, overwhelmed mode that most of us spend most of our time in. It creates—and can also be caused by—that feeling you have when you're rushing from one place to the next, trying to get a million things done in too short a time, and feeling like your to-do list never ends. Think of SOS-O as constantly going pedal to the metal—your foot is pressing down on the accelerator, and you can't seem to get it off. You start to think that the only way you're going to stop is when you finally hit a wall (which can happen—it's SOS-E!).

Here are the common symptoms of being stuck in the ON position:

- Afternoon fatigue, caffeine or sugar cravings, usually at about 3:00 to 4:00 P.M.

- Allergies, food reactions, hives

- Anxiety, irritability, or depression

- Cravings for sugary, salty, or fatty foods, or carbs (starches, baked goods)

- Difficulty with focus or memory ("brain fog")

- Difficulty sticking with a diet or exercise plan, trouble with "willpower"

- Digestive problems

- Eczema

- Fatigue after eating

- Fatigue, exhaustion, chronic overwhelm

- Feeling "tired and wired"

- Hormone problems of any type, including PMS, infertility, endometriosis, polycystic ovarian syndrome, bothersome menopausal symptoms

- Insomnia

- Low sex drive

- Stubborn weight, being overweight, or difficulty gaining weight

- Waking up tired even if you've slept all night

Conditions associated with SOS-O include:

- High blood pressure

- High cholesterol

- Insulin resistance, metabolic syndrome, or diabetes

- Hashimoto's thyroiditis

- Osteopenia or osteoporosis

- PCOS, endometriosis, and infertility

Driven to Exhaustion: SOS-E

If SOS-O is pedal to the metal, SOS-E is the crash and burn. You've hit the wall; you're burned out. It's the feeling of being wiped out, in disrepair, in overwhelm so deep you can't climb out. It happens because your brain dials down the overdrive reaction to protect you from chronic overload, and with it, dials back your cortisol and adrenaline production. It's the ultimate negative feedback loop. You end up in SOS-E, feeling deeply exhausted, your reactions low in everything from metabolism, mood, mental focus, and memory, to immunity, hormones, and thyroid—to save energy.

While most of us can carry on in a state of SOS-O (so effectively does the body accommodate many types of stress), somewhere along the line, if the stress overwhelms your coping abilities, whether physically, mentally, or emotionally, you end up feeling spent or "fried." Your body's ability to tolerate stress malfunctions, and your immune system follows. You get sick with colds and infections, you feel wiped out and can't think clearly. Because your immune system starts working against you, instead of for you—which you'll learn more about in the next chapters—autoimmune conditions arise. For example, Hashimoto's disease is an autoimmune condition wherein one suffers a low-functioning thyroid due to an immune attack on this gland, and is the most common example of an autoimmune condition with roots in SOS. All autoimmune conditions, however, are associated with fatigue. Below are the common physical and emotional consequences of being driven to exhaustion.

- Allergies
- Autoimmune disease
- Decreased concentration and memory
- Depression
- Excessive need for caffeine
- Fatigue, exhaustion, fatigue on waking
- Frequent colds, bronchitis, sinus infections, urinary tract or yeast infections, cold sores, or herpes outbreaks
- Increased aches, pain, inflammation
- Increased fear and apprehension
- Loss of ambition, low motivation
- Low blood pressure
- Low blood sugar symptoms
- Low sex drive
- No appetite in the morning
- Scattered thinking
- Short fuse, irritability

- Slow recovery from illness
- Sugar and carb cravings
- Tendency to feel better or have more energy toward evening

SOS AND YOUR THYROID

The thyroid and adrenals influence many of the same functions and profoundly impact each other. Because they are so interconnected, you often can't effectively treat one without ensuring the health of the other. They are thrown into imbalance by the same five Root Causes, and diagnoses in both are often missed by conventional medicine.

Let's turn our attention specifically to the role of the thyroid gland in women's health, and to how the thyroid and adrenals interact.

What Exactly Is the Thyroid, Anyway?

Your thyroid is a butterfly-shaped gland weighing about an ounce, in the front of your neck. Like the adrenals, the thyroid plays a central role in the control of your metabolism, mood, hormones, and cognitive function. It is your body's thermostat, turning the dial up—or down—on your body's energy expenditure and metabolism, growth, and reproductive functions based on the feedback your brain gets from your internal environment. It's involved in hundreds (or more) of biological functions, including brain development and function, breathing and heart rate, nervous system functions, body temperature, muscle strength, skin health, and hormones that govern menstrual cycles and fertility, mood, weight, and cholesterol levels.

Your thyroid determines how efficiently you burn calories, how easily you lose weight, how much energy you have, whether you have regular bowel movements and regular periods, whether you have PMS or cyclic breast lumps, whether you can achieve and maintain a healthy pregnancy and produce breast milk after your baby is born, whether your mood is depressed, anxious, or joyous, the quality and capacity of your brain to learn, remember things, and focus, and so much more. It does all of this through the production of two main thyroid hormones: triiodothyronine (T_3) and thyroxine (T_4). While T_4 is produced by the thyroid in much greater quantities than T_3, the latter is the active form of the hormone and is made by the conversion of T_4 to T_3 throughout your body, especially in a healthy, functioning liver.

The thyroid knows how much thyroid hormone to produce and when, through signals that, much like with your adrenals, start in the brain. In this case, thyroid-stimulating hormone (TSH), which is made by the pituitary gland in the brain, regulates thyroid hormone production by signaling the thyroid when it's time to get busy. When thyroid hormone levels in the blood are low, the pituitary releases more TSH. When thyroid hormone levels are high, the pituitary decreases TSH production. This is called a feedback loop: a positive feedback loop leads to more production of thyroid hormone; a negative feedback loop puts the brakes on thyroid hormone production. As you might imagine, given how many functions are regulated by thyroid hormones, when the thyroid is disrupted, or your body isn't getting enough thyroid hormone, a whole host of symptoms and problems will ensue, due to hypothyroidism.

UNDERSTANDING HYPOTHYROIDISM AND HASHIMOTO'S

Hypothyroidism refers to decreased thyroid function or decreased action of the thyroid hormones in the body. Hypothyroidism is, by far, the most prevalent form of thyroid disease in the United States, accounting for 80 percent of thyroid problems and affecting at least one in ten women, or at least twenty-eight million individuals. Hypothyroidism comes in two main forms: nonautoimmune thyroid disease, usually simply called *hypothyroidism,* and the autoimmune form called *Hashimoto's thyroiditis,* or more commonly, *Hashimoto's.*

Hashimoto's disease is the most common form of all thyroid disease in the United States (in many places in the world the nonautoimmune type is more common due to iodine deficiency), accounting for at least 90 percent of all hypothyroidism. It affects women far more than men—75 percent of those affected are women. Women are at least seven times more likely to develop Hashimoto's than men, and it can have a tremendous and devastating impact on a woman's quality of life.

In Hashimoto's, the immune system attacks the thyroid gland—which is why it's an autoimmune condition. Large numbers of white blood cells called *lymphocytes*, immune system cells, accumulate in the thyroid and make antibodies that start to damage the thyroid, interfering with its ability to produce thyroid hormones. Without adequate thyroid hormone, many of the body's functions slow down, sometimes drastically. It is the presence of antibodies in the blood that determines whether you have Hashimoto's versus nonautoimmune hypothyroidism.

Nonautoimmune hypothyroidism can be caused by a number of factors, including nutrient deficiencies, excess iodine exposure, excess exposure to certain foods (including green drinks with certain vegetables, as I'll discuss later) that can dampen thyroid function, and various challenges that prevent the body from effectively converting inactive thyroid hormone to the active form, or inability of the body to effectively use thyroid hormone. This is similar to insulin or cortisol resistance; the cells of the body can become resistant to thyroid hormone, meaning they stop responding to it. If it can't bind to and trigger the cell to do its work, you can end up with symptoms of hypothyroidism. Chronic or substantial stress can also suppress the pituitary gland enough to interfere with thyroid hormone production, as it does sex hormone production, yet one more reason to get out of SOS.

In some cases, which can occur with either form of hypothyroid condition, the body is making enough thyroid hormone, but the active form of the hormone, T_3, is converted to an inactive form called *reverse T_3* (RT_3), which the body stores rather than uses, and which leads to symptoms of hypothyroidism.

All of this will be discussed in chapter 7.

Hypothyroidism can also be due to more serious problems in the hypothalamus and pituitary. This is rare, but it should be investigated with your doctor if you have symptoms of hypothyroidism but your labs appear to be normal by the standards discussed in chapter 7.

For simplicity's sake, unless I am discussing one or the other specifically, throughout this book I am going to refer to nonautoimmune hypothyroidism and Hashimoto's collectively as hypothyroidism. The symptoms of hypothyroidism are the same, regardless of the origin of the problem.

Hypothyroidism: An Internal Energy Crisis

The symptoms of hypothyroidism include:

- Anxiety
- Brain fog (poor memory and concentration)
- Carpal tunnel syndrome
- Cold intolerance
- Constipation
- Depression
- Dry skin
- Fatigue
- Goiter (swelling in the front of the neck)
- Hair loss
- High cholesterol
- Hormone imbalances, including PMS, irregular periods, cyclic breast tenderness, and low sex drive
- Impaired memory
- Infertility
- Insomnia
- Low immunity, including frequent colds and infections
- Menstrual disturbance
- Miscarriage, especially with any of these other symptoms
- Muscle weakness
- Nerve pain
- Postpartum depression, low breast milk production after baby's birth

- Slow heart rate

- Slowed mental processing

- Slowed physical movements

- Swelling or puffiness around the eyes

- Weight gain

Untreated, hypothyroidism has been associated with weight gain, high cholesterol, cognitive decline and dementia, and heart disease.

Hypothyroidism Is Underdiagnosed and Undertreated

Cara, thirty-eight, had been gaining weight for months even though she hadn't changed her diet or exercise. She was tired all the time and could tell that her mental concentration was off. Moisturizing couldn't kick the dry skin that was making her itchy, and constipation was now becoming a regular problem. She was more anxious than usual and unable to tolerate stress. Her doctor told her she was probably just depressed from being a mom with young kids, and that even though her thyroid test number was close to the upper edge of normal, it was still normal, so he wouldn't treat her. She could come back in six months for a recheck, but in the meanwhile, he recommended she start a diet and consider Prozac.

One year of suffering later she landed in my medical practice. I ordered some tests, and within a week, Cara and I had the answer: Hashimoto's. Over the next few months we worked together to find her Root Causes, which included gluten intolerance and Epstein-Barr virus. With a few adjustments we found the right medication for her, and within weeks, her energy was back. She again felt happy and hopeful, her mind was focused, and she began to drop the weight she'd picked up.

Clearly this wasn't just "all in her head"—and there was a solution, just as there is for you.

Unfortunately, as I'll discuss in chapter 7, most doctors don't routinely order a full panel of thyroid tests and so miss a thyroid diagnosis, leaving millions of women without answers. As Marina, forty-nine years old, told me: "It has been a very long and frustrating road trying to convince my endocrinologist that even though my labs were 'normal,' I still experienced every classic symptom of hypothyroidism. After a while I really did think it was 'in my head,' like I was told. I learned to live with the incredible fatigue, mental and physical sluggishness, and, oh, the unfounded sadness! It really has been difficult to cope with these symptoms on a constant basis and having to be my own health advocate all along the way—researching, investigating, questioning—even begging physicians, hoping to open their minds."

Of the estimated twenty-eight million Americans with known thyroid disease, as many as 50 percent *more* women may have the disease without knowing it. Consider, for example, that it is estimated that as many as 30 percent of women being treated for depression may actually have hypothyroidism as the underlying cause, which, if treated, could alleviate their depression. Further, at least 15 percent of all those on thyroid replacement medicines (an estimated 1.6 million individuals), almost all women, still have hypothyroidism despite being on medication, because of lack of treatment of the underlying causes, inadequate or incorrect medication treatment, dismissal of symptoms, or lack of appropriate follow-up testing by doctors to assess thyroid health status with appropriate adjustment of treatment as needed.

The SOS-Thyroid Connection

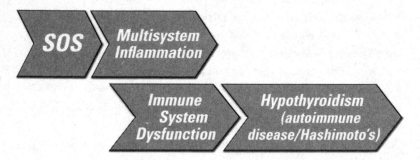

The impact of SOS on the thyroid can be profound. Anytime your body is under prolonged stress, your body will go into an energy-conserving mode much like when we turn down the thermostat in our homes in an energy crisis. The responsibility for going into this mode falls to the thyroid, which responds by slowing down thyroid hormone production and, with it, all of your body's energy-expending functions from metabolism to reproduction.

Additionally, chronic SOS can cause your immune system to become confused, leading to autoimmunity, including Hashimoto's, the most common of many autoimmune conditions that may develop. Finally, all the same Root Causes that lead to SOS can also independently lead to Hashimoto's, so reversing these Root Causes of SOS is also essential in the effective treatment of Hashimoto's, and hypothyroidism generally.

In chapter 3 you'll take a questionnaire that will help you to determine whether you have hypothyroidism, and you'll be directed to which tests can help you determine whether you have Hashimoto's or nonautoimmune hypothyroidism. The SOS Solution will get you out of SOS, reverse the five Root Causes, and help you get your thyroid function back in gear.

INFLAMMATION: THE SECRET LANGUAGE OF SOS

Your immune system acts as a constant surveillance system. Inflammation is the chemical and cellular response that is mobilized when that surveillance system registers something it doesn't like. In minute amounts, inflammatory reactions are turning on and off all day, as your body responds in real time to the millions of potential threats you might encounter. The problem is that our modern life exposes us to so many triggers so often that our inflammatory responses go into overdrive. The wear and tear you experience from diet, pollution and toxins, and stress leads to chronic inflammation. Your immune system becomes activated, sounding the alarm that something needs to be done, and when your body is always on the defensive, you run into problems. Excess inflammation is a common denominator connecting the damage caused by the five Root Causes, and is present in most chronic health problems.

Inflammation is often described as a fire because one of the most recognizable signs is heat, along with swelling, redness, and pain—for example, the symptoms of a splinter you've put off removing. When it's functioning

If You've Been Treated for Graves' Disease or Thyroid Cancer, This Book Is for You, Too

If you've had remediation for Graves' disease (autoimmune hyperthyroidism), whether you've had your thyroid removed or received radioactive thyroid treatment (thyroid ablation), or if you've had your thyroid removed as part of thyroid cancer treatment, you, too, are likely to be functionally hypothyroid, and thus the recommendations in this book apply to you, too. The same Root Causes that lead to Hashimoto's are those that can also lead to Graves' disease, so though you've had conventional disease treatment, this doesn't mean you've eliminated the Root Causes, leaving you with the risk that they can show up in other areas of your body. Therefore, I recommend that you, too, follow the SOS Solution, to protect and nourish your health. However, if you have had loss of your thyroid, you will actually be dependent on thyroid medication, and will not be able to stop taking it, even if you heal your Root Causes.

optimally, that fire remains contained, like a fire in a stone fireplace. But should that fire escape from the fireplace and start burning down your house, as happens with chronic inflammation, you have a major problem. Out of control, inflammation damages everything in its path. Once inflammation gets a chronic foothold, the result is a domino effect of mounting inflammation, which over time can become a self-perpetuating runaway train causing everything from obesity, diabetes, heart disease, and fatigue to fertility problems, depression, dementia, and even autoimmune disease.

AUTOIMMUNE DISEASE: IMMUNE SYSTEM MUTINY

Autoimmunity occurs when your body's immune system starts attacking your own cells because it mistakenly tags them as a virus, bacteria, or other invader, a process called *molecular mimicry*. The attack can happen in almost any body part—your gut lining in Crohn's disease and ulcerative colitis; your joints in rheumatoid arthritis; your skin in psoriasis; and in the case of Hashimoto's, your thyroid. Often the damage becomes widespread, symptoms show up in distant systems, as happens, for example, with celiac disease, and is why autoimmune diseases are associated with a wide array of local and generalized symptoms, notably pain, fatigue, and depression. Autoimmune diseases may begin after an infection and can also result from an overly permeable digestive system that allows food or gut bacterial proteins called LPSs (short for lipopolysaccharides) to reach your intestinal immune system, where they are seen as foreign invaders, or they can be a result of an extreme time of stress.

According to conventional medicine, once you have an autoimmune disease, it's a self-perpetuating and permanent process that carries on even after the trigger has been eliminated. But this is not always the case. There is research—on celiac disease, for example—showing that by removing a trigger, we can arrest the autoimmune process.

A big part of the SOS Solution is hitting the brakes on runaway inflammation and immune system confusion. As you cool down inflammation, aches and pains you've had for years can disappear, sleep will come more easily and be refreshing, your thinking will be clear, and you will have the energy to live life the way you want to.

2

THE FIVE ROOT CAUSES OF ADRENAL AND THYROID DYSFUNCTION

| Chronic Emotional and Mental Stress | Food Triggers | Gut Imbalances | Toxic Overload | Immune Disruption and Stealth Infections |

WHEN YOU LOOK AT A TREE, you see only the parts above the ground, but beneath the soil's surface spreads a massive network of roots, often more extensive than the entire branch system, the health of which is essential to the health of the tree. Conventional medicine tends to see only the aboveground parts, the symptoms and nameable diseases, treating these as if they were the problems when in fact they are only symptoms of problems in the roots. In this chapter, we're going to look at what's below the surface of your medical symptoms and conditions, and uncover the Root Causes that led to them in the first place.

The Root Causes of SOS and Hypothyroidism

1. Chronic emotional and mental stress

2. Food triggers, blood sugar imbalances, and nutritional insufficiencies

3. Gut imbalances

4. Toxic overload

5. Immune disruption and stealth infections

ROOT CAUSE 1: CHRONIC EMOTIONAL AND MENTAL STRESS

Your body hears everything your mind says.

—Naomi Judd

Have you ever been so stressed out that you wished you could blink yourself straight to a sunny beach? Maybe you'd settle for a hammock in a quiet backyard. Have you caught yourself thinking, "I'm so overwhelmed I can't take it anymore," "I feel like I'm at my breaking point," or "I'm working so hard to meet everyone's needs that there's just no time to stop and breathe"? If so, welcome to the United States of Stress!

The United States of Stress

To be clear, and we'll talk more about this soon, when I use the word "stress," I'm talking about feeling stressed out, or chronically overwhelmed. For two years in a row the annual stress survey commissioned by the American Psychological Association found the following:

- Seventy-five percent of all Americans have moderate to severe stress.

- A full 25 percent experience severe stress.

- At least 43 percent of all U.S. adults suffer adverse health effects due to stress.

Maybe not so surprising. But check this out: *Women top the charts in all stress-related statistics,* including having more physical symptoms as a result of stress than men. Not only do women experience their own stress, but in addition we tend to internalize our partner's stress, and also world stress—what we read in the news, and feelings of terror and social vulnerability—more than men.

Learning to recognize when you're stressed out and turning it around are crucial to getting—and staying—out of SOS. But—and I am stating this loud and clear—when I'm talking about being stressed out, I am in no way implying that your symptoms are "in your head." As women we've been called overly sensitive, overly emotional, and overreactive. Women have told me even their doctors have accused them of this. So we learn to ignore our symptoms and our stress—stuff it, tough through it, and suck it up—lest we sound complaining or overreactive. Stress is a real medical phenomenon, and not one to be dismissed.

You know the *feeling* of stress, anxiety, pressure, overwhelm, irritability, weepiness, frustration, anger, and so on, but what is stress, really? It's all the physical, mental, and emotional reactions we have when we're carrying more of a load than we are able to bear. The feelings and thoughts associated with being stressed out are your inner GPS telling you that you're overwhelmed. Listening to the language of stress and knowing that it is affecting your sleep, hormones, weight, and brain can help you to recognize when you're in SOS. Let's look at some of the ways stress might be affecting you—without your even realizing it.

No Peace Without Good Sleep

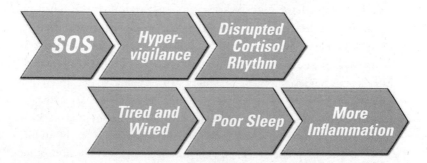

"I know I shouldn't because I'm not sleeping well," Lindsey said, "but I can't get through the afternoon without that second cup of coffee. By 3:00 in the afternoon I'm exhausted, and I've still got to make it to the end of the workday. So I drink the coffee, then I'm wired at bedtime. Then I stay up too late, usually catching up on email and puttering around on Facebook. In truth, I enjoy that time to myself after the kids and my husband have gone to bed, but when I finally do get into bed, around midnight, I just lay there awake, staring at the ceiling, irritated and anxious, knowing that I'm going to be even more tired tomorrow."

Sleep is when your body restores itself: tissue rebuilds, accumulated toxins are eliminated, and your brain consolidates your day's experiences and turns them into new knowledge. But the vast majority of us are living with a sleep debt, so we're missing out on those restorative benefits. Moreover, poor sleep messes up your cortisol rhythm and affects everything: your weight, food choices, personal choices, mood, hormones, immunity, mental clarity, memory, cognitive function, sex drive, and even pain levels. Women who sleep fewer than five hours each night weigh more, even when they consume fewer calories, than women who sleep for at least seven. When you are sleep-deprived, ghrelin, your "hunger hormone," increases, while the hormone that tells your brain you're full, leptin, gets suppressed—so you end up being unable to control "fatigue eating."

Lindsey aptly described one of the most common symptoms of elevated cortisol—feeling tired and wired—and she isn't alone with this sleep problem; 49 percent of American women say they lay awake in bed at night, unable to sleep. SOS triggers adrenaline release, causing hypervigilance, which keeps you alert and acutely aware of your surroundings. You feel like you're in an action thriller and you're on night watch.

Even just one night of disturbed sleep can raise your nighttime cortisol, which in turn blocks the production of the sleep hormone melatonin, creating a vicious cycle that makes it harder to fall and stay asleep, and harder to wake up easily in the morning. Melatonin is critical for the natural detoxification that is supposed to happen while you're sleeping, so disrupted rest means you're not breaking down accumulated toxic chemicals and hormones, including those in your brain, but also other hormones, especially estrogen. So too little sleep or not enough quality sleep can mean brain fog, memory and focus problems, PMS, breast pain, mood swings, and other hormonal problems.

Melatonin is also suppressed by the blue light emitted by electronics; so if you're wired and hanging out on your computer instead of doing more helpful sleep-promoting practices, you're compounding the problem. When sleep patterns shift, so does your gut flora—and not for the good. You'll learn more about what this means for your health later in this chapter.

Finally, inflammatory cytokines, though they are coursing through your blood with the intention of protecting you from infection, not only make you tired, irritable, and achy the same way they do before you get the flu, they also upset the rhythm of the region in your hypothalamus that acts as your circadian clock. When this happens, your wake and sleep cycles become flipped, leading to increased nighttime wakefulness and increased daytime sleepiness. Chronic inflammation likely explains why women with autoimmune conditions experience circadian rhythm disruptions and more than normal amounts of fatigue. Insomnia also can cause decreased morning cortisol, causing you to feel groggy and tired in the morning and into your day.

What happens when you're tired all the time? Like Lindsey, you run the risk of ending up on a treadmill of getting more wired and more tired. You feel irritable and depressed. You can't focus at work. Your memory takes a hit. Your coping skills go down. You feel more overwhelmed, and late morning and late afternoon you head straight in the direction of the nearest sugar and caffeine for energy and a dose of feel-good chemicals that sugar releases in your brain.

Studies show it can take a week or more for the cognitive and physiological consequences of poor sleep to wear off—even after increasing sleep—so reclaiming restful sleep is going to be one of the first things on the agenda when you start the SOS Solution.

Can't Eat Just One? Stress Blocks Willpower

Being in control of your food choices is key to keeping your weight healthy and inflammation at bay. But at least a third of women state that lack of willpower is their number one obstacle to making the best health choices, and more than half say that for their willpower to improve, they'd have to feel less fatigue. SOS sabotages willpower. Over time, cortisol rewires the neural circuitry in your frontal cortex, the part of your brain responsible for what is called *executive function*, or good decision making. When this happens, your willpower goes out the window, and with it control over food choices, often along with your good intentions to get exercise, eat less sugar, and "have only one" of whatever it is. No wonder just telling yourself to eat less and exercise more doesn't usually work.

SOS May Be Why Your Diets Haven't Worked

If you're in SOS, it's likely that chocolate, ice cream, cookies, or a couple of glasses of wine at night have become a routine you're having trouble shaking. I've had more than a few patients with a secret ice cream or cookie stash, and it's a direct result of SOS. Sugar and fat are the molecules that get burned up rapidly to fuel the stress response. When the emergency is over, your body needs to refuel itself, and its favorite fuels? Yup! Sugar, carbs, and fat. Stressed women not only eat larger amounts of high-fat, high-sugar foods, but when we do, we're more prone to abdominal obesity and insulin resistance compared to less stressed women who eat the same foods.

Your brain practically ensures that when you are under constant stress, you'll go for sugary, fatty, and salty foods by releasing a flood of feel-good nervous system chemicals such as serotonin and dopamine that calm your nervous system with every bite as they also bring cortisol back into normal range. That's why they are called comfort foods—they are literally comforting your nervous system. This comfort comes at a price. We become addicted to the foods that are bringing comfort, and since these are typically sugary and fatty foods, we eat more of them, causing us to pack on belly fat and VAT, or *visceral abdominal fat*, a type of hidden fat that produces inflammatory cytokines that wreak havoc on the entire body. This further drives inflammation and perpetuates SOS. Talk about a powerful vicious cycle that makes it hard to eat healthily or lose weight. It doesn't help that the food industry makes tasty treats available and desirable at every turn, so hard to resist that it's nearly impossible to prevent your primitive brain from tossing that Ben & Jerry's right into your shopping cart while your rational brain is telling you, "Don't do it." It also doesn't help that women, more than men, are likely to eat sugary, fatty foods when we're stressed out—and since we're more likely to do the grocery shopping, we're also more likely to be exposed to the temptations on every shelf.

Stress Dials Down Your Thyroid Function

When you are under prolonged stress, your SOS response is to dial your thyroid function down to conserve energy. Your thyroid puts a temporary hold on anything but the bare necessities of energy production, dramatically slowing down metabolism and any other functions that require a lot of energy, such as sex drive and reproduction. Your adrenals act like a wise accountant telling your thyroid, "Hey, the budget's a little tight right now, so better to not spend. In fact, why don't you sock that money away for a rainy day?" Concerned, your thyroid complies by cutting back on the production and use of active thyroid hormone (free T_3) and puts what does get produced into a savings account in the form of inactive reverse T_3 (RT_3). Acute stress—for example, when you have a fever or infection—naturally causes this to happen for a few days so that you have energy on hand for your healing process. Chronic stress makes this a more regular state, and in time can lead to chronic thyroid function suppression, causing you to become hypothyroid.

Like the straw that broke the camel's back, it's been documented in the medical literature that an illness in the family, the death of a loved one, a move, a new baby, or a change of job can push you over the edge into the onset of hypothyroid symptoms. Hashimoto's has also been described in association with chronic anxiety or stress, or a history of childhood trauma. Stress uses up important nutrients—for example, selenium and magnesium—depriving the thyroid of what it needs for hormone production or protecting itself from inflammation, thus creating another pathway whereby stress leads to thyroid problems in SOS. Stress also inhibits both the ability of the body to convert inactive thyroid hormone (T_4) to the active form (T_3) and the ability of the active form to get into your cells. Cortisol makes the thyroid hormone receptors on your cells resistant (less sensitive) to the active form of thyroid hormone, such that cells don't uptake thyroid hormone, and then it can't do its job within the cells to activate the thyroid's many functions in your body and brain. So even if your thyroid function is normal, you can still experience symptoms of hypothyroidism as a result.

Cortisol also reduces your ability to clear estrogen from your system through your liver. Guess what? Increased estrogen increases the production of a carrier protein called *thyroid-binding globulin* (TBG), which does exactly what it sounds like—binds onto thyroid hormone. This form of thyroid hormone is not active, so your thyroid function goes down even when your thyroid is pumping out the stuff like it's supposed to—and your lab tests might also look normal, so your doctor misses the diagnosis.

SOS, Stress, and Brain Strain

Think back to when a teacher called on you unexpectedly in class and suddenly your mouth went dry, your heart was thumping in your ears, you froze, and you couldn't remember a thing you studied the night before. Now magnify that reaction to understand the impact of chronic stress on your mind and mood.

Stress affects cognitive functioning. When you're in SOS, your brain is "wired" to be alert for danger—so your brain's focus is heightened to threats in your environment. It's in the process of searching for triggers or memories that relate to danger—it's not focusing on making new memories unless those memories are going to be lifesaving in the future. Changes in your brain due to the prolonged effects of cortisol make you more likely to cement and replay negative, worrisome, or distressing memories (this is how traumatic memories get stored and how post-traumatic stress disorder develops), while making it harder to learn and store new information.

Over time, cortisol exposure alters nerve connections in parts of your brain (i.e., the hippocampus and temporal lobes), suppressing short-term memory. This can prevent you from remembering what you've just read or studied, and also impacts word finding (you know, that thing that's on the tip of your tongue that you just can't recall?). Repeated stress can cause the nerves in these regions to shrink and die, reducing the thickness of parts of your brain that control emotional regulation, willpower, and decision making. The hippocampus also helps to regulate the stress response, inhibiting the response of the HPA axis to stress (a negative feedback loop). When hippocampal functioning is impaired, it's harder for us to tamp down the stress response, another example of the self-perpetuating nature of SOS.

Elevated levels of cortisol enhance memory for emotionally arousing events, pushing us toward seeing life with jaundice-colored glasses, while reducing our memory for information unrelated to the source of stress.

Did You Forget Something?

"Brain fog," flagging memory, and decreased focus and concentration are worrisome symptoms because you may think that you are developing dementia. Some women find this the scariest of their symptoms. Cognitive challenges can also make getting your work done really difficult, may lead to considerable delays in completing projects, and may impact your word finding, leading to embarrassment in meetings and conversations. Memory challenges can make even common tasks such as parking your car fraught with anxiety as you worry about whether you'll remember where it is, and tiresome as you come up with ways to compensate. While any sudden changes in your mental focus or concentration or severe progressive changes do warrant a conversation with your doctor, most of the time reversible causes of SOS are the culprit.

How does SOS affect your memory and focus? In several ways.

The brain was, until recently, thought to be generally impermeable to and separate from what's going on in the rest of your body, thanks to a filtering layer of tiny blood vessels that make up the *blood-brain barrier* (BBB). We now know, however, that the BBB is not impermeable to much of what's going on in the rest of the body, and that particularly, the inflammatory cytokines that move into gear when the stress response gets activated, get into your head. And when they do, they cause a phenomenon called *brain-flammation*, which is just what it sounds like: inflammation in the brain (or "inflame in the membrane," as I end up humming in my head). This is why SOS is the primary culprit in foggy thinking, poor concentration, and poor memory, as well as in fatigue, anxiety, irritability, and, notably, depression.

Stress also hastens the appearance of certain biological markers of brain aging—in other words, when SOS goes on for too long, it can ultimately be one of the causes of dementia. In one study of 800 Swedish women age thirty-eight to fifty-four, 153 women developed dementia during the following thirty-eight years, with Alzheimer's dementia diagnosed in 104 of the cases. Those women who were chronically "stressed out," jealous, moody, anxious, or worried showed the highest risk of developing dementia. As if that's not enough, chronic high blood pressure due to elevated HPA axis activation can eventually reduce blood flow to the brain, ultimately reducing cognitive function.

Shedding Light on Depression and Anxiety

The statistics on depression and anxiety in women are staggering. Women experience major depression and anxiety disorders twice as often as men, and depending on the study, between one in four and one in six women is on an antidepressant—two and a half times more than men—and many women are now on antianxiety medications, including potentially dangerous and addictive benzodiazepine drugs prescribed like candy by too many doctors! If you're experiencing either depression or anxiety, you can feel like you're stuck in an endless and hopeless cycle of despair that's impossible to get out of. It's not impossible.

While there are many life circumstances that can lead to depression and anxiety, including past traumas and difficult situations, the same cytokines that cause fatigue and brain fog by crossing the blood-brain barrier also play a leading role in causing depression, through a process called *neuroinflammation*. Studies show that at least 30 percent of all cases of depression are due to chronic inflammation, and as you've seen, chronic stress and its cousin, poor sleep, breed inflammation. Negative mental loops can be caused, and cause SOS, and have been shown to raise cortisol, and then you're really in a vicious cycle.

Numerous studies have shown a significant increase in circulating inflammatory chemicals, including C-reactive protein, IL-6, and TNF-α in even otherwise healthy individuals with depression. A recent study showed that PET scans of the brains of individuals with depression showed significant inflammation, and one's level of depression correlates with the amount of inflammation.

One might wonder whether inflammation is "the chicken or the egg" in depression. Enough studies have been done now to show that it is the inflammation that is triggering the depression, though chronic depression does create a vicious cycle that also triggers SOS, often because of the poor health choices we make when we are chronically depressed. Depression is not a one-size-fits-all experience, and differences in how women experience depression fall on a spectrum of lethargic and fatigued to agitated and anxious, corresponding with underactive or overactive adrenal function. These corresponding pathways act as bridges to chronic diseases as well. While the goal of inflammation is to protect us from harm in the long run, chronic

Trauma and Early Origins of SOS

Love is what we were born with. Fear is what we learned here.
—Marianne Williamson

Experiencing a threat to your survival at any time in your life, but particularly when you're young, can leave you more sensitive to stress, anxiety, and worry, causing your stress response to kick in at a lower "set point" than people who haven't experienced trauma. Your primitive brain centers, particularly your amygdala and hippocampus, stored those troublesome memories in deep memory banks to protect you from anything that resembles a similar threat going forward and pulls them out at lightning speed—often unnecessarily. So you may also be on heightened lookout for anything to go wrong at any time. You may want to live more optimistically, but find yourself more often "waiting for the other shoe to drop," and plagued by more symptoms than your current lifestyle easily explains. You may have patterns that you've had a hard time shaking off.

If the trauma involved a depressed, absent parent, or an alcoholic parent whose moods you couldn't trust awaiting you when you returned from school each day, then as an adult you might experience dread each day on your way home from work, and not understand that your sense of anxiety is based on past experience. If the trauma was generalized instability and stress, lack of love, a borderline personality or narcissistic parent, bullying at school, or any trauma you experienced out in the world—any of these can create a general sense of lack of safety and lead to an overall hardwiring of your brain that the world is not a safe place. It creates a very low set point for your stress response.

Essentially you became programmed to be in SOS and tend to be on the lookout for the worst as a personality default—because your brain thinks this will keep you safe. The upside of this is that you are also likely to be a highly sensitive person—able to read facial expressions, social cues, and people's body language, for example, quite exquisitely. And the good news is that your brain can be rewired, via a very nice aspect of the human brain called *neuroplasticity*. By creating new thought patterns, reframing your beliefs, and establishing new, healthier ones, you can keep the upside while letting go of the downside, SOS.

Note: Reading about trauma or a stressful past can cause buried trauma to surface. This can be very hard. Please call a trusted friend, and if needed, seek a professional who can help you to sort through your memories and feelings.

immune activation and inflammation come at a high price—potentially our mental health.

SOS and Your Hormones— Not Tonight, Honey, I'm in Survival Mode

Hormone disruption is a major side effect of being in chronic overdrive, and is a warning sign of SOS. When you're stressed, cortisol steals the building blocks you need to make estrogen, progesterone, and testosterone. This is why you might skip a period when you experience a stressful event in your life, or lose interest in sex when you're stressed out or exhausted all the time. And that's not all. Being stuck in the stress response means you end up dealing with PMS, PCOS, irregular periods, ovarian cysts, endometriosis, fertility problems, cyclic breast lumps and tenderness, premature ovarian failure, and exacerbated menopausal symptoms, to name a few of the common hormonal problems I see as a result.

It's not surprising, then, that one in eight women in the United States seeks fertility counseling, more than five million women in the United States have PCOS, and one in ten has endometriosis, not to mention the millions of workdays women lose due to PMS and the impact of low libido on relationships.

PCOS and Endometriosis— Yup, They're Related to SOS, Too

SOS leads to a number of common "women only" problems that can have a serious impact on health and quality of life. The hormonal imbalances, insulin resistance, and inflammation associated with SOS can form the underpinnings, for example, of endometriosis and PCOS.

Endometriosis is a potentially painful chronic disorder in which tissue that normally lines the inside of the uterus—the endometrium—grows outside of the uterus, commonly on the ovaries, the bowel, or the tissue lining the pelvis. Just like the lining inside your uterus, it is triggered by your monthly hormonal cycles to thicken, break down, and shed with each menstrual cycle. This shedding, akin to the bleeding you have during your menstrual cycle, causes the blood in the abdominal cavity to become trapped, where it irritates surrounding tissue, and eventually causes the formation of scar tissue and adhesions that cause the abdominal organs to get stuck together, often leading to chronic abdominal and pelvic discomfort, constipation, and urinary and fertility problems. Fundamentally, it is a problem associated with dysregulation in the immune system and chronic inflammation, which are also tied into the core imbalances in SOS.

Polycystic ovarian syndrome (PCOS) is one of the most common metabolic and hormonal conditions among women, affecting as many as 5 to 10 percent of women of childbearing age, and 40 percent of women with insulin resistance or diabetes. Less than 50 percent of these women are properly diagnosed, thus PCOS has been called the "silent killer" because, untreated, it has been linked to an increased risk for developing type 2 diabetes, high cholesterol, high blood pressure, and heart disease. It occurs as a result of insulin resistance, which in turn also leads to elevated testosterone.

Cortisol and adrenaline also aren't the only hormones that your adrenal glands are producing when the stress comes knocking. When the stress response gets activated, your adrenal glands produce another hormone, called DHEA/DHEAS, as well as androstenedione. These hormones buffer the brain from the impact of cortisol. But when these get elevated due to chronic stress, PCOS can result. High testosterone levels can cause disturbing symptoms: hirsutism (excessive hair growth, especially on the face), male-pattern baldness, and acne. It also can prevent ovulation and thus is responsible for about 70 percent of all cases of infertility due to lack of ovulation. The good news is that it can be reversed, and getting out of SOS is a major ticket out of PCOS.

Stress and Your Immune System

When you're in SOS, whether because of stress or physical triggers, your inflammatory cell production increases. Your body is staying prepared for all possible threats, including those that could require fast activation of your immune system. This immune system overactivation increases your risk of developing inflammatory reactions—for example, eczema, hives, food intolerances, and allergies. You may also find yourself with chronic low-grade inflammation, which can be responsible for fatigue, weight gain, brain fog, migraines, low blood pressure, anxiety and panic attacks, cognitive function changes, insomnia, aches and pains, weight gain, depression, and conditions such as chronic fatigue syndrome, fibromyalgia, and PMS.

Over time your immune system can become confused by the mixed message of constantly being told to fight an infection when there's no infection present. Your body's immune response can turn from friend to foe, leading to a mutiny wherein the immune system turns against and attacks your own cells and organs, thus leading to any number of autoimmune conditions. Your brain also becomes desensitized to the signal that it's supposed to turn off inflammation; autoimmunity can become a runaway train.

A rebound effect can also eventually occur whereby elevated cortisol, which suppresses inflammation, can inhibit your infection-fighting responses so much that you become more vulnerable to infections—so you get sick more often than you should, or, for example, have trouble fighting off seasonal infections such as colds, flu, or bronchitis. It also makes you more susceptible to both infection with and reactivation of certain viral infections, particularly the Epstein-Barr virus (EBV, a virus in the herpesvirus group, along with chicken pox, and also the virus responsible for mononucleosis), which may cause severe fatigue and is considered a possible "stealth" cause of autoimmune conditions.

The elevated cortisol and the overproduction of inflammatory cytokines that accompany SOS also directly suppress thyroid function and active thyroid hormone production. And as mentioned above, when your immune system's messages get confused, they can go rogue and attack your own tissues—including your thyroid—leading to Hashimoto's.

The awesome thing about stress (yes, I did just say that) is that you can learn to reframe and transform your response to it so that it no longer makes you sick and tired. In fact, believe it or not, I'm going to show you how to harness stress to make it work for you. You can learn to say no, learn to put your own oxygen mask on first so you can help others, and learn some skills that keep you chill when things get hot. Chapter 5 is going to give you the skills you need to reduce stress as much as possible and to stay on top of those inevitable stresses that happen in life.

ROOT CAUSE 2: FOOD TRIGGERS OF SOS

What you eat—and what you don't eat—profoundly affects your health. Let's look at the big dietary triggers we'll take on in the SOS Solution that can be at the root of SOS and thyroid problems: blood sugar imbalances, high-sugar and high-carb diets, hidden inflammatory food triggers, and the phytonutrient gap.

Blood Sugar Imbalances, Hungry Fat Cells, and SOS

Have you ever suddenly felt anxious, exhausted, shaky, overwhelmed, or irritable, only to bite into a muffin or doughnut, down a handful of M&Ms, or knock back a mocha latte and suddenly feel your inner calm almost immediately restored? When your blood sugar is low because you've been too busy to eat, or you haven't been eating the right foods, your brain, which needs glucose to survive, sends out an immediate signal telling your whole body that you've gone into survival mode and that sugar is the only antidote that's going to keep you from crumpling to the ground and dying right this minute. You urgently feel the need to have something sugary, fatty, or carbohydrate-dense. When you give in to the craving, you feel better. You sigh and your shoulders relax. All of the survival hormones and chemicals that were making you feel jangled get tucked safely back into your cells, where they belong.

Unfortunately, that good feeling doesn't last for long, and the internal crisis cycle vengefully reignites. About an hour later you're foggier than ever, sleepy, "hangry," and probably beating yourself up because on top of

Apple or Pear: What Your Body Shape Can Tell You About SOS

Your body shape can reveal a lot about what's going on in your body, particularly whether you are apple- or pear-shaped. Pear-shaped women are narrow on the top and in the middle, and broad on the bottom. While women with pear shapes may be apt to have some hormonal problems, it is usually associated with nonserious problems. However, being apple-shaped—that is, wide around the middle—even if you are a slim apple (or what Dr. Mark Hyman calls "skinny fat"), is an indication that there's trouble with your cortisol or your insulin, and that you've got inflammation. A waist circumference of more than thirty-five inches puts women in the danger zone for disease risk—metabolic syndrome, diabetes, high blood pressure, heart attack—and death (for men it's greater than forty inches). This is due to all of the reasons I've shared with you in previous chapters about the dangers of belly fat.

The fastest way to figure out if you are an apple or a pear is to grab a tape measure and calculate your waist-to-hip ratio (WHR). First, circle your waist with the tape measure, just above the level of your navel, and look at the number in inches. Next place the tape measure around your hips—at your actual hips, where your legs join into the sockets of your pelvis, which is usually at the widest part of your fanny. Again, note the number in inches. To calculate the ratio, you put the waist number in the top of a fraction, and the hip measurement in the bottom—or if you hate math or have too much brain fog to think clearly, simply look online for a waist-to-hip calculator and plug the numbers in. The calculator will do the work for you. A normal waist-to-hip ratio for women is 0.80 to 0.84. Greater than 0.85 means obesity and can spell trouble.

I recommend calculating the waist-to-hip ratio now, and then repeat it once every two weeks to trend your progress until it's in the normal range. However, if taking measurements isn't your thing, no worries—you'll notice when you can button your pants more easily and you can fit back into that favorite skirt or slacks. I find this to be as valuable as lab testing for trending results.

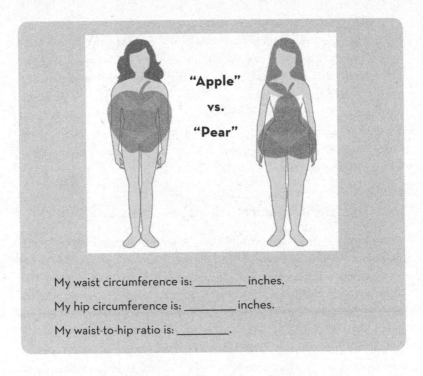

My waist circumference is: _____ inches.

My hip circumference is: _____ inches.

My waist-to-hip ratio is: _____.

it, you've sabotaged your diet. You're in survival mode again, which is why at 5:00 P.M., when you're at the grocery store checkout, that "natural" peanut butter cup or that dark chocolate almond bar seems irresistible, and practically is, because the primitive part of your brain that's craving glucose can't say no. Your brain is going to choose survival over whether you can fit into your "skinny jeans"—every time.

Symptoms of low blood sugar include shakiness, irritability, intense hunger, sweating, fatigue, light-headedness, nausea, and loss of mental clarity, and some women even faint. If you experience these with any frequency, it's important to eat more protein and fat and always to keep an emergency stash around. We'll revisit this in the SOS Solution Reboot, covered in chapter 4. If your blood sugar yo-yos often enough, you end up in SOS. Your cortisol revs up, you gain weight, and your brain stops listening to the hormone leptin, made by your fat cells, that tells you you're full. So you keep eating. This is called *leptin resistance*, and like its cousin, insulin resistance, causes chronic low-grade inflammation.

Further, under SOS, your brain amps up the release of a chemical called *neuropeptide Y* (NPY), which is like Miracle-Gro for your fat cells, and even more so when it gets together with junk food. So the standard Western diet, high in unhealthy fats, starches, and sugar, massively compounds the problem. All of these hormonal and chemical messengers make you pack weight around your middle to store—because your brain is thinking, "Hey, this gal isn't eating very much—are we in a famine?" It can get to the point where you're not even in charge of your appetite and the food you're eating. Who is? Hungry fat cells.

The Flip Side: Too Much Sugar, Carbs, and SOS

We all love a little sugar now and then. Even our ancestors liked it, but their sweet tooth was satisfied with seasonal berries and possibly occasional access to honey. The Western diet has taken our love for sugar too far for our own good. The average American eats about 160 pounds of sugar and 200 pounds of white flour each year. That's a staggering combined 1 pound a day. If you're not sure how much that is, look at a 5-pound bag of flour next time you're at the supermarket. Better yet, put it up next to your waist to see how much you'd be adding to your body in just five days! Frighteningly, 81 percent of Americans now consume more than the highest daily acceptable level of sugar every single day.

Over the past three decades, the rates of chronic disease have paralleled the increase in sugar and carbohydrate consumption, especially refined carbohydrate products (white flour, white rice, pasta, baked goods, cereal, pastries, etc.), and the results are stark: for the first time in human history the rates of obesity now exceed malnutrition worldwide. But even "normal weight" individuals are 40 percent more likely to suffer from chronic diseases as a result of metabolic problems and chronic inflammation that can be traced to high rates of sugar consumption. Sugar and refined flour products spike insulin and trigger release of inflammatory cytokines, which in turn lead to the formation of free radicals that are toxic to your cells and are proinflammatory.

When you're stressed out, your body increases its cortisol output in response to sugar consumption at a greater level than it otherwise would in times of calm. In other words, more stress, more sugar, more cortisol.

Trouble Gaining Weight?

For a small number of women, rather than experiencing the typical weight gain associated with SOS, the initial and immediate appetite suppressant effects of acute stress become the predominant feature, and may persist chronically. Thus you may lose weight or have trouble gaining it—even though you may still have cravings and even binge out on certain foods.

While not being able to gain weight sounds like a problem most women would like to have, if you're struggling with being underweight, you know it's not as good as it sounds—or necessarily looks. It can leave you looking gaunt, cause dry skin and hair loss, and can wreak havoc on your hormones, which rely on some fat stores for their production, leading to problems with fertility, libido, and mood, to name a few. If being underweight is a problem that you're struggling with, the SOS Solution will reset your cortisol and with it your appetite and ability to get to your healthy body weight.

Because of its effects on ghrelin, leptin, and the reward (addiction) centers of your brain, cortisol then keeps you wanting more sugar. This, in turn, literally blunts your taste for healthy foods, a result of this combination of hormones on reward centers of your brain. The healthy stuff just doesn't taste as good as the sugary, fatty, salty, and carb-rich options.

Further, regular and high levels of sugar consumption can lead to detrimental changes in your gut flora, which in turn can lead to systemic inflammation, leaky gut, and problems with nutrient absorption. Proper absorption is no small matter, since it is the vital way that every single cell in the body is nourished. When absorption doesn't happen properly, the body becomes undernourished and sick. In addition to the sugar-induced nutritional deficiencies that keep your immune system from its best performance, sugar also inhibits proper immune response, so you get sick more often. Studies have also linked high sugar consumption to cognitive decline—Alzheimer's disease is now referred to by some as type 3 diabetes because of evidence that chronic inflammation and oxidative damage may be factors in its onset.

The Common Trigger Foods

Many of my patients are surprised to discover that they're sensitive to some of the foods they eat regularly—and often crave the most. When you are intolerant of or sensitive to foods you're eating, you become chronically inflamed. This can happen because:

- You have an inherent inability to digest that food, as is the case with lactose intolerance;

- You have either an inherited or acquired autoimmune response to a food, as is the case with celiac disease, an autoimmune condition; or

- You have developed a gut problem called leaky gut, making your immune system overly reactive to that food (you'll learn about leaky gut under "Root Cause 3").

In the next chapter you'll complete a questionnaire to help you figure out if you have hidden food triggers, and you'll uncover which they are when you do the SOS Solution Reboot in chapter 4. The following are the most universally common food triggers.

Gluten: For Some, It's Public Enemy Number One

Gluten refers to specific proteins in wheat, barley, and rye that give bread that chewy, elastic quality and make those nice air pockets that make bread rise. It's also hidden in a surprising number of products: salad dressings, soy sauce, other sauces, ketchup, beer and a number of other alcoholic beverages, and even deli meats where it is used as a "glue" to hold meat cuts together, to name a few. Some body products and cosmetics—including some lipsticks—also contain gluten. Additionally, a number of foods, including corn, oats, millet, coffee, and dairy, though they don't contain gluten, may "cross-react" with gluten, causing many of the same symptoms.

Celiac disease, an autoimmune condition that can cause serious systemic inflammation due to the consumption of gluten, which was previously thought to be rare, is now proven to be much more common, affecting one in a hundred Americans. Historically, it was thought that consuming gluten was only a problem for people with celiac disease; however, gluten sensitivity, though not an autoimmune condition, can also cause significant chronic inflammation and symptoms for the millions of people

Muscle Up Your Metabolism

Muscle doesn't just make you look buff—it's metabolically active, meaning that it burns calories even when you're not exercising. In fact, it is so metabolically active that it burns fat while you're at rest—a really great reason to exercise and build some more muscle. The magic is in your mitochondria, "organelles" within muscle cells that act as miniature powerhouses. More muscle means more mitochondria. But here's the thing: chronic activation of the stress response causes you to break down muscle, and when your adrenal function is low, your DHEA and testosterone production decline as well, and guess what they're responsible for—building muscle. So to build muscle, you want to not only power up your exercise, but also power down SOS.

suffering—sometimes without knowing the cause—from this condition.

Celiac has been associated with more than fifty-five medical conditions and numerous nutritional deficiencies (especially iron, B_{12}, folate, and vitamin D) due to poor absorption through the gut. About 10 percent of people with celiac disease also develop another autoimmune condition—as many as 10 percent of those with celiac are also found to have Hashimoto's. Studies have also demonstrated considerable improvement in and even resolution of subclinical hypothyroidism and Hashimoto's, via improvement in lab results, on a strict gluten-free diet.

It was after switching several of my patients to a gluten-free diet a number of years ago that I became a believer in gluten-free eating for those who are sensitive. Patients were reporting dramatic improvements—and even complete resolution—of symptoms such as brain fog, hypothyroidism, and rheumatoid arthritis just a few weeks after removing gluten from their diets. Their responses were sometimes so significant and fast that I hardly believed them! While I do not put every patient on a gluten-free diet, it is a commonly effective first-line approach in my medical practice and is a central part of the SOS Solution Reboot. Following this program, you'll discover whether gluten-free is best for you.

For some women, grains and even legumes are triggers. This is either due to sensitivity to the foods themselves, or due to microbiome or blood sugar imbalances that impact carbohydrate breakdown in your gut, leading to production of by-products that cause fatigue, brain fog, bloating, or other symptoms.

Other Common Food Triggers

A number of additional foods commonly act as chronic inflammatory triggers, though these vary widely among individuals. These include dairy, corn, soy, nuts, nightshades (tomatoes, bell peppers, potatoes, and eggplant), and yeast (baker's yeast, brewer's yeast, and vinegar).

Dairy, which in small amounts can be a healthful part of the diet when organic, is not well tolerated by large numbers of people. For some, inherent enzyme deficiencies in the intestinal lining prevent digestion of the sugars in dairy, causing sometimes severe and immediate diarrhea, gas, and cramping, though in some it may cause constipation, a less obvious association. This is known as lactose intolerance. Yet others are sensitive to proteins in dairy; caseomorphins, for example, can lead to brain fog and depression, and have even been associated with actual addiction to dairy products, which is why you may find cheese so appealing, you may crave it, and may binge out on it when you do have it. Dairy, even when organic, can impact women's hormone balance as well, and inorganic dairy can contain significant amounts of antibiotics, hormones, and environmental toxins, all of which preferentially accumulate in the fat in dairy. Leaky gut and IBS often suggest intolerance to dairy, but can cause any number of symptoms, including anxiety, depression, and acne. When proteins in dairy (especially casein and caseomorphins from cow milk products) migrate across the intestinal lining and reach the intestinal immune system, they can trigger chronic low-level inflammation. Because they are such a common trigger, I ask everyone to go off of them completely during the Reboot and pay attention to whether symptoms clear up.

Some people are sensitive to eggs, but often tolerate them when they are baked. Some tolerate the yolks better than the egg white, and some the whites better than the yolks. However, because they are a rich source of not only protein, but also the important nutrient choline, which is a boon to brain function, I include eggs in the diet unless you have symptoms when you eat them. Similarly, many people just don't digest soy well, yet soy and other beans and legumes, which also can cause sensitivity because of a component called lectins, are an important part of a vegetarian diet. In fact, the health benefits of beans and legumes are significant and include weight loss, lower cholesterol, and better heart health even if nothing else in the diet changes much.

Nuts are a common food allergen, but additionally, when overconsumed, as I've seen happen in Paleo diets where they become a staple food for some, I've seen exacerbations in inflammation, particularly joint pain. Corn also can be hard to digest, and may be a cross-reactive food for you if you are gluten-intolerant; further, most corn in the United States is genetically modified, and some have postulated that it is the use of glyphosate, an agricultural chemical contaminant in corn and other grains, that makes these harder to digest now, thus contributing to the increase in grain intolerances we see in our culture.

Finally, some don't tolerate yeasts—including in breads, vinegars (with the exception of apple cider vinegar in most cases), and alcohol. If it's just red wine and balsamic vinegar you don't tolerate, this can be due to sulfates rather than yeast, but if you suffer from Candida overgrowth, you might not tolerate yeast-containing products until that is cleared up, or at all.

While I don't recommend that everyone take all of these out of their diets indefinitely, in the SOS Solution Reboot you'll remove many for a short time to see which might be triggers for you personally.

Artificial and Processed "Foods" Aren't Foods, So Don't Eat Them

Processed foods have been found to cause an incredible list of health problems, including gut lining damage and impairment to the mechanisms that protect your DNA, and they can confuse the immune system over what to attack, leading to chronic inflammation and autoimmune disease. Seven additives cause the greatest harm: sugar, salt, emulsifiers, organic solvents, gluten, microbial transglutaminase, and nanoemulsions. All highly processed, artificial foods (sometimes called "Frankenfoods") should be removed from the diet. They all cause more harm than good.

Artificial sweeteners are also a problem. A recent study found that regular use of the artificial sweeteners aspartame (i.e., Equal, NutraSweet) and sucralose (Splenda) is correlated with Hashimoto's. Past studies have also found a harmful impact on the gut microbiome and blood sugar metabolism, swaying gut flora in the direction of the gut bacteria species that promote obesity.

I agree with food activist and journalist Michael Pollan: If your great-grandmother wouldn't recognize it, or you can't pronounce what's on the food label, don't eat it.

The Phytonutrient Gap: A Bigger Problem Than You Might Realize

For so many women, sugar-laden and refined carb foods have become quick substitutes for good nutrition, and we're paying the price. As a result of this and other massive changes in the American diet over the past sixty years, at least 80 percent of Americans are not getting the daily nutrients they need for even basic health from their diet. Instead, most Americans are overfed and undernourished, getting too many calories from poor-quality foods, and not getting enough important nutrients from high-quality foods. *The phytonutrient gap* is the term used to describe the difference between the nutrients you need for optimal health, and the nutrients you're actually getting.

The biggest deficit is of important vitamins, minerals, and protective phytochemicals (*phyto* means "plant") that are found in fruits and vegetables and that protect your cells from damage and support healthy natural detoxification. For example, in 2009, the World Health Organization published a report stating that 75 percent of Americans consumed less magnesium than needed. Some say that we have a nationwide magnesium deficiency. Low magnesium contributes to type 2 diabetes, metabolic syndrome, elevated C-reactive protein (a major blood marker of inflammation), hypertension, atherosclerosis, migraine headaches, anxiety, sleep problems, depression, menstrual cramps, heart palpitations, chocolate cravings, and restless leg syndrome. Low magnesium is also a risk factor for Hashimoto's.

Most of us are not overtly deficient enough to develop the most serious symptoms that tell your doctor you have a nutritional deficiency (though in truth, most doctors aren't on the lookout for these). Instead, you develop nutritional insufficiency, skirting under the radar of a diagnosis but low enough to have subtle symptoms that can contribute to big diseases, for example, low zinc, vitamin D, vitamin A, and selenium are all associated with Hashimoto's; magnesium, vitamin D, and chromium are all needed to

Food Immunology 101

Food allergy: A sudden and potentially life-threatening reaction to certain foods, most commonly peanuts, tree nuts, or shellfish, though there can be others, mediated by IgE antibodies, and possibly requiring medical attention. These allergies may require lifelong avoidance of the triggering foods, though many food allergies—for example, to dairy and eggs—may be outgrown by adulthood. However, food allergies can also arise at any time, including during adulthood.

Food intolerance: This usually refers to an inability to digest specific foods due to genetic or acquired lack of enzymes required for doing so—for example, lactose intolerance due to lactase insufficiency, or histamine intolerance due to insufficiency of one or more histamine-degrading enzymes. These may be circumvented by avoiding those foods, supplementing with the missing enzymes, or in certain cases, as might occur with histamine or fructose intolerance, taking specific steps to repair damage to the gut lining or flora that may have precipitated or worsened the intolerance.

Food sensitivity: In this case, you're neither allergic nor inherently intolerant of the food, but you feel worse when you eat it and better when you don't. This is often due to blood sugar problems when related to carbohydrate-rich foods, low digestive enzymes or stomach acids when it comes to fatty foods or nonspecific foods, or gut dysbiosis, again especially when it comes to carbohydrate-rich foods. Food sensitivities can often be cleared up by healing the gut with the 4R Program for Gut Health (see chapter 6), though sometimes it's best to just avoid the triggering food or foods.

regulate blood sugar, and insufficiencies are associated with elevated blood glucose, insulin resistance, and diabetes; low magnesium can cause cardiac arrhythmias; zinc and vitamin A are essential for the health of the gut lining; and the list goes on . . .

The awesome thing about the SOS Solution is that it is specifically designed to bridge the phytonutrient gap. However, certain medical conditions—Hashimoto's and celiac disease are prime examples—can

| Common Nutritional "Insufficiency" Signs and Related Conditions* ||
Nutrient	Sign
Essential fatty acids (omega-3)	Dry eyes, depression, cognitive function problems, dry skin
Iodine	Goiter (neck swelling where the thyroid is located), hypo-thyroidism
Iron	Fatigue, hair loss, pale skin or conjunctiva, weakness, shortness of breath, poor appetite, rapid heart rate, more frequent colds and upper respiratory infections
Magnesium	Leg or other muscle cramps, eye or facial twitching, constipation, restless leg syndrome, rapid or irregular heartbeat, elevated blood sugar, sleep disturbances
Vitamin B$_{12}$	Fatigue, weakness, constipation, loss of appetite, numbness and tingling in the hands and feet, difficulty maintaining balance, depression, poor memory, soreness of the mouth or tongue
Vitamin D	Depression, Hashimoto's, elevated blood sugar, diabetes, obesity; bone pain and muscle weakness can indicate inadequate vitamin D levels, which are commonly low in U.S. adults
Zinc	Frequent colds and upper respiratory infections, white spots on your fingernails, loss of sense of taste or smell, delayed wound healing

* This table is only a representative sample of common insufficiencies and common symptoms associated with these; it is not exhaustive.

prevent you from absorbing nutrients through your gut. So can leaky gut and gut dysbiosis, both of which are incredibly common, and which I'll talk about soon. Insulin resistance and diabetes can lead to increased excretion of certain nutrients, such as magnesium, and chronic stress can make you need extra B-complex. This is the importance of doing a total nutrition tune-up with the SOS Solution. As you can see, just getting enough nutrients from your diet isn't always enough.

ROOT CAUSE 3: GUT IMBALANCES

If you've ever been told that your symptoms are all in your head, guess again—they could be in your gut. Michelle, forty-two, was experiencing recurrent yeast infections, chronic gas, bloating, loose stools, and anxiety, and recently began feeling fatigue with mild aching in her fingers. She noticed that certain foods that she could previously eat with no problem made her feel worse. Eating grain made her tired, and sugar was making her crazy—but she was craving both. Her doctor told her that her symptoms were due to stress, and prescribed a medication for the yeast infections. But I knew something else was going on when she came to see me.

A review of her history revealed that Michelle was in great health until she got a staph infection on her honeymoon in the Bahamas. After more than twenty rounds of antibiotics, she noticed symptoms and hadn't been the same since. Her labs were normal, so her story pointed to gut and microbiome damage from antibiotics. We dove into the SOS Solution Reboot and gut repair program to restore her gut flora to normal. Her digestive symptoms cleared up quickly, and with it so did her fatigue. The repair also restored her normal vaginal flora, and she stopped having yeast infections. After a few months Michelle was able to reintroduce grains, but because she liked how she felt without it, kept sugar out of her diet.

The Guts to Be Healthy

Michelle's story illustrates how important gut health is to overall wellness. In fact, science emerging on a nearly daily basis now illustrates that we've only begun to understand the significance.

The lining of your digestive system forms a protective barrier internally, much as your skin does externally. From tip to tail, your digestive system is lined with cells that produce a variety of enzymes that break down your food, stomach acid that creates a pH inhospitable to harmful organisms you can pick up from food and your environment, and collections of immune cells and nerves that communicate with your entire body, including your brain. A healthy digestive system extracts and synthesizes the nutrients you need from your food, is a protective immune system barrier between your external and internal worlds, and detoxifies and eliminates waste.

Your intestinal ecology is made up of an estimated one hundred trillion diverse microorganisms, collectively called the microbiome. To give you perspective on the volume this number represents, the average adult's microbiome weighs more than two pounds (one kilogram), about the weight of your brain. These organisms have a profound impact on nutrient absorption, detoxification, the health of your gut lining, even your moods, appetite, food cravings, and mental function, and when out of balance can lead to inflammation, neuroinflammation, obesity and diabetes, hormonal problems, anxiety, depression, and brain fog. Your microbiome extracts calories and nutrition from your food, detoxifies chemicals and hormones, and synthesizes vitamins and iron for absorption. Healthy forms of bacteria prevent gut hyperpermeability—which I discuss in the next section—through the production of short-chain fatty acids and butyrate, which keep the intestinal lining healthy and intact. Conversely, unhealthy forms of intestinal organisms release toxins that increase intestinal permeability by disrupting the integrity of the intestinal lining.

Two major problems can arise in your digestive tract that can throw you into physical and emotional turmoil: leaky gut and dysbiosis.

Leaky Gut: When Your Guard Is Down

If unfolded and laid flat, your intestinal lining would cover two tennis courts. Made up of several layers, it is meant to allow peaceful coexistence with your intestinal guests—the trillions of bacteria, yeasts, and other organisms that live there—without triggering a massive immune reaction to them, while at the same time providing a selectively permeable barrier that lets the nutrition you need from your food (which some of those little buggers even help to manufacture) into your body. The surface layer provides a physical barrier, with lots of rich mucus to protect the lining from inflammation and nutrients that feed the microbiome, and extensive fingerlike projections called villi in the small intestine that provide an enormous surface area for nutrient absorption.

Another layer provides an immune barrier. It turns out that about

70 percent of the body's immune system is in the gut lining, in lymphatic tissue called *gut-associated lymphoid tissue* (GALT), which communicates with both your immune and nervous systems, including your brain. Therefore, inflammation in the intestinal lining can affect your entire immune system and even your mood. The various layers work together to selectively allow nutrients through to the bloodstream, while preventing harmful protein fragments and other particles from bacteria and foods from escaping the gut and having contact with the sensitive immune tissue and your bloodstream. Much of this action is happening in one thin cell layer of your intestines called the *epithelium*, which is punctuated by "gates" called *tight junctions* that let nutrients through but keep harmful particles and invaders out.

Leaky gut occurs when there is damage to the gut lining as a result of stress, certain medications (especially antibiotics and NSAIDs such as ibuprofen), environmental toxins, nutritional deficiencies (especially zinc and vitamins A and D), microbiome disruption, and inflammatory food triggers (especially gluten), any of which can lead to permeability of these tight junctions.

When the integrity of the gut lining is breached, the ability to maintain a discrete border crossing station is disrupted and the intestinal lining becomes more permeable. This is technically called "intestinal hyperpermeability," but I will refer to it by its more common name, "leaky gut." Leaky gut allows food particles, fragments of bacteria and other organisms, and other small intestinal waste products that are hanging out in your gut waiting to be eliminated (or in the case of bacteria, live there all the time) to cross into the immune-system rich layer of your intestinal lining, triggering immune reactions there, and then even into your bloodstream, where big inflammatory trouble begins.

Though bacteria can happily coexist within the intestine, fragments from their outer coats, especially a fragment called LPS, are toxic to the rest of the body. So too are proteins and other particles from your food. So when any of these migrate across the inner protective barrier of your gut and into your circulation, the body recognizes them as foreign invaders—just as it would any bacteria, virus, or foreign body—and begins to mount an attack. Immune cells are dispatched to neutralize the invaders, and inflammation goes rampant. Leaky gut is a well-established cause of chronic systemic inflammation, insulin resistance, weight gain, and even obesity. Sometimes

Your Microbiome Determines Your Stress Set Point—from Birth

The development of the microbiome, from the time of your birth, via the proper microbial colonization that naturally occurs during vaginal birth and breast-feeding not only influences the development of your immune system, but sets the tone for how well the HPA axis is able to respond to stress and whether you're more likely to find yourself in SOS as an adult. While this isn't something you can change retroactively, your microbiome and stress response can be improved upon with the SOS Solution. Knowing whether you were born on time or prematurely, vaginally or by cesarean, were breast-fed, or received antibiotics in the first couple of years of life, or whether your mom struggled with symptoms associated with microbiome disruption—all of which impact the type of organisms you get colonized with—can help you to understand your gut-related physical symptoms and your stress tolerance, particularly if you're prone to being highly sensitive, anxious, or reactive.

This emerging information on the role of the microbiome in immune system and HPA axis development also sheds light on the importance of avoiding unnecessary antibiotics when we are pregnant, doing what we can to increase our likelihood of vaginal birth (women in the United States have a one in three chance of a cesarean section), breast-feeding, and avoiding unnecessary antibiotics for our kids.

the body starts to get confused and immune cells start to attack your own cells. Autoimmune disease is also a well-established result of leaky gut. While many women with leaky gut have obvious digestive system symptoms, such as gas, bloating, constipation, or loose stools, or symptoms after eating, such as fatigue, mood changes, or rapid heartbeat, sometimes the symptoms are much less obvious. A few of the many symptoms and conditions directly associated with leaky gut and the chronic inflammation it causes include:

- Fatigue

- Food intolerances

- Irritable bowel syndrome

- Celiac disease (celiac can be both cause and result of leaky gut)

- Hashimoto's

- Crohn's disease and ulcerative colitis

- Rheumatoid arthritis

- Allergies, hives, eczema

- Arthritis, joint aches and pains

- Obesity, heart disease, diabetes, and, as a result, nonalcohol fatty liver disease (NAFLD)

Even when the bacteria or other organisms are cleared from your system, the autoimmune response can persist indefinitely, until steps are taken to break the cycle. Reversing leaky gut, as you'll learn to do in chapter 6, is one of the steps that can calm immune system chaos and get you out of SOS— and sometimes even reverse autoimmune disease.

Dysbiosis: Trouble in the Garden

Your digestive system is colonized with microorganisms from your mouth to your anus; each region of the gut has its own unique flora, in varying amounts. *Dysbiosis* is the technical name for disruption in your microbiome. You can have overgrowth of unfriendly species, loss of helpful species, or most commonly, a combination of both. It can occur in any area of the gut; most commonly it occurs in the small and large intestine. Like leaky gut, it is caused by:

- Stress, which changes the milieu of the gut, as well as blood flow to the gut lining, impacting the health of the intestinal lining and the type and quality of gut flora you grow

- Certain medications (see page 212), especially antibiotics that can wipe out enormous numbers of gut flora species even with just one dose, antacids that reduce stomach acidity that protects against bacterial overgrowth in the upper small intestine (when this overgrowth occurs, it is called small intestinal bacterial overgrowth), and medications that damage the gut lining (for example, ibuprofen and Tylenol)

- Deficiencies of gut-protective nutrients (especially vitamin A, zinc, iron, and vitamin D)

- A diet high in unhealthy carbs, sugars, and bad-quality fats, and low in fiber, fresh fruits, and vegetables, and lacking traditionally fermented foods such as sauerkraut, yogurt, and kimchi

Eating a diet of highly processed foods for just ten to fourteen days can reduce your microbiome diversity by 40 percent, while those who eat a traditional whole-foods diet are up to 40 percent more resilient to stress and mental illness than those who eat a processed foods diet. It's no wonder then that a shift in the Western diet for the worse in the past few decades has corresponded directly with an increase in chronic and autoimmune diseases and obesity.

Recent research has uncovered a connection between industrial food additives and autoimmune disease. It appears that these additives (discussed in the section on environmental toxins below) damage the epithelial lining of your intestines, and this too can create leaky gut, which then activates an autoimmune cascade. Conversely, a diet rich in high-fiber, antioxidant-rich vegetables, slow-burning carbohydrates, good-quality protein, and excellent fats, along with a small amount of naturally fermented foods, provides the "ingredients" needed for a healthy intestinal lining and microbiome. You'll learn all about these in chapter 4.

While medications may sometimes be necessary and even lifesaving, most have unintended consequences, and when it comes to antibiotics, proton pump inhibitors (PPIs), NSAIDs, and acetaminophen, the consequences are damage to your gut ecosystem and infrastructure. More than 70 percent of the antibiotics prescribed in the United States are unnecessary, and on top of this unnecessary insult, 80 percent of all antibiotics produced in the United States end up in our meat as a result of being fed to cattle to make them grow fatter, faster.

Antibiotics destroy the gut flora responsible for about 90 percent of your metabolic activity, hormone detoxification, nutrient synthesis, and protection of your intestinal lining, which is meant to protect against leaky gut. Even just one course of treatment can irrevocably wipe out entire species of important gut microflora. Many women have had the experience of taking an antibiotic for bronchitis or another infection, only to then spend months battling a vaginal yeast infection. This is because the antibiotic wipes out the *Lactobacillus* and *Bifidobacterium* species that keep *Candida* (yeast) in check.

PPIs (antacid medications such as Prilosec) and NSAIDs induce leaky gut and have been associated with the development of autoimmune disease, while acetaminophen damages the delicate lining of the stomach and can lead to gastrointestinal bleeding and problems with the absorption of nutrients needed for gut health. Small intestinal bacterial overgrowth, or SIBO, a common result of PPI use, has been associated with a number of extraintestinal manifestations including obesity, rosacea, restless leg syndrome, infertility and pregnancy complications, and joint pain.

Because the microbiome is involved in so many aspects of our health, ranging from regulating nutrition and calorie extraction from food, to communicating with our brain about what's going on in the gut through the production of neurotransmitters and other chemical messengers, a lot can go wrong when the microbiome is disrupted. Here are some examples:

Dysbiosis makes you fat: Different species of gut flora use energy in different ways—some, especially in the strain called *Firmicutes*, are able to extract a lot of calories from food, meaning that if you're loaded up with this type, you might store fat even if you're not overeating. In contrast, *Bacteroides*, another species, doesn't guzzle up the calories—so when you have a preponderance of these guys, you're apt to be leaner. The case for this was made super strong when it was shown that fecal transplants (yes, harvesting and transferring poop) from lean mice into obese mice made the fat mice lose weight. Guess what? The same thing has been shown in humans, along with a reduction in insulin resistance.

My microbiome made me eat it! Sugar and carb cravings: This may sound crazy, but whether you love chocolate or don't crave it at all, whether you go for kale or cake, may be a factor of what's going on in your gut microbial community! Your gut microbiome can actually manipulate you into eating certain foods that specific organisms in there need to survive and thrive. It does this in two ways: it creates cravings for foods that they specifically need for their own growth by making our brain register those foods as tastier and more appealing; and they produce toxins that make us feel unwell and alter our mood, through affecting various neurotransmitter levels, until we eat the foods that satisfy them. They literally hijack the messages going from the gut to the brain along the vagus nerve.

Anxiety and depression: Beneficial species of gut flora produce butyrate, which reduces anxiety and depression, among a number of protective relationships between healthy gut flora and mood. When the microbiome, or the intestinal lining, is perturbed, butyrate production drops. It's no wonder that studies that have restored beneficial gut flora (through the consumption of yogurt) have resulted in reduced levels of anxiety in study participants. The gut has two major communication methods: the enteric nervous system, sometimes called "the second brain," and your microbiome. This second brain is a network of approximately a hundred million neurons that are embedded in the lining of your gut and communicate using more than thirty-five neurotransmitters; in fact, much of your serotonin is produced in your intestines.

About 95 percent of the information passing through one of the largest nerves in your body, the vagus nerve, goes from the gut to the brain, not the other way around, as had long been thought. It may be that many of the emotions you experience originate not in your brain, but reflect the state of what's going on in your gut. We now know that disruptions in your gut can lead to unhappy moods and thoughts. It has been experimentally demonstrated that stimulation of the vagus nerve similarly to what might happen with gut disruption, can cause depression. In the SOS Solution Reboot section I'll show you how you can begin to change your mind and mood by healing your gut.

Brain fog: In addition to affecting your mood, the health of your microbiome can affect your mind, causing brain fog. This happens as a result of the chemicals and gasses that are produced by fermentation in your gut—which are determined by your particular microbial community and the foods you eat that cloud your thinking. For example, a high-sugar or highly refined carbohydrate diet, in the setting of intestinal dysbiosis, can lead to the production of by-products that can make you feel drunk, groggy, "drugged," fatigued, and foggy after a meal, or all the time if that's most of your diet, or you have significant dysbiosis.

Hormonal chaos: Healthy gut flora contain bacteria with genes that are specifically capable of breaking down and helping your body to eliminate estrogen, and constitute what is called the *estrobolome*. They are critical for transforming plant compounds called *lignans*, from vegetables and legumes, into *phytoestrogens*, plant hormones that protect your body against the risks of excess estrogen. As such, they prevent excess estrogen from recirculating from the intestine. When the microbiome is damaged, estrogen recirculates in a particularly toxic form. This increases a woman's risk of becoming estrogen dominant, and increases risk of breast, ovarian, and endometrial cancers. Women with more diverse gut bacteria, as is found in diets with high fiber, high vegetable, low sugar, and no unhealthy fats, have a reduced risk. Because estrogen and cholesterol are related to each other chemically, it is likely that obesity, high cholesterol, and changes in microbiome colonies are all related to each other, and may also connect the dots on why obesity is linked to higher risk of breast cancer.

Elevated estrogen levels can inhibit thyroid function by causing an increase in sex hormone–binding globulin (SHBG), a protein in your blood that binds a number of hormones, rendering them unavailable for use until needed. Unfortunately, SHBG also binds to thyroid hormone, making it unavailable, too.

Chronically elevated estrogen is also a risk factor for gaining weight, so may be yet another reason for that muffin top, and because high estrogen blocks progesterone, you may experience fertility problems, miscarriage, mood, and sleep problems related to low progesterone. Further, elevated cortisol also blocks progesterone receptors, the places on your cells where progesterone "docks," and like a key in a lock, allows it to perform its jobs. So even if your blood levels are normal, your body and brain can be registering low progesterone, making you feel anxious, depressed, and irritable;

Your Gut Influences How You Think and Feel

The connections between mind, mood, and microbiome are so strong that there's now a whole area of research in "psychobiotics"—studying the potential for using probiotics for mental health problems.

A study at UCLA found that eating a cup of yogurt twice daily for four weeks led to reductions in anxiety in twenty-five women, based on before-and-after brain scans while looking at a series of images of happy and unhappy facial expressions. The researchers concluded that the probiotic organisms in the yogurt favorably change the intestinal microbiomes of the study subjects, which changed their brain chemistry. Another study, done in 2015, found that among forty-five individuals given a prebiotic, a carbohydrate that feeds healthy gut flora, there was reduction in cortisol, stress, and anxiety, with a shift in thinking from negative to more positive thoughts. Beneficial species of gut flora produce butyrate, which reduces anxiety and depression; conversely, when the microbiome or the intestinal lining is perturbed, butyrate production is decreased. Healthy gut flora can reverse anxiety and depression, and with them, SOS.

affecting your sleep and your menstrual cycles; and upsetting the balance of your estrogen level, making you estrogen-dominant and more prone to heavy periods and lumpy, painful breasts, impacting your fertility, and increasing miscarriage risk.

Don't despair: prebiotics and probiotics can repair the microbiome, help you lose weight, and reverse your risks, and you're about to learn how to use them in chapter 4.

ROOT CAUSE 4:
ENVIRONMENTAL TOXINS

Lydia, fifty-six, a petite, fit blond firecracker, came into my office looking for alternative treatments for her rheumatoid arthritis. Otherwise symptom-free, she'd been living in Southeast Asia for five years, and was diagnosed with rheumatoid arthritis when her joints started to swell painfully. Over a period of three years, her joint pain and swelling got progressively worse, and she also began feeling fatigued and generally unwell. Though it hadn't stopped her from managing her multimillion-dollar corporation, it had slowed her down and forced her to now take afternoon naps. Her rheumatologist suggested an immune system-suppressing medication to slow the disease and minimize potential damage to her joints. But when Lydia read the potentially life-threatening side effects of the medication, she thought, "Heck no!" and decided she'd try a holistic approach first.

When I reviewed Lydia's health history and food journal, I noticed that she frequently consumed fish. When I asked her about this, she told me that she ate fish, especially tuna, often twice daily because that was the animal protein she trusted the most to be safe to eat in Thailand. Because of the heavy contamination of fish with mercury, I asked Lydia to take all high-mercury fish completely out of her diet (see page 146 for more about mercury in fish and which are safe to eat). I also put Lydia on a combination of herbs and supplements to reduce joint inflammation and to help bind and eliminate the mercury from her system. In three months her blood levels of antibodies for RA were down to a third of their original level. She continued the program and after another three months was so improved that her rheumatologist concurred that there was no need to start the medication.

Mercury is just one of countless environmental toxins that have seeped their way into our air, water, and food. When researchers studied the salmon caught in Washington's Puget Sound, they discovered that the fish housed a cocktail of more than eighty-one pharmaceuticals, including Prozac, Advil, Benadryl, Lipitor, cocaine, Cipro (and other antibiotics), Flonase, Aleve, Tylenol, Paxil, Valium, Zoloft, Tagamet, OxyContin, Darvon, nicotine, and caffeine—all drugs and toxins that may have been destined for our dinner tables! The researchers also found residues of personal care products, anticoagulants, fungicides, and antiseptics in the fish.

The same contaminants are found widely in drinking water. Not only do decontamination methods fail to remove most of them, but also decontamination facilities have consistently managed to avert regulations to raise their standards. Indoor air is now considered more polluted than outdoor air due to the volume of toxins in home building materials, furnishings, electronics, and the hundreds of individual chemicals in our household cleaners, fuel sources, insecticides, body products, perfumes, and cosmetics. Of the more than eighty thousand chemicals in circulation, 90 percent have never been tested for safety in human health, and fewer than two hundred known to be toxic to the nervous system have been tested for safety in vulnerable populations such as children or older adults.

Just how great is our exposure? Researchers from the Environmental Working Group found that 287 environmental chemicals were detectible in the umbilical cord blood of newborns, all "downloaded" through the mom's blood, through the placenta, during pregnancy. What about adults? In its 2009 study on human exposure to environmental chemicals in the United States, the Centers for Disease Control and Prevention (CDC) found that of the 212 chemicals they were looking for, virtually all 2,400 survey participants had measurable levels of those chemicals in their blood or urine. In this survey they added 75 more chemicals than in a previous study—and all were present. The chemical load each of us is carrying is called our *body burden*.

And every single one of us has been exposed, even if we live in a seemingly pristine place. No matter where we live, we're not immune to exposure. These chemicals persist in the environment for decades, and have been found thousands of miles from where they were originally used, transported by air, water, birds, large migrating animals, and in the foods we're sending around the world. Pesticides used in Mexico have been found in polar bears in the Arctic! These chemicals are so persistent that even pesticides that were banned in the 1970s still make their way into our foods through soil and animals, and can routinely be found in blood samples of adults and children alike. Since humans are the highest up on the food chain, we're getting the greatest exposure through eating animal products. Women have more fatty tissue than men, so we accumulate at even higher levels.

Even minuscule amounts of known toxins have a profound effect on our health, far greater than many scientists—and governments—had predicted. Individual chemicals are combining in our bodies to form new compounds that have never been studied. We have become living labs while agricultural, industrial, and pharmaceutical companies profit, thanks—in huge part—to their lobbyists, who persistently work to prevent better safety standards from being implemented by the federal government. In some cruel irony (or vicious profiteering), some of the same companies that make the herbicides, pesticides, and other toxins also manufacture the drugs used to treat the diseases caused by them.

Our increasing exposure to toxins has paralleled the rise in cognitive problems, from brain fog to Alzheimer's, hormonal problems including early puberty, endometriosis, PCOS, infertility, premature ovarian failure, and breast cancer, autoimmune diseases, and diabetes. Our personal exposure actually began just after World War II, when many of our grandmothers were pregnant. How? It has been shown that toxin exposure going back one and two generations impacts our personal epigenetics—so if your grandmother got exposed to the insecticide DDT when she was a kid, for example, as many did while chasing trucks that were spraying the chemical to eradicate mosquitoes, it can partly explain why you're struggling with symptoms now, even though you're doing your best to be healthy.

Agricultural chemicals (herbicides, pesticides, and antibiotics), industrial waste, heavy metals, hormone-disrupting plastics, solvents, and flame retardants permeate our air, water, food, soil, clothing, furniture, body products, cleaning products, and electronic devices, and we absorb them. They bind to cells in our immune, nervous, and endocrine systems, and especially to delicate tissue such as our thyroid, damaging their function. They increase inflammation and oxidative stress, cause "brain-flammation," and alter genetic expression. Chronic low-dose exposure dramatically increases risks for metabolic syndrome, prediabetes, and cognitive decline, including impaired memory and attention, and may double the risk of developing Alzheimer's disease.

Sound familiar? Yes, they put us into SOS!

And if you are struggling to lose weight or improve your blood sugar—and nothing you try seems to work—toxins, again, may be to blame. Called obesogens and diabesogens, these toxins trigger changes in your cells that increase fat and cortisol, alter insulin production and secretion, and lead to insulin resistance, metabolic syndrome, and diabetes.

Loss of detoxification resilience leads to chronic inflammation and can result from exposure to environmental toxins. When this happens, we feel suboptimal and fatigued, and are at increased risk of more serious problems—topping the list, autoimmune conditions. If perfumes and other strong chemical odors bother you, if you have symptoms that you aren't clearing your estrogen well, for example, chronic or cyclic breast tenderness, frequent (more often than four weeks apart) or heavy periods, or uterine fibroids, or if you have an autoimmune condition, are tired all the time, or have chronic fatigue, you could very well have detoxification overload. This happens when there's a mismatch between what you're being exposed to and what your body is able to clear through your natural detoxification pathways in your liver and gut.

The following is a rundown of the worst offenders.

Hormone-Disrupting Chemicals

Endocrine-disrupting chemicals (EDCs) are particularly sneaky because they are readily absorbable and mimic our hormones. But they are *not* our hormones and are found in human tissue at much higher concentrations than "endogenous" (made by your own body) hormones. As a result, they can overstimulate, block, or disrupt the hormones' natural actions by sending mixed messages throughout your endocrine system. Xenoestrogens ("foreign" estrogens) mimic estrogen, and thyroid-disrupting chemicals (TDCs) do just that. EDCs cause inflammation, weight gain, and insulin resistance, and stimulate cells to grow when they shouldn't—causing problems such as early puberty in girls, endometriosis, and breast cancer in women. TDCs can compete with iodine, preventing it from getting into the thyroid cells, where it is needed for the formation of thyroid hormone, change the shape and function of the thyroid gland, block the production of thyroid hormone, inhibit the ability to turn inactive T_4 into active T_3, prevent the transport of thyroid hormone throughout the body, and prevent binding of active thyroid hormone to thyroid receptors, all of which have been shown to have the same predictable harmful downstream effects as hypothyroidism.

Fluoride and Other Halogens

I know we've all been sold on the wonders of fluoride, but fluoride, along with chlorine and bromine, are members of a chemical group called halogens, which also includes iodine. They share a similar structure that allows them to interfere with thyroid function. Chlorine and fluoride are found in drinking and bathing water, where we ingest and breathe them in; chlorine is also found in pools, spa water, bleach and cleaning products, while fluoride is found in toothpaste, a number of pharmaceuticals, Teflon, and nonstick cookware. Bromine is in flour products used in baked goods and bread; it is also found in flame retardants, and as an additive in sugary beverages that contain brominated oil. Interestingly, fluoride was used in the medical treatment of hyperthyroidism in the 1950s because of its known inhibitory effect on thyroid function, so it's no surprise that some studies have found that fluoride may reduce thyroid function.

Heavy Metals

The harmful effects of heavy metals on the endocrine system, immunity, and brain function have long been known because of problems with infertility, Hashimoto's, and neurological diseases in factory workers who have been exposed. They appear to have a particular impact on women's reproductive function. They have an affinity for the pituitary, which is the relay station for messages to the adrenals, thyroid, and ovaries, and when deposited there, communication to all three is interrupted, leading to fertility and other gynecologic problems, thyroid problems and SOS, and all of the downstream effects on your cholesterol, weight, heart, and brain.

The most studied thyroid-disrupting heavy metals that we're commonly exposed to are mercury, lead, and cadmium, though there are many more, all of which are now abundant in our water, soil, food, and air largely due to industrial environmental contamination. All of these metals seem to affect the thyroid in one of several ways: they interfere with iodine transport into the thyroid, interfere with deiodination (the process whereby T_4 becomes T_3, the active form of thyroid hormone) in the liver and other tissue, and block the thyroid receptors from accepting thyroid hormones.

Mercury exposure has been associated with cellular autoimmunity, and mercury accumulates in the thyroid gland at particularly high levels in women and has been shown to dramatically increase antithyroglobulin antibodies, a possible sign of thyroid gland damage caused by an

Endocrine Disrupters in Your World*		
The Disrupter	**Where It's Hiding****	**What It Does**
Bisphenol-A (BPA)	Plastics in food and beverage containers, plastic wrap, drinking straws, baby bottles, plastic toys, dental sealants, receipts (Connecticut banned their use in these because women of childbearing age handle most of the grocery and other receipts and thus have the highest exposure), and airline tickets	Disrupts hormones, disrupts the immune system, stimulates autoantibody production; causes weight gain, insulin resistance, and diabetes
Dioxins	Also banned but persistent in the environment and show up in our foods, especially meat, dairy products, and fish, as well as breast milk	Cancer-causing, disrupts hormones
Organo-phosphates, organo-chlorides	Your food in the form of herbicide and pesticide residue, computers (where it leaches out as we handle them), refrigerators, flame retardants, and waste dumps	Disrupts hormones, disrupts the immune system, disrupts the microbiome, stimulates autoantibody production; causes weight gain, insulin resistance, and diabetes
Parabens	In thousands of foods, cosmetics, and pharmaceuticals	Disrupts hormones
PBDEs	PBDEs are flame retardants and are in a shocking number of household items, including most furniture, mattresses, bedding, drapery, rugs, computers, and televisions; they are also in children's sleepwear, car seat covers, and nursing pillows	Disrupts hormones, major impact on thyroid due to containing bromine, blocks effect of T_4 on brain development and function

The Disrupter	Where It's Hiding**	What It Does
PCBs	Banned in the 1970s, but persistent in water, air, and soil	Disrupts hormones, disrupts the immune system; causes weight gain, insulin resistance, and diabetes
Phthalates	Most body products, including shampoos, nail polishes, and soaps, fragrances and perfume, food packaging, IV tubing, PVC tubing, shower curtains, vinyl flooring, plastics with a #3 recycling number, detergents and household cleaning products, to name just a few of the thousands of places phthalates can be found	Disrupts hormones; causes weight gain, insulin resistance, and diabetes
Triclosan	Antibacterial hand and dish soaps, toothpastes, hand sanitizers, and deodorants	Disrupts hormones

* Note that chemicals in many of these groups have multiple different names, and not all are required to be listed as ingredients in personal care products, foods, household items, baby products, or furnishings.

** These are just representative examples; they are in many more related sources, and are also in air, water, soil, and residue we track into our homes from walking outside.

autoimmune disease. Most of the mercury having this impact likely comes via fish consumption.

Cadmium exposure reduces T_4; lead appears to reduce FT_3, T_3, and T_4; and each carries with it a substantial risk of harm to numerous other aspects of our health, particularly neurotoxicity, which can increase our risk of developing degenerative diseases, notably Alzheimer's, and whose low-level impacts long before disease manifests may cause any number of nervous system conditions, including poor concentration and memory. Of note, heavy metals have estrogenic activity as well, so are disrupting hormones at many levels.

Mold Exposure and Illness

Within a week of doing the "good deed" of clearing out her mother-in-law's basement of old books, piles of stored clothes, and furniture that Daria found notably covered in mold and mildew, she developed a fiercely painful "lump" in her throat, and within a few weeks, now struggling with intense fatigue, was diagnosed with new-onset Hashimoto's with sky-high antithyroid antibodies (see page 381). Prior to the basement cleanup, she had no symptoms of a thyroid problem whatsoever.

While the majority of fungi are not harmful to immunologically healthy individuals (they can be deadly for the immune-compromised person), a number of species, including those found in indoor environments, can cause illness, including asthma, chronic allergic rhinitis, and other respiratory symptoms. However, the role of fungal exposure in autoimmune and other chronic illness—for example, chronic fatigue syndrome (CFS)—is not scientifically proven. Yet Daria is just one of many patients I've worked with who reported the onset of autoimmune disease or other chronic illness, particularly CFS, associated with mold exposure. Therefore I don't dismiss the possibility of a connection though there is scant scientific evidence for this connection.

My recommendation is that if you are struggling with chronic symptoms or conditions and have exhausted other causes, and certainly if you have respiratory symptoms, and you have known or suspected mold exposure in your home or workplace, see an allergist, rheumatologist, or an integrative or functional medicine doctor skilled in the proper assessment of fungal exposure via appropriate testing. If appropriate based on those results, explore home (or office) evaluation to see whether indoor remediation is indicated.

ROOT CAUSE 5: STEALTH INFECTIONS

Melanie, forty-two, was acutely ill when she came to see me. Her symptoms started several days after her mother's funeral, a very stressful time for her.

Her neck became swollen and highly painful to touch. In the emergency department she was told she had a viral infection, she was given ibuprofen, and no medical testing was performed. Over the next few weeks she became deeply fatigued and intensely anxious. Her primary care doctor eventually did thyroid testing, which showed she had Hashimoto's, and he started her on Synthroid, the most common thyroid medication on the market, but it didn't help at all.

When I first saw Melanie, her thyroid labs had worsened, as had her symptoms. She felt awful, though her doctor had been increasing her medication steadily for weeks. Based on the severe swollen glands, fatigue, and lack of response to the medication, I suspected that she might have an infection. Sure enough, testing (see page 386) came back positive for active Epstein-Barr infection, likely a reactivation of the mono she'd had in college in her early twenties. Over several months, with the herbal and supplement treatments I share with you in chapter 6, her energy returned, her anxiety resolved, her thyroid labs began to return to normal, and she was also able to come off of thyroid medication.

Chronic infections can keep your body in a chronic state of low-level alarm, or mild SOS, which makes me think of them as stealthy—they are slipping under the radar barely detected and unexpected. Chronic stress can reduce your body's ability to respond effectively to infection, altering its ability to keep infections contained. That's why stress can lead to reactivation of dormant infections, causing cold sores and herpes outbreaks in the herpesvirus family (as in EBV).

Epstein-Barr virus and another infection, cytomegalovirus (CMV), are stealth infections associated with multiple autoimmune diseases, including rheumatoid arthritis (RA), Sjögren's syndrome, multiple sclerosis (MS), and lupus. There is enough evidence to suggest that it's important to have viral labs checked if you do have Hashimoto's, particularly if you also have painful swollen glands or a known exposure, or if you've been started on medication and aren't getting better. *Yersinia enterocolitica*, a bacterium that affects the intestine, has also been identified in patients with Hashimoto's, though it is not certain that it causes it. Of note, Lyme disease is a great imitator of Hashimoto's, so it should be excluded by proper testing if there is fatigue, joint pain, swollen glands, or Lyme-related symptoms.

Several theories raise possibilities for infections that can cause autoimmune disease. In the *molecular mimicry theory*, the immune system remembers specific proteins on the viruses and then looks for similar proteins as targets for an attack; in the case of Hashimoto's, the thyroid becomes that target in a case of mistaken identity for the virus. This can happen even after the body has cleared the organism. Another possibility is called the *bystander effect,* in which a virus either enters the body's cells and the immune system attacks the cells along with the virus, or the virus stimulates the release of specific immune cells that are primed to attach to the body itself. What's clear is that autoimmune conditions are on the rise, they are especially common in women, and there is a role for infection in triggering autoimmunity. Further, it's clear that SOS disrupts the immune system and, with that system being chronically overwhelmed and exhausted, makes it more difficult for your body to contain infection and inflammation. Supporting the immune system directly and staying out of SOS are important strategies to consider as we look for solutions to the autoimmune epidemic we're facing.

PLANT NEW ROOTS

The SOS Solution lets you find and weed out any unhealthy roots that are affecting your wellness, and plant new roots of health, happiness, and connection, good sleep and effective ways to reduce stress, a nourishing and delicious diet, proper digestion, and the ability to detoxify from environmental burdens and to have robust immunity. In the next chapter you'll use self-assessments to identify which of the five Root Causes are affecting you personally, and once you have those results in hand, we're going to get you on the SOS Solution and turn your health around.

3

WHAT'S YOUR TYPE? DECODING YOUR ROOT CAUSES

I'T'S TIME TO MAP OUT what's going on inside of that wonderful body of yours. The dual purpose of this chapter is to learn how your symptoms connect to SOS and the five Root Causes so you can become more aware of your various stress points and learn how to be especially attentive to keeping those related systems strong, and also to allow you to customize your SOS Solution to your specific needs. While the SOS Solution is universal—you do not have to individualize it to make it work for you—going through the questionnaires will allow you to customize the program to understand more about, and to target, your specific imbalances. Your unique patterns can be super interesting to discover; you might have an "aha moment" or two as symptoms and systems come together before your eyes.

Using this chapter is easy. Though there are quite a lot of questionnaires, they can be completed in about fifteen minutes total. Here's what you do:

1. **Fill out the questionnaires** by checking off symptoms that apply to you. Go through each questionnaire even if you think you're not having any problems in that category—you might be surprised to discover that symptoms you chalked up to "just

When in Doubt, Get Checked Out

There is a time and a place for medical care. If you have a new onset of fatigue, meaning it's suddenly appeared in the past few months, weeks, or days, and you can't really explain it, if you're feeling particularly run down, have had recent significant weight loss without dieting, are having major changes in your mental clarity or memory, have had recent changes in your bowel habits—for example, new onset of constipation, changes in your stool caliber, loose stools, or blood in your stool—or if you suspect symptoms of an autoimmune disease, I recommend that you work with your primary care provider to get proper testing. At a minimum this includes:

- A complete blood count (CBC) to make sure your red and white blood cell count is normal
- A blood chemistry panel to make sure your liver and kidneys are working properly
- Glucose, hemoglobin A1C, and insulin testing to make sure you're not fatigued because of diabetes, a common cause
- Antinuclear antibody (ANA) and specific autoimmune antibody testing to check for autoimmune disease
- Lyme disease testing if you've had a possible exposure, as well as testing for other possible infections

Additionally, your doctor should do a complete physical exam, and for women over fifty, check for healthy heart function. Although you can start the SOS Solution at the same time, *when in doubt, get checked out.*

life" actually are important and even have a pattern. If you don't like to write in your books, you can download copies of the questionnaires at avivaromm.com/adrenal-thyroid-revolution.

2. **At the end of each questionnaire, tally your score.** Each check counts as one point.

3. **Read the comments and recommendations in the results section of each questionnaire.**

4. **Use the questionnaires to track your progress** in the "before" and "after" columns to make this easy. My recommendation is to take the questionnaires now, and then again after you do the Reboot for fourteen days, but before you start the section on Repair. This is because the SOS Solution Reboot itself so effectively clears up a lot of symptoms that repeating these questions at that time will give you a sense of how much repair of systems you'll need in Week 3: Repair. I'll remind you to retake these questionnaires at the end of the Reboot.

Dr. Romm, I Have So Many Patterns! Is That Normal?

It's very likely you'll discover that you have several—or even all—of the five Root Causes playing a role in your health, and this might seem a little scary. Never fear! I promise it doesn't mean that you're a hopeless wreck or that you're falling apart. It has to do with the complex world we're living in, leading to a host of exposures you didn't know were causing problems. Don't worry. All of the women I treat started out struggling with a host of Root Causes. Your symptoms are your allies; they tell you where your body's "pain points" are. Knowing your imbalances gives you the road map to healing them.

THE QUESTIONNAIRES

Decode Your SOS Type: Overdrive or Exhaustion?

Harkening back to chapter 1, SOS occurs in two main patterns: SOS with Overdrive and SOS with Exhaustion or, commonly, a combination of both, with one set of symptoms more predominant. Take the questionnaires here to see which pattern you fall into.

Are You in SOS with Overdrive (SOS-O)?

Check the box next to any symptoms you relate to. Each check counts as one point.

Symptoms	Before Reboot	After Reboot
I have trouble falling asleep; I often feel "tired and wired"		
I fall asleep and then wake up a couple of hours later		
I feel tired in the morning, even after a full night's sleep		
I wake up hungry during the night		
I feel tired during the day; I often hit a slump at about three to four o'clock in the afternoon		
I need coffee to start my day; I sometimes need another cup in the afternoon		
I crave sweets, coffee, or chocolate (or salty foods or carbs) (especially in the afternoon)		
I often feel stressed or overwhelmed; I've been under stress for weeks (or months or years)		
I feel anxious, worry a lot, or often think something "bad" is about to happen		
I jump at loud noises		
I feel I have no food willpower		
I stress-eat		
I have irritable bowel syndrome (IBS)		
I have low (or no) sex drive		
I'm too irritable		
I'm overweight, especially around my middle ("muffin top")		
I have trouble gaining weight		
Sometimes I'm really blue or even depressed		
I feel like I never accomplish enough; I'm often pushing myself to do more		

Symptoms	Before Reboot	After Reboot
I look more wrinkly than I think I should for my age		
My memory is not great; I have trouble with my focus		
My menstrual cycles are irregular		
I've had trouble getting pregnant in the past, or I've had a miscarriage		
I have polycystic ovarian syndrome		
I've been told I have high cholesterol		
I've been told I have bone loss (osteopenia or osteoporosis)		
I get sick easily; coughs and infections tend to linger		
I have hives (or allergic reactions, asthma, or seasonal allergies)		
I've been diagnosed with an autoimmune disease		
I've been told that my blood sugar is high; I have metabolic syndrome (or insulin resistance or diabetes)		
SCORE		

If you scored:

0-3 points: Good news! You're not in SOS with Overdrive; you're probably under the normal amount of stress that one might expect just from being human and living life. Keep up the good work of staying out of SOS-O and go through the whole SOS Solution to revitalize your health.

>3 points: You're in SOS-O. Do the whole SOS Solution, but you can customize your plan from the start by adding in relaxing herbal and nutritional supplements and tips on pages 166-67, sleep tips on page 189, adaptogens from page 248, or a combination of these. Make sure to thoroughly read chapter 5, "Reframe," and incorporate relaxation practices into your daily life. If you scored greater than 8 points, add in the SOS testing on page 387, and make sure to also get thyroid testing (see page 261).

Are You in SOS with Exhaustion?

Check the box next to any symptoms you relate to. Each check equals one point.

Symptoms	Before Reboot	After Reboot
I often feel really exhausted; I might describe myself as "burned out," "crispy," or "fried"		
I wake up at three to four o'clock in the morning; sometimes it's hard to fall back to sleep		
I wake up tired even when I've gotten a good night's sleep		
I feel anxious a lot		
Everything feels overwhelming these days; it's hard to get motivated to do any of it		
I'm getting sick way more often than I think I should		
I'm having cold sores (or herpes outbreaks, yeast infections, or urinary tract infections)		
I crave sugar (or carbs or salty foods)		
I don't have much tolerance for exercise; I get wiped out pretty quickly		
I'm depressed, weepy, and emotionally exhausted		
My motivation and drive are really low		
My hormones are all over the place, and my cycles are really irregular		
I have no sex drive		

Symptoms	Before Reboot	After Reboot
I've been diagnosed with an autoimmune disease		
I've been told I have low blood pressure; sometimes I get dizzy, especially when standing up from a lying-down position		
Sometimes my heart races		
My memory is not what it was		
I've been diagnosed with chronic fatigue syndrome (or fibromyalgia)		
I sometimes feel confused (or unable to make decisions)		
My wounds seem to take a long time to heal		
SCORE		

If you scored:

0-3 points: Good news! You haven't crossed over into SOS-E, or you're probably experiencing the normal amount of fatigue that one might expect just from being human and living life. The SOS Solution will be perfect for your needs. The SOS Solution will get you back on track and feeling great again.

>3 points: You're in SOS with an exhaustion pattern. Do the whole SOS Solution, but you can customize your plan from the start by adding in relaxing herbal and nutritional supplements and tips on pages 166-67, sleep tips on page 189, adaptogens from page 248, or a combination of these. Make sure to thoroughly read chapter 5, "Reframe," and incorporate relaxation practices into your daily life. If you scored greater than 8 points, your body is experiencing a lot of wear and tear. You'll want to add in the SOS testing on page 387, and make sure to also get thyroid testing (see page 261).

But Wait, I'm a Combination of SOS-O and SOS-E

Because cortisol has a diurnal rhythm, you can be in SOS-O during one part of the day, and SOS-E in another, while being predominantly one type or the other. The SOS Solution is designed to bring you back into healthy balance by resetting your normal cortisol rhythm, so you don't have to worry too much about fitting neatly into a pattern to make this program work for you.

Do You Have Hypothyroidism? "Test, Don't Guess"

The million-dollar question: Do you have Hashimoto's? Or if you already know you have hypothyroidism, are persistent symptoms telling you that your thyroid is still sending out a call for help and some extra TLC (thyroid loving care!) and healing of a Root Cause? A better medication or a different dose?

The thyroid questionnaire will give you a great deal of information, but when it comes to thyroid health, my motto is "Test, don't guess." Therefore, with the thyroid questionnaire comes a special set of scores and instructions:

If you score more than 3 points, or if you have a history of thyroid problems and are having any possible hypothyroid-related symptoms, it's essential to get thyroid testing as soon as possible (see page 261) so the test results come back, ideally, in the first couple of weeks while you're on the SOS Solution Reboot.

This way, you'll already be tackling your Root Causes, but you'll also be able to target the most appropriate thyroid treatment plan to help you get your thyroid function back on track, outlined in great detail in chapter 7. While all of the other steps of the SOS Solution are essential to follow, adding in specific thyroid recommendations, including the right medication at the right dose if needed, can be a game changer for your energy, metabolism, hormones, mind, and mood.

Check the box next to any symptoms you relate to. Each check equals one point.

Symptoms	Before Reboot	After Reboot
I feel sluggish; even my limbs feel heavy sometimes		
I'm often fatigued and run down; sometimes I have zero energy		
I've gained weight in the past few months, and I can't figure out why		
I'm having trouble losing weight, even though I've tried dieting and exercise		
I have insomnia, have trouble falling asleep, wake up too soon after I go to sleep, or wake up at three to four o'clock in the morning		
My memory and concentration aren't what they were		
I'm feeling blue; I'm struggling with depression; I've lost my sense of joy and pleasure		
I often feel anxious or worried, and fear that something bad is going to happen		
My bowels are generally sluggish; I have a bowel movement less than once daily		
I feel cold all the time; I have to wear sweaters even when nobody else is		
My skin is dry (or itchy or rough)		
My hair or nails are dry, coarse, and brittle		
I've been losing a lot of hair; my hair is thinning		
My cholesterol is high		
I've got puffiness around my eyes, and my face gets puffy		
I've noticed that the outer thirds of my eyebrows are thin (or have virtually disappeared)		

Symptoms	Before Reboot	After Reboot
I crave sugar and carbohydrates		
I've had fertility problems		
I have PMS or heavy periods, or I've skipped periods completely		
I've had trouble getting pregnant (or have had a miscarriage in the past)		
I have (or have had) postpartum depression (or trouble producing breast milk)		
I catch every bug that goes around		
I tend to have a low body temperature		
I get a lot of joint aches and muscle weakness		
I have celiac disease or another autoimmune condition		
I've been diagnosed with carpal tunnel syndrome, tendinitis (or plantar fasciitis)		
I get numbness or tingling in my hands or feet		
SCORE		

If you scored:

0-3 points: Good news! You *probably* don't have Hashimoto's, or if you already know you do, you've got a good handle on the symptoms. Complete the rest of the questionnaires, and follow the SOS Solution to optimize your health and address other contributing patterns and Root Causes. However, if after two weeks on the Reboot, you still have symptoms—even if just a couple—on the thyroid questionnaire when you repeat it, it is reasonable to get thyroid testing.

>3 points: There's a good chance that your thyroid function is slow, though other causes can produce similar symptoms. I recommend that you get thyroid testing (see page 261) and start the SOS Solution while waiting for your results. If your results come back positive, continue the SOS Solution but also jump over to chapter 7, "Recharge," for specific additional recommendations. If your tests come back normal, continue on with the rest of the SOS Solution.

The Root Cause Assessments

Now you're going to complete questionnaires that will help you identify which of the five Root Causes have been putting you into SOS and/or Hashimoto's. Before you start, though, take a minute and put your SOS-O, SOS-E, and hypothyroidism scores, and any individualized plans, onto the charts provided on pages 119–20.

Root 1: Chronic Mental and Emotional Stress

Could Stress Be Affecting Your Health?

Check the box next to any symptoms you relate to. Each check equals one point.

Symptoms	Before Reboot	After Reboot
I get headaches		
I have IBS; stress makes me have to run to the bathroom		
I get stomachaches		
I'm pretty sure I'm a perfectionist		
I often have back, neck, shoulder, or other muscle tightness or pain		

Symptoms	Before Reboot	After Reboot
I get jaw pain; I clench or grind my teeth		
I can't get to sleep; I often have interrupted sleep (or I wake up too early)		
I'm often nervous or anxious (or worried)		
I'm often tearful or on the verge of tears		
I'm often edgy or feel like I'm ready to explode		
I often feel powerless, helpless, dependent, or vulnerable		
I have negative thoughts about myself or my body several or many times a day		
I'm under constant or frequent pressure; I feel overwhelmed and overloaded		
I can never meet my own standards or someone else's; I know I'm a perfectionist		
I've lost the pleasure in my life; life feels "flat" and I'm bored		
I use food to calm my stress or change my mood		
I use cigarettes or alcohol (or other substances) to calm my stress or anxiety		
I feel guilty for no reason		
I've been nagging a lot lately; I'm critical of others, I pick fights, and I have no stress tolerance		
I shop to ease my stress		
SCORE		

If you scored:

0-3 points: Good news! You're handling life's emotional stresses well. Keep up the great work and enjoy the SOS Solution for optimizing your health and balance, and work on minimizing the stressful triggers you have control over.

>3 points: Okay, right now you might be feeling like stress is your middle name. I've got your back, sister! You might want to start your SOS Solution by reading chapter 5, "Reframe," and jumping right into the stress busters. You can swing back to the Reboot after you've gotten started on restoring deep, refreshing sleep or relaxation practices— and also supplements—that will soothe your mind and moods. Sound amazing? Heck, you can even jump over there right now and pick a couple that you like. I highly suggest the Quickie (page 199)—it's fast, it feels awesome, and it's not what you think I'm talking about at all. Circle back when you're done; I'll be waiting.

Root 2: Food Triggers

Do You Have Food Triggers or a Phytonutrient Gap?

Check the box next to any symptoms you relate to. Each check equals one point.

Symptoms	Before Reboot	After Reboot
I'm tired often, or feel "drunk" or "drugged," especially after eating (FT)		
I have food sensitivities (FT)		
I skip meals a few times a week because I'm too busy to eat (PG-MAG)		
I get leg or foot (or other) muscle cramps (PG-MAG)		
I get twitching around my eyelids/eyes (PG-MAG)		
I am sensitive to loud noises (PG-MAG)		

Symptoms	Before Reboot	After Reboot
I grind my teeth (PG-MAG)		
I have restless leg syndrome (PG-MAG, iron)		
My heart skips beats sometimes or flutters (palpitations) (PG-MAG, iron)		
I get migraine headaches (PG-MAG, FT)		
I get menstrual cramps (or PMS) (PG-MAG)		
I'm indoors most of the time (PG-VIT D)		
I'm a vegan (or vegetarian) and don't supplement with vitamin D or vitamin B_{12} (PG-MAG, iron, VIT D, B_{12})		
I get numbness or tingling in my hands or feet (PG-B_{12})		
I have osteopenia or osteoporosis (PG-MAG, VIT D, CA)		
I have insulin resistance or metabolic syndrome (or diabetes) (PG-MAG, VIT D, FT)		
My skin is dry and itchy (PG-EFA)		
I have dry eyes (PG-EFA)		
I crave sweets but have an energy crash a few hours after I eat them (FT, PG-MAG)		
My hair or nails aren't healthy (PG)		
I drink soda or fruit juice more than once a month (PG)		
I eat mostly processed or packaged foods (PG)		
I bruise easily (PG-VIT C)		
My gums bleed when I brush (or floss) (PG-VIT C)		
I'm often constipated or get loose stools after eating (or have IBS) (FT)		

Symptoms	Before Reboot	After Reboot
I get sick (or have colds) easily, and infections linger (PG-ZN)		
I get hives or have eczema or allergies (or asthma) (FT)		
My heart sometimes races after I eat certain foods (FT)		
I get cracks at the corners of my mouth (PG-B-complex, FT)		
I get white spots on my fingernails (PG-ZN)		
I have a stressful relationship with food (PG)		
SCORE		

Key: B_{12} = vitamin B_{12}, CA = calcium, EFA = essential fatty acids, FT = food trigger, MAG = magnesium, PG = phytonutrient gap, VIT C = vitamin C, VIT D = vitamin D, ZN = zinc.

If you scored:

0–3 points: Good news! Sounds like you're not struggling with food-related symptoms. Your nutrition sounds like it's in good order, and maybe a little guidance can improve a few symptoms. Pay attention to any improvements you notice during the Reboot, because your food intolerances/sensitivities can show up in symptoms that weren't on this questionnaire.

>3 points: There's a good chance you've got food sensitivities or are low in important nutrients—particularly iron, vitamin D, magnesium, or vitamin B_{12}. The Reboot will help you figure out which foods are triggers for you, while the testing information on page 381 can help you to identify specific nutritional deficiencies. If any tests come back positive, see page 381 for which foods and supplements will get you to optimal levels. The Daily Dose Supplements (pages 166-67) will get you started on replacing the nutrients you're most likely to be low in. Follow the Reboot as strictly as you can, paying close attention to how you feel when you have removed foods, as well as any symptoms that recur when you add them back in.

Are Blood Sugar Imbalances Causing SOS?

Check the box next to any symptoms you relate to. Each check equals one point.

Symptoms	Before Reboot	After Reboot
I often skip meals because I am too busy		
I sometimes become weak, dizzy, or shaky because I haven't eaten in a while; I find myself famished before I even realize I'm getting hungry, or I sometimes need sugar or carbs fast because I'm so hungry		
I'm hungry again after dinner, before going to bed		
I crave sweets or carbs		
I wake up hungry in the middle of the night		
I skip breakfast more than one day a week		
I eat a low-calorie diet but can't seem to lose weight		
I've been diagnosed with insulin resistance metabolic syndrome (or diabetes)		
I'm overweight, especially around my middle (or have a muffin top)		
I have PCOS		
I frequently get yeast infections		
I get tired shortly after I eat something sugary or with carbs		
I get angry or irritable, then realize I'm hungry		
I get headaches when I forget to eat		
I exercise less than three times each week		
I've been told I have hypoglycemia		
SCORE		

If you scored:

0-3 points: Good news! Sounds like you're doing a great job keeping your blood sugar steady and your metabolism in peak performance. If you do have any symptoms, pay special attention to learning to balance your blood sugar with the SOS Solution Reboot.

>3 points: Time to take action. Like the 63 million Americans struggling with their blood sugar, you're not alone. Since blood sugar imbalances and insulin resistance put you at higher risk for diabetes and heart disease, I recommend that you start on the SOS Solution while setting up appropriate blood sugar, insulin resistance, and cholesterol testing (see page 381), and if your test results come back elevated, continue the SOS Solution while adding in specific supplements for blood sugar support on page 250.

Root 3: Gut Disruption

Do You Have Gut Imbalances?

Check the box next to any symptoms you relate to. Each check equals one point.

Symptoms	Before Reboot	After Reboot
Immediately after eating, I start sneezing or develop congestion (LG)		
I have heartburn (gastroesophageal reflux disease [GERD], reflux, acid indigestion) (GI)		
I have celiac disease (GI)		
I crave bread (or sugar or alcohol) (M)		
I've been told I have SIBO (SIBO/M)		
I have yeast overgrowth (Candida) (M)		
I get anal itching (M)		
I have chronic vaginal yeast infections (M)		

Symptoms	Before Reboot	After Reboot
I had Group B Strep (GBS) infection during pregnancy (M)		
I get indigestion when I eat fatty foods (M)		
I've been told I have leaky gut (intestinal hyperpermeability) (LG/M)		
I have incomplete bowel movements (M)		
I've taken antibiotics more than once in the past three years (LG/M)		
I frequently had antibiotics as a child (or in my teens, twenties, or more recently) (LG/M)		
My SOS or Hashimoto's symptoms started after a bout of food poisoning (or travel diarrhea) (LG/M)		
I've had food poisoning or travel diarrhea in the past five years (LG/M)		
I take ibuprofen (or other NSAID drugs) or Tylenol regularly (weekly or more often) (LG/M)		
I often have loose stools (M/GI)		
I feel "drunk," drugged, or tired after eating (M/GI)		
I notice that I sometimes have undigested food in my stool (M/GI)		
I get full very quickly when I eat; I can eat only a very small amount at a sitting (SIBO/M)		
I get nauseated after I eat (SIBO/M)		
I regularly need antacids (SIBO/M)		
I have food sensitivities (LG/M/GI)		
I get symptoms when I eat gluten or dairy (LG/M/GI)		

Symptoms	Before Reboot	After Reboot
I have seasonal allergies (or food allergies, asthma, or eczema) (LG/M/GI)		
I feel down, irritable, moody, or weepy after I eat certain foods (LG/M/GI)		
I get a skin rash, hives, or eczema after I eat certain foods (LG/M/GI)		
I have Hashimoto's (or rheumatoid arthritis, psoriasis, or another autoimmune disease) (LG/M/GI)		
I get constipated; I have a bowel movement less than once a day; my bowels are sluggish (M/GI)		
I take medications for reflux or acid indigestion (or have to take digestive enzymes or other supplements to digest my food) (LG/M/SIBO)		
SCORE		

Key: GI = gluten intolerance / celiac, LG = leaky gut, M = microbiome, SIBO = small intestinal bacterial overgrowth.

If you scored:

0–3 points: Good news! Your digestive system seems to be in good health, or you have only very mild symptoms. Since the SOS Solution, especially the Reboot and gut repair, can bring your digestive system back into balance without you having to do anything additional, my recommendation is to complete the first two weeks of the program, then retake this questionnaire.

>3 points: Your gut is asking for some help. Start on the SOS Solution and make sure to complete the 4R Program for Gut Health on page 211. If after three weeks of sticking with the Reboot and the 4R Program for Gut Health you still have more than five symptoms on this questionnaire, I recommend seeing a local integrative or functional medicine practitioner for appropriate testing (see page 381 for gut health testing recommendations) and additional support.

Root 4: Environmental Toxins

Does Your Detoxification System Need Extra Help?
Are You in Toxic Overload?

Check the box next to any symptoms you relate to. Each check equals one point.

Symptoms	Before Reboot	After Reboot
I suffer from regular (or frequent) headaches		
I have allergies and sensitivities		
I am fatigued with no good reason for feeling this tired		
I have trouble with memory and focus		
I have a bowel movement every other day or less often		
I'm bothered by perfumes (or strong scents or chemical odors)		
I'm sensitive to household cleaning products		
My skin is sensitive to perfumes, soaps, and detergents		
When I drink coffee or have caffeine, my heart races and I feel anxious or wired		
I have more than two mercury amalgam fillings		
I drink fluoridated water; I use fluoride-containing toothpaste		
I went through puberty or started my period before age ten		
I have PMS (or heavy, painful, or irregular periods)		
I have breast tenderness or breast lumps regularly		

Symptoms	Before Reboot	After Reboot
I regularly drink from plastic water bottles (or heat my food in plastic containers)		
I have chronic fatigue syndrome (or fibromyalgia)		
I don't sweat easily		
I regularly take acetaminophen (Tylenol or similar)		
I wear makeup every day, and usually don't buy the "green" or organic types		
I use perfumes, or products with perfumes in them, like my shampoo, soap, and hair spray		
I use conventional household cleaning products		
I live in a newly built house that is very airtight		
I eat inorganic meat or dairy more than once a month		
I eat inorganic produce (fruits and vegetables) most of the time		
I eat seafood regularly, and don't select only low-mercury sources		
SCORE		

If you scored:

0–3 points: Good news! You don't have obvious symptoms of toxic overload, and your detox systems seem to be in good working order, or if you are dealing with a small amount of overload the SOS Solution will help you to detoxify your body—and your life—and to naturally boost and support your body's detoxification systems.

>3 points: You're probably dealing with a fair amount of toxic overload, and your detoxification system needs support. The SOS Solution will help you to reduce your overall toxic exposures and will naturally boost and support your body's detoxification systems. You'll want to go through the SOS Solution, continue to avoid toxic exposures going forward, and make sure to emphasize the healing foods and herbs I recommend throughout the program and especially in chapter 6, "Repair." If you scored more than 8 points, you're dealing with a fair amount of toxic overload or your detoxification system is missing the nutrients and energy it needs to get the job done. If after four weeks of following the recommendations in this program you continue to have a high toxic load score, consider finding a local integrative or functional medicine practitioner to help you test for your total toxic body burden.

Root 5: Stealth Infection

Do You Have a Stealth Infection?

Check the box next to any symptoms you relate to. Each check equals one point.

Symptoms	Before Reboot	After Reboot
My symptoms began after I had a viral (or other) infection		
I'm tired more often than I think I should be		
I'm exhausted all the time		
My muscles feel heavy and tired		
I have aching or swelling in my joints		
I've had mono (Epstein-Barr virus [EBV]) in the past		
I currently have mono or EBV virus		
I have chronically (or currently) swollen lymph glands		
I have Hashimoto's thyroiditis		
I have GERD or have been treated for *H. pylori* infection		
I've had cytomegalovirus (CMV) in the past		
I've had a herpes infection		

Symptoms	Before Reboot	After Reboot
I get cold sores often (or when under stress)		
I've been bitten by a deer tick and haven't been properly treated (or I have Lyme disease)		
SCORE		

If you scored:

0-3 points: Good news! You are unlikely to have a stealth infection. Keep up the good work of supporting your immune system, and enjoy following the SOS Solution.

>3 points: There's a good chance that a stealth infection is a contributing factor in your symptoms. Do the SOS Solution and repeat this questionnaire once you've completed the program and have followed the stealth infection recommendations for at least four weeks. If you continue to score in this range when you repeat the questionnaire, getting tested for the common stealth infections is recommended.

ARE YOU READY FOR THE SOLUTION?

You did it! You finished the first part of this book! I hope that by now you've breathed a huge sigh of relief hearing that you're not alone, that your symptoms are not in your head, that there are real reasons that explain why you've been feeling like you have—frazzled, frumpy, forgetful, foggy, or on a hormonal roller-coaster ride you're ready to leave—and that there's a doctor who cares and has gathered the solutions you need together for you.

Together, let's take you off the roller-coaster ride of symptoms you've been on. This is a really exciting time when you can put your new knowledge into action, kiss your old symptoms good-bye, and finally get the results you've been looking for.

So what's next? *The SOS Solution.*

How do you do it? It's actually super easy—I've laid out the blueprint for you in a series of chapters that contain the five SOS solutions for each of the five Root Causes.

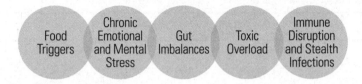

The next chapter brings you into the start of the SOS Solution, with the Reboot. It is the place for everyone to start. In this phase, which actually lasts through the plan until you reach the Replenish phase in week four, you'll eliminate food triggers, bridge your phytonutrient gap with the Daily Dose Supplements women need the most but are almost always short on receiving, and get your blood sugar healthy and steady. During this first week, I'll also introduce you to Replenish Self-Care, inspiring meditations, reflective practices, and awesome activities that will help you do everything from pick your priorities in life so that you're not chronically overloaded, to meditations that will help you cool down from stress while resetting your nervous system to CALM.

Before we start on your Reboot and the entire SOS Solution, please read below for what you'll need to begin for self-care.

Personal Pattern Tracker

Now it's time to create a map of your patterns, pathways, and progress. Fill out your score for each category using your tallies from each of the previous questionnaires. Repeat the questionnaires after two weeks on the Reboot, and again at the end of the four weeks of the SOS Solution to refine your plan and address any remaining symptoms or imbalances.

Personal Pattern Tracker			
Pattern or pathway	**Score Today Date __/__/__**	**Repeat Score 1 Date __/__/__**	**Repeat Score 2 Date __/__/__**
SOS-O			
SOS-E			
Hypothyroidism			
Stress			
Food triggers			
Blood sugar			
Gut disruption			
Environmental toxins			
Stealth infection			
My waist-to-hip ratio (see page 64)			

My Patterns and Plans at a Glance

Use this chart to get a picture of your patterns from most significant to least, based on your above scores, what steps you'll take next, and which tests are recommended, if any.

My Patterns	My Customized Next Steps	Recommended Testing
My primary SOS pattern is:		
I fit the hypothyroid pattern: Yes No		
My Root Cause pathways, from highest to lowest score:		
1.		
2.		
3.		
4.		
5.		
6.		
7.		

Replenish Self-Care Repair Kit: What You'll Need

Ideally, you'll want to have the following items on hand before you start your Reboot in order to practice your daily dose of self-care, an important part of the overall plan.

A journal: Any notebook will do, or you can purchase a lovely book intended as a journal if you'd prefer something a little more special.

Epsom salts and lavender (or other) relaxing aromatherapy oil: Purchase two bags of Epsom salts from your local pharmacy—they're inexpensive and make a great muscle-relaxing, magnesium-rich bath soak anyone can take; and a one-ounce bottle of good-quality lavender essential oil (see "Resources" on page 393) to have on hand for Replenish Baths.

A skin dry brush: Dry brushing stimulates and removes toxins from the largest organ of your body—your skin. You can find a natural bristle dry brush at most pharmacies and natural food stores. They are inexpensive and can amplify the detoxification work you'll be doing in this program. It feels great, too. Instructions are on page 232.

Herbal teas: My favorite blends include relaxing herbs such as chamomile and lemon balm; stimulating digestive-aid teas with cinnamon, ginger, and cardamom; or tart herbs such as rose hips and rooibos. See "Resources" for where to purchase and how to learn more about herbs.

Optional: Candles, music

Get Ready to Succeed

I know it can seem that your body is your enemy when you are struggling with so many symptoms and trying your best to keep up with your daily responsibilities, especially if all you really want is to crawl under the covers and sleep for a week. You might be feeling angry at your body, as if it has betrayed you, and sometimes wish you could trade yourself in for a new model—or get your old you back. I get it. But I promise you that your body isn't your enemy. Survival Overdrive Syndrome is, believe it or not, your body's sane response to a crazy world. Your body is doing exactly what it's supposed to do under stress. Your symptoms are signal flares, SOS signals, that help is needed. The SOS Solution is an opportunity to hit the pause button and listen to your body, change your habits, and turn things around.

Here are some tips to get you started on your way to success:

Put yourself on the front burner: As women, we too often put ourselves on the back burner—we don't see investing in ourselves as having value. This plan is about learning the importance of doing exactly that—because investing in yourself is one important and powerful step we can take to start listening to our bodies and valuing how we treat ourselves so we stay out of SOS. You deserve to do this.

Don't procrastinate: "I'll start tomorrow" rarely works, but I also want you to plan for success, so be practical and patient with yourself. If you have a massive deadline in two weeks, or it's right before the winter holidays when Grandma will be baking all of your favorite cookies, or you're on the first day of a trip to Italy (seriously, are you not going to drink wine and eat bread in Italy?), how is that going to go? You don't have to do this plan perfectly to succeed—just get started and do your best. You just have to do it! There's no race to the finish here, and all the improvements you make will be good improvements.

Set clear expectations: If you've got a partner or kids, or friends you hang out with a lot, let everyone know that you'll probably be eating a little bit differently than they will, and that you might be weaving some new foods into the family routine or pal get-together. You might be taking a walk after dinner instead of watching TV. You might be writing in your journal in the evenings and ask that your quiet time for doing so be respected. And you're not going to be keeping treats and temptations in the house, and you ask them to respect that, too (if you're single, then say everything I just recommended to yourself, as a reminder). And ask for help. Your partner, a sister, or a friend might really love to do the program with you—or might be willing to cheer you on, remind you of your goals, and keep the stuff away from you that you're trying to avoid.

SOS Rx: Safe Supplement Use

Throughout this book you'll find recommendations for herbal and nutritional supplements. While natural supplements can provide many health benefits, just because something is natural doesn't mean it's safe. Also, while adverse reactions are rare, they can occur in anyone—even to a supplement that doesn't cause reactions in most people. Therefore, having some guidelines for safe use is important. Before you start the supplement plans in this book, here are the key safety rules:

- Don't start supplements if you're on prescription medications without the guidance of a licensed primary care provider, preferably the one prescribing those medications. Not all herbs, supplements, and medications go well together.

- More is not better: Do not exceed the recommended doses, which also means do not duplicate supplements from one section of the book to another. Taking an herb or supplement as directed for one Root Cause or symptom covers you for each time it's recommended, unless otherwise directed—for example, if your core Daily Dose multivitamin contains 400 IUs of vitamin D_3, but 2,000 IUs are recommended for a specific Root Cause, you'll "supplement the supplement" to make up the difference. I recommend looking through each section that applies to you, and whenever possible choosing those supplements that appear in more than one place to minimize the number of different supplements you'll be taking, which will make your plan easier and also more economical. You'll find a printable version of all of the supplements used in this book, organized by category, at avivaromm.com/adrenal-thyroid-revolution. Use the list to prevent taking supplements redundantly, and bring it to the store with you for easier supplement selection.

- If you develop a rash, nausea, headache, or any other new symptom within a few days of starting a supplement, with no other explanation for the symptom, discontinue the supplement.

- The symbol ⊘ next to any supplement or group of supplements means that it is not safe for use in pregnancy. However, unless otherwise specified, the absence of this symbol does not mean I am condoning a supplement's use in pregnancy. Unless otherwise specified, the recommendations in this book *are* generally safe as directed while breast-feeding, but if you notice any changes in your baby's digestion, a rash develops, or you notice any other symptom after starting a supplement, discontinue taking that supplement.

- To identify reliable products, look for the GMP (Good Manufacturing Practice) seal on your products, and if you can, purchase products from major retailers that obtain third-party testing on their products and that are as free as possible from binders, fillers, excipients, and artificial colors and flavors. For more information on safe supplement selection, go to the federal government's Office of Dietary Supplements at ods.od.nih.gov.

Celebrate your wins and the small gains: Celebrating our wins is something we often forget to do! But your brain not only likes celebrations, it also likes rewards. They inspire you to reach higher, and they validate the hard work you've done to achieve something. I recommend counting a win at the end of every day and building some rewards for yourself into your plan, because these will keep you motivated. The reward can be as simple as a little extra "you time," or something more fancy—like that special dress you've been promising yourself.

Enjoy the scenery: A question I get all the time is "How long does it take to see improvement?" It's our adult version of "Are we there yet?" You are as unique as the next woman reading this book; your body will respond at its own pace. So having patience with yourself is super important. Enjoy the process. Getting healthier will happen.

Phone a friend: There's an African proverb, "If you want to go fast, go alone; if you want to go far, travel together." With the SOS Solution, traveling together—and celebrating together—will actually help you to travel farther, faster. I highly recommend having fun with the plan with a friend or group of friends. To help you make the most of this plan now, and for a lifetime, I've created a whole host of resources that you can take advantage of. If you choose to do this program on your own, know that you are not alone; there are millions on this journey, too! You can join my online course and use this book in a guided format, you can join the online community to meet other awesome women trying to take their health back too and get a bit of extra support and handholding, and you can access additional health tools and top-tier nutritional coaching from my personal team to get small-group or individualized support. Just come hang out over at avivaromm.com /adrenal-thyroid-revolution.

Dream big: Don't make feeling better an option for yourself—make it your big dream. Don't make self-care an option; make it your daily lifelong commitment. Don't make becoming who you want to be—and loving who you are—goals for the future; start right now. Believing in you is what your brain wants to hear you doing—and that's a major step toward getting out of SOS.

You'll be amazed by your results, which aren't miracles but results of a proven solution for getting better and staying better—and along the way, transforming what you believe about yourself. You can go from feeling that you are in a downward spiral of one problem after another, into a life where you actually love your body and realize how much healing your body is inherently capable of without relying on experts and medications at every turn. You'll realize you are your own best healer, with a sense of empowerment in your ability to take care of your health—a game changer for also taking control of other areas of your life!

All right, Lovely, let's Reboot!

Part 2

THE SOS SOLUTION

REBOOT

Remove Food Triggers, Restore Self-Healing

| Reboot: Remove Food Triggers | Reframe: Chronic Emotional and Mental Stress | Repair: Root Causes and SOS Damage | Recharge: Your Adrenals and Thyroid | Replenish: No More Running on Empty |

We are indeed much more than what we eat,
but what we eat can nevertheless help us be
much more than what we are.

—ADELLE DAVIS

YOU KNOW WHEN you have too many programs open on your computer and it goes into that annoying spin with that wheel icon? It's overloaded with information, and all you can do is shut down and reboot. When you're in SOS, you're a bit like that—you've got so many inputs and so much information coming in from all directions your body goes into overload trying to process it all. You need a Reboot.

The Reboot is the first twenty-one days of the SOS Solution. It gives you a chance to restart from the overload that has you in a spin, starting with getting your body out of any confusing messages it's getting from unhealthy foods or foods that are a unique SOS trigger for you, while replacing the nutrients that give your body the messages you need to vitalize your intrinsic self-healing capacities—which you do have even if you've been led to believe that you don't.

Most of us think of food as calories and nutrients at best—and food as reactions or emotional captivity at worst. But what those calories and nutrients are really doing is providing information to your cells, which in turn informs your mood, brain function, hormonal balance, and energy. What you put into your body literally forms the building blocks of your life, which in turn affects your mental clarity, emotions, confidence, relationships, career, and happiness. The wrong food sends your body into information overload.

The Reboot inherently improves detoxification. You'll be doing your best to remove toxins from your food, going organic whenever possible, as well as from your environment, while adding in the phytonutrients your body needs to enhance your natural detoxification processes.

The Reboot will get you off the roller coaster of sugar, caffeine, and other "pick-me-up" food addictions while giving you the energy you need to do this with surprising ease. Many women find this phase so effective at relieving symptoms and improving their energy, sleep, and mood that the rest of the plan becomes a matter of fine-tuning rather than heavy lifting. That's also why the Reboot comes first in the plan.

The Reboot is based on the two principles I shared at the beginning of the book:

1. **Eliminating** obstacles to health—in this case, food triggers (gluten, for example, and other foods that cause intolerances); hidden toxins in your food and food packaging; and foods that cause your blood sugar to be imbalanced (sugar, fast-burning and processed carbs).

2. **Replacing** what your body needs for healing—in this case, those foods and nutrients that your body needs for optimal wellness and activating self-repair (vegetables and fruits rich in phytonutrients and phytochemicals), those that keep your blood sugar steady and boost metabolism (good-quality proteins and fats), and those that reset your cortisol (proper carbohydrate cycling).

REAL, FRESH FOODS ACTIVATE YOUR SELF-HEALING CAPACITIES

Your body has an amazing capacity for self-repair, which means you can look younger and feel more energized. You can learn how to eat to nourish yourself so that you feel awesome from your cells to your soul, and importantly, without a crazy amount of effort. As you make important changes in what and how you eat, you'll begin to:

- Repair SOS damage to your gut, immunity, and detoxification systems by adding nutrient- and antioxidant-rich food that soothes inflammation
- Naturally balance your hormones
- Think more clearly and sleep better
- Begin to heal your adrenals and get your thyroid hormones back on track
- Make it nearly impossible for your body not to reach its best
- Feel lighter, brighter, and more at ease in your own skin again

The result? Your cortisol rhythm can spontaneously reset. Your metabolism will get a recharge. Inflammation will disappear, and you will be rid of the symptoms that are preventing you from feeling like your best version of yourself. In addition, you will learn a whole new way of eating that allows you to say good-bye to dieting forever, while recovering a level of energy you may have forgotten could be yours. Further, if you make this plan your lifestyle, you'll be amazed to learn that you can reduce, or become free of, numerous medical conditions, and with them, some of the medications you might wish you didn't have to take.

At the end of the 21-Day Reboot you'll transition fully to the Replenish Lifestyle, keeping the core principles you'll learn about during the Reboot, while experimenting with adding back some of the foods you removed, to see which you tolerate. These steps together will allow you to naturally create the most personalized diet that is right for you.

NOT JUST ANOTHER DETOX PLAN

We believe in counting our blessings. Not points, carbs, or calories.
—DANIELLE DUBOISE AND WHITNEY TINGLE, SAKARA LIFE

Your body is genius at moving you toward health; you just need help clearing out what's getting in the way of what your body knows how to do. Each minute your body is working through a variety of pathways to naturally detoxify contaminants from the environment, foods you eat, and hormones you produce or ingest (for example, oral contraceptives). The Reboot emphasizes the foods and nutrients that support your natural detoxification system while helping you steer clear of foods, ingredients, and even food packaging that add to your toxic burden.

Most detoxes are about restricting calories. At first and for a short while you might lose weight on those plans and feel better, but after just a few days, your brain starts to register a problem—hunger—and kicks you into SOS. Your hunger hormones have a little chat and decide that it's time for you to pack on some weight and hold on to it. Your metabolic thermostat—your thyroid—gets dialed down in the process to make sure you're not burning too much fuel. That's why you can be on a low-calorie diet and not lose weight—or you might even eventually gain it—making restrictive eating plans counterproductive.

As women we spend enough time in a struggle with food, worried about having symptoms if we eat the wrong foods, gaining weight, even "being judged" when eating in public if not on the latest diet. Food has lost its pleasure. We eat our food with a dose of guilt and shame, as well as confusion about what we really should be eating. My hope is that the SOS Solution will change the food conversation in your head so you can once again enjoy the real foods that will bring your body into its own natural balance and healthy size and shape—which are different for every woman at every stage of life. It's about truly loving yourself and making the changes you want to from that perspective, and eating fresh, high-quality, real foods.

Food should satisfy your body, delight your senses, please your taste buds, and be something you want to share because food is life: it's social, it's pleasure, and all of that is also health. That said, if you're used to standard American fare, your taste buds have become accustomed to an artificial-flavor, high-salt, high-sugar sensory overload, and it may take a week for your taste buds to unlearn old habits and become acquainted with new and delicious but sometimes acquired ones. Also, remember that SOS inflates the taste pleasure you get from sugar and salt. So as you change your diet and come down from living in SOS, simple, good, natural foods, properly seasoned as you'll learn to do with the Replenish recipes, will become your new favorites, and you'll wonder how you ever ate all that artificial stuff.

Healthy also doesn't require $16 juices, thousands of dollars a month in supplements, esoteric food ingredients, or fancy kitchen paraphernalia. If you can afford those, all power to you, but if you can't, that's okay. The program works when you eat simply of the deliciously fresh foods that are included in this plan—and that's completely within your reach. The SOS Solution is for real women, on real budgets, with real lives—like you and me. That said, it does take an investment in yourself to get well. If you don't pay now, eventually you might pay later. The cost of disease is high. Keep in mind how much you could be saving in health care in the long run, not to mention how much you'll immediately start saving on lattes and eating out—which can be thousands of dollars a year if you do the math. At my website you'll find additional resources for eating well on a budget. Visit avivaromm.com.

THE HEALTHIEST DIET IN THE WORLD

The food plan in this book is based on the ancestral—or traditional—Mediterranean diet, which is the only way of eating that has been scientifically proven to:

- Prevent and reverse metabolic syndrome and diabetes
- Prevent and reverse high blood pressure and high cholesterol
- Reduce toxin exposures
- Reset cortisol and reduce inflammation
- Improve fertility
- Prevent cognitive decline and Alzheimer's dementia

That is because it includes abundant anti-inflammatory, nutrient-dense foods rich in the phytochemicals your body craves for optimal detoxification, metabolism, and healthful longevity. Those following a traditional

Mediterranean diet not only have at least a 30 percent lower likelihood of developing heart disease, diabetes, and dementia, but also, in a study of more than ten thousand women, they were 40 to 50 percent more likely to live into their sixties and seventies without developing *any* chronic diseases, memory problems, or mental health problems, and without any major physical limitations.

Eating a total of eight servings of fresh veggies and fruits each day is associated with a higher level of mental well-being. A diet rich in plant nutrients can keep brain-draining inflammation at bay, improve the health of the mood-friendly gut microflora, and support detoxification of environmental chemicals, and internal and environmental hormones that can affect your mind and mood. Even in your fifties and sixties, it is not too late to prevent and even reverse many chronic diseases.

It's also the only way of eating that contains all of the components that health experts agree are health-promoting, regardless of the diet camp they're in: whole fresh foods, plenty of vegetables, good-quality protein, good-quality oils, nuts, and seeds, and slow-burning carbs in modest amounts, all in moderation. And it's the only way of eating that can be easily adapted to your needs whether you're vegan, vegetarian, Paleo, gluten-free, dairy-free, or have another personal preference or health need. There are only two things you need to know to get started: how to follow a Mediterranean-style diet, and how to personalize it to your health. That's exactly what you're going to learn in this chapter.

HERBIVORE, CARNIVORE, OMNIVORE: BALANCE YOUR ENERGY EQUATION

I live with an omnivore's dilemma. Having spent nearly two decades and three and a half pregnancies (including nine years of breast-feeding) as a vegetarian, and much of that as a vegan, I understand the philosophical, spiritual, environmental, and health reasons for making those choices. But as a doctor taking care of women, while I see many vibrant and healthy vegans and vegetarians, I see just as many who are having a hard time keeping their blood sugar steady and thus end up hungry a lot, shaky, and eating a lot of carbs, fruit, and energy bars to fill up.

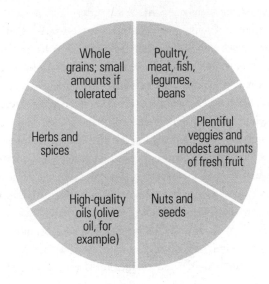

On the other hand, excess meat consumption, particularly red meat, is associated with a host of health problems. Numerous studies show that vegetarians have lower rates of diabetes, cholesterol problems, and even cancer largely due to healthier digestion and lower overall rates of estrogen dominance.

Women who eat more red meat and less fish and vegetables have higher rates of endometriosis, breast cancer, and colon cancer. A plant-based diet contains resistant starches that help keep blood sugar steady and also improves the quality of your microbiome, which, as you now know, means better physical and mental well-being. More meat consumption is associated with less fiber consumption, which increases your levels of harmful estrogens and breeds the wrong bacteria in your microbiome.

High-protein foods keep you energized, keep your blood sugar steady, and also provide the amino acids your body needs to transport hormones and manufacture important detoxification agents in your body, such as the important detoxifier, glutathione. Here's my take on it: Try to let go of dogma coming from all directions and listen to what your body needs. If you're tired all the time, unable to lose weight, can't get your blood sugar under control, are having mood swings, cravings, hormonal problems, or any other symptoms that just won't budge, and you're an ardent vegetarian, consider the addition of modest amounts of animal protein over the next three weeks and see what happens. Your body might need a missing element it's just not otherwise getting from your vegetarian diet. Conversely, if you're hard-core Paleo and are struggling with a lot of inflammation, hormonal problems, low energy, intense cravings, or sleep problems, for example, you may need to liberalize your diet to include some grains and legumes, and make sure you're getting enough vegetables. I don't want to trample on your personal beliefs—my role here is just to point out what might help—and I've seen changes in diet flip energy on and symptoms off like hitting a light switch. So think about it—even if you just try it for the next twenty-one days. Flexibility and variety are two of the most important "ingredients" for a healthy diet and keeping your energy balanced.

If you are currently following a vegan/vegetarian lifestyle, and prefer to continue avoiding meat or animal products, you can absolutely continue to do so. Follow the plan, substituting in the vegan recipes you'll find in the Reboot and Replenish Menus and Recipes for the meat recipes.

HERE'S HOW YOU'LL REBOOT

- **Prepare:** Pick a date to start the Reboot. That can be right now if you're ready to kick some of your food habits immediately. Or wait until you've done the kitchen makeover, below, which can take one to three days, depending on how well stocked your kitchen is already.

- **Take out the hidden food triggers:** During the first week, and for the entire 21-Day Reboot, remove all of the foods in the section "Foods to Remove: The SOS Food Triggers," starting on page 138.

- **Add in the Replenish foods** starting on day one and for the entire 21-Day Reboot, using the Replenish Meal Plans as a guide.

- **Add your Daily Dose Supplements.**

- As often as you can, **notice and record how you feel** after a meal or a snack; the goal is to learn how different foods make *your* body feel so you can personalize your lifestyle for the long run. Do certain foods make you feel energized? Light? Focused? Those are YES foods for you. Do some leave you tired, sluggish, bloated, achy, or foggy? Those are the NO foods—at least for now.

THE REBOOT, WEEK BY WEEK

Here's a chart of what you'll be changing with your food, week by week.
You'll have a daily planner and recipes, day by day, to guide you.

	What You Eliminate	What You Emphasize	Supplements
Week 1: Reboot	All Reboot NO foods Grains and legumes Foods you personally don't tolerate Nightshades Nuts Fruit if it gives you gas or bloating	All Reboot YES foods except those you are eliminating If you are vegan or vegetarian, use energy vegetables and wild red rice or black rice instead of grains for this one week, and avoid beans as well during this time, though chickpeas and legumes (e.g., lentils) may be included as they are often well-tolerated	Daily dose
Week 2: Repair	Continue to eliminate: All Reboot NO foods Foods you personally don't tolerate Nightshades Fruit if it gives you gas or bloating	All Reboot YES foods except those you are eliminating Plus add back in: + ½ cup of grains at dinner each evening (if tolerated) + 1-2 servings of legumes/day + 1 oz. of almonds or walnuts/day	Daily dose + Repair
Week 3: Recharge	All Reboot NO foods Foods you personally don't tolerate Nightshades Fruit if it gives you gas or bloating	Continue above	Daily dose + Repair + Recharge

PRE-REBOOT KITCHEN MAKEOVER (ONE TO THREE DAYS BEFORE YOU START)

Take Back Your Kitchen

Taking back your kitchen is a powerful vote in favor of your health. Cooking at home dramatically improves weight loss and health, doesn't have to cost more, and can be done creatively so that you learn to save time. Getting your kitchen set up doesn't have to cost a fortune, and you don't need much, but you will need some healthy cooking basics (pots, cutting boards, vegetable knives, measuring cups and spoons, for example), especially stainless steel pots and glass storage containers. Please visit my website, avivaromm .com/adrenal-thyroid-revolution, for a list of cooking supply basics if your kitchen is not set up for prep, and suggestions as to where to purchase them affordably.

Now's the time to clear out sugary treats, chips, snacks, and the NO foods in the next section. You have to chuck it all to make it hard to eat them!

You'll also definitely want to recycle or toss and replace these kitchen items that can leach toxins into your food:

- Plastic food storage containers
- Plastic water and other beverage containers
- Teflon (or other nonstick) cookware
- Nonstick and spray oils
- Antibacterial kitchen soap

FOODS TO REMOVE: THE SOS FOOD TRIGGERS

For the next three weeks you will be excluding the foods listed below. My experience is that it's best to just rip off the Band-Aid—go cold turkey, eliminating all inflammatory hidden food triggers at once. If your brain is resisting the idea of giving up your favorite foods (coffee drinkers, see below), I promise that you'll have plenty of delicious, energy-boosting foods to eat during the next twenty-one days. When you start to feel the kind of energy you haven't had in years, you'll want to keep going.

The Reboot NO Foods

Completely Eliminate All Artificial Ingredients and Poor-Quality Oils and Fats

Artificial colors and flavors	Food preservatives
Fake dairy substitutes ("creamers")	Fried foods
Fat substitutes (margarine, olestra, etc.)	Processed meats
Food additives	Trans fats
Food coloring and dyes	Vegetable oil, corn oil

Completely Eliminate Sugar and White or Refined Carbohydrates

Artificial sweeteners and sugar substitutes (Equal, NutraSweet, etc.)

Fruit juice and soda

High-fructose corn syrup

Sugar (this includes natural sugars such as honey, maple syrup, etc.)

Avoid Gluten and Cross-Reactive Grains

Barley	Oats
Corn	Rye
Millet	Wheat

· Avoid Dairy Products

You can use almond and coconut milks (unsweetened) for recipes that call for milk, and in your tea. Coconut yogurt is a nice alternative to dairy yogurt during the Reboot. You'll find a surprisingly rich and creamy homemade frozen dessert, as well as an "I Can't Believe It's Chia" pudding, if the ice-cream gremlin starts calling your name and you can't ignore it.

Cheese	Ice cream
Cottage cheese	Kefir
Cream cheese	Milk (dairy)
Cream, half-and-half	Yogurt (dairy)

The Reboot NO Foods

Avoid Common Food Triggers If You Know You Are Sensitive or Are Uncertain

These three food categories are not a problem for everyone, but if you suffer from joint pain and swelling, or rheumatoid arthritis, or other auto-immune disease, nightshades and nuts may be a trigger for you—omit them from any of the recipes during the Reboot. You can experiment with adding them back in during the Replenish if they don't seem to be a trigger for you.

Nightshade vegetables (tomatoes, eggplant, peppers, and potatoes). They are marked as such (NS) in the recipes. If you see them as a vegetable addition, simply omit. If you see canned or crushed tomatoes, swap with vegetable or organic chicken broth; if you see tomato paste, omit except in tagines or curries—and then swap with coconut cream to thicken.

Nuts, especially peanuts

Soy (if you do choose to include soy, choose only organic, non-GMO)

Yeasted products (wine, beer, and other alcoholic beverages, vinegars, yeasted bread, products containing vinegar, such as mustard) (Apple cider vinegar is usually still well tolerated on a yeast-free diet, so substitute it anywhere you see other vinegar if you are avoiding yeast on your personalized plan.)

Avoid Alcohol and Caffeine

Alcohol (wine, beer, mixed drinks, hard liquor—all of it)

Caffeine (coffee, black tea, chocolate, green tea, and maté)

Avoid Your Personal Food Triggers

Foods that you tend to crave and your personal "comfort foods" (more sneaky culprits and code for "cravings")

Foods you know trigger symptoms

Foods that you eat day in and day out (if you have leaky gut, your body may be temporarily reactive to them)

How Strict Do I Have to Be?

If you're a scientist doing an experiment, the only way to be sure of your results is to do the experiment 100 percent. Same here—the Reboot is your chance to be your own experiment, to get curious about what

Six Tips for Keeping It Simple in the Kitchen

1. Plan Ahead

How many times have you stood in front of your open fridge or pantry and wondered what you're going to eat for dinner? This plus hunger and fatigue are a recipe for a take-out call to the nearest pizza joint or Chinese restaurant. I think ahead to my week's worth of meals on Sunday, and then follow it up with my grocery shop, shopping list in hand. I've done this for years, and it's so simple once you get in the habit. If you have kids, it will transform your life. And it will save you money and from eating take-out more than you want to.

2. Set Reasonable Expectations: Don't Make Every Meal Gourmet

Real food is simple, satisfying, and delicious—and can often be prepared relatively quickly. None of this requires elaborate, complicated, fancy, or gourmet. Enjoy simplicity.

3. Canned (or Bottled) Beans Are Cool

Purchase only cans that say BPA-free, or buy precooked beans in glass bottles (more expensive, though).

4. Frozen Is Fair Game

Fruits and veggies should ideally be fresh, but frozen options, as long as they have no added ingredients (sugar, salt, preservatives) are an excellent alternative for when you need to prepare something fast and need ingredients that are prepped for you.

5. Prep Ahead or Cheat with "Precut"

Having some time each weekend or an evening each week where you plan out your menus, shop, and prep your food ahead of time may sound time-consuming, but in the end, I promise, it will actually add time to your life. I recommend prepping as you unpack your groceries—for example, wash and cut your veggies before you even put them in the fridge, and store them in a glass storage container so they're ready for use.

6. Batch Cook, Repurpose, and Make Enough for Leftovers

Plan your meals so that you're repurposing or getting leftovers for the week. Preparing several days of your whole grains ahead of time also saves time, as does making a large salad ahead of time (don't dress it ahead of time; it will get soggy!).

makes your body work best for you. You want to go 100 percent. That said, life happens. You get stuck at work unexpectedly and have to eat what's brought in. It's your kid's birthday and you cave and have a piece of cake. If you go off the plan, don't throw in the towel; just keep going, add in a couple of extra days if you can, and make note of what happened and why in your journal. Notice how you feel—physically and emotionally—and what happened that led you to step off the plan for a minute. Then figure out what you can do to avoid that obstacle next time. Common hidden obstacles include:

- Hidden food triggers lurking in, for example, ketchup, mayo, yogurt, pickles, salad dressings, sauces, deli meats, canned goods, soups, and milk alternatives. This is an especially big problem when eating out, so be watchful.
- Grabbing something fast (hint: keep an emergency Snack Stash on hand; see page 160).
- Parties: If you do have to eat out or go to a party, eat ahead of time and then just order a veggie appetizer. If you're going to a potluck, bring a dish that works for you and stick to that.
- Social drinking: If everyone's having a drink, order sparkling water with a splash of cranberry juice. Nobody has to be the wiser.

And if you do go for it and have a drink, eat the cookies, whatever, no worries—just pick back up where you left off with the Reboot. This is a no-failure plan. Just keep going. Self-love here, please.

Sugar, Salt, Fat: How Do I Handle Cravings?

> *Between stimulus and response there is a space.*
> *In that space is our power to choose our response.*
> *In our response lies our growth and our freedom.*
> —VIKTOR E. FRANKL

Each day we have literally hundreds of "food thoughts" and have to make many in-the-moment decisions that affect our health, such as when we reach for that pint of Ben & Jerry's or down that bag of cookies or chips almost automatically. Here are my recommendations for handling cravings.

Give your body what it's asking for: If you crave fat, sugar, or salt, it's because you're in SOS and your body is craving the extra support and energy, or you're struggling with another Root Cause, for example, dysbiosis or a phytonutrient gap. Of course, chowing down on a Snickers bar is not a sustainable solution. Keep satisfying alternatives on hand to fill the craving need, for example:

- Dry-roasted nuts with Himalayan or sea salt when you want something salty
- Baked homemade sweet potato fries for the chips attack
- Frozen berries, "Soft Serve" (page 378), or a small bar of 72 percent dark chocolate so you can have a few squares if you just really want something sweet

Avoid triggers: Avoid settings that trigger cravings—for example, sitting down in front of the TV with a big bag of chips, shopping when you're hungry, showing up hungry to the holiday potluck that's overflowing with everything tempting.

Change the conversation in your brain: The best way I've found to change the food conversation in the brain is to form new habits. One of these is giving yourself Permission to Pause. Here's how: when it comes to a food craving, or a binge on the brink, simply give yourself ten golden seconds to shift your thoughts and emotions into mindful awareness of *how you want to feel.* Is eating that going to get you there? Before opening the fridge or cabinet, take a breath and get curious about how you're feeling and what's driving your "snack attack." Ask yourself:

- Am I really hungry?
- Do I really want this right now?
- How will I feel later if I eat this?
- What does my body need right now?
- Is there an alternative I can choose? (Check out the "No-Crash Emergency Stash and Replenish Snack Recommendations" on page 160 for a healthy alternative, call a friend, go for a brisk walk, dance it out.)
- What am I *really* hungry for? (Could be something interesting to do, love, interaction, mental stimulation.)

Indulge Now and Then

I bet you didn't expect me to say indulging is healthy! But I promised that this plan is not about food deprivation. You have to have an honest conversation with yourself about food, and find the balance between reaching how you want to feel and making yourself neurotic about food.

It's a fact that our brains rebel against overrestriction. It raises your cortisol and makes you more likely, not less likely, to binge out. It sets you up for failure. So does beating yourself up when you eat something "not on your plan." Therefore, please indulge now and then if you need to. Just don't do it on things that make you feel sick, as in your personal food triggers, if you can help it. Enjoying food sets you up for success. Food can be a joyous part of your life that makes you feel really great—and great about yourself. If there's a food you love and it's not something you have an intolerance to, then my philosophy is to eat it, savor it, enjoy every bite, and bathe in the afterglow of a desire satisfied.

Hunger in Your Soul

I don't believe in guilty pleasures,
because I don't believe in feeling guilty.

—KATHRYN BUDIG

Sometimes cravings are coming from an unmet need or desire that's easier to subdue with food than to face or do something real about. We fill gaps in love, satisfaction, and inner peace with food, and we use food to calm our anxieties, fears, and depression. The great writer Maya Angelou said, "There is no greater agony than bearing an untold story inside you." It is this very agony that can lead to cravings as we try to quiet the voice of that story, the agony of unfulfillment. If this resonates with you when you get quiet and deeply honest with yourself, then do this practice: Carve out five minutes and ask yourself this one question: "What am I really hungry for?" Listen for whatever answer comes to you, and pay attention to that message. Knowing the truth can start to set you free from the food craving and redirect your attention to creating what you're really seeking for deeper fulfillment.

"Dr. Romm, I've Gone Gluten-Free Before, and It Didn't Help"

Sometimes someone will say, with some amount of frustration at the suggestion that they try going gluten-free, "Dr. Romm, I've gone gluten-free before and it didn't help." If this is also the case for you, there are a number of reasons why this can happen:

- You didn't go gluten-free for long enough—it can take up to three months to see a dramatic difference.
- You didn't go *completely* gluten-free—you were letting a little gluten slip into your diet, or were getting inadvertent contamination.
- You are sensitive to gluten cross-reactive foods. These can be triggers, so if you're sensitive you have to take these out, too, to get results.
- Gluten isn't your problem—you have one or more of the other Root Causes at play, giving you other options to work on.

EATING FOR LIFE: THE REBOOT YES FOODS

You might be thinking, "Well, she's now put my entire diet on the 'can't eat it list,' so what am I going to eat?" Don't worry; there's plenty! I think you'll be pleasantly surprised to find that the Reboot and Replenish Plans give you more and better food options, not fewer. And these are the high-fiber, energy-rich, nutrient-abundant foods that are going to get you out of SOS and get you feeling like yourself again.

I've provided three weeks of meal plans so you never have to stand in front of the fridge wondering what to eat. You can select any options you like—just be mindful of where you are in the Reboot. Don't get stuck on traditional meals—you can have a breakfast frittata for lunch or dinner, or a wrap for breakfast. If you just don't have time to prepare breakfast, sub in a smoothie. However, if smoothies cause you any bloating, you may need a warm meal for breakfast to get your digestive fire going, or you may have some fructose intolerance. In that case, select any of the warm breakfast alternatives, and omit fruit during the 21-Day Reboot.

Meat, Poultry, and Fish

Protein provides the building blocks for all of the structures in your body. It's a major source of food energy, keeps your blood sugar steady, giving you about two hours of fuel per serving, and provides the amino acids and sulfur-rich compounds you need for peak detoxification. Meats are also rich in vitamins B_6 and B_{12}, zinc, selenium, and a metabolism-boosting nutrient, coenyzme Q_{10}. Lean, free-range, grass-fed, organically grown meats, non-GMO plant proteins, and wild-caught or organic farm-raised fish are preferable. During the Reboot, I recommend having red meat no more than once weekly starting in week two, only in portion sizes discussed later in this chapter, instead emphasizing low-mercury fish, poultry, and eggs.

Examples of animal proteins include:

- Beef
- Chicken, skinless
- Eggs

- Fish (low in mercury; see below)
- Lamb
- Turkey

Make Mine Low in Mercury, Please

To avoid excess mercury, most of which comes from eating fish, only low-mercury varieties should be eaten, or an omega-3 essential fat supplement can be taken instead; these are tested and consistently found to be safe. For printable guides and apps on the low-mercury fish you can eat, please see "Resources," page 393.

Beans and Legumes

Legumes and beans are plant-based sources of protein that also provide the powerful protective phytoestrogens that block and reduce the effects of more harmful environmental endocrine disrupters and help your body eliminate toxic breakdown products of estrogen. They are rich in zinc, folate, and amino acids to support detoxification, especially DNA-protective methylation. During week one you'll eliminate all but the least inflammatory ones: garbanzos and lentils.

Additional beans and legumes that can be included in moderation, or if you are a vegetarian, after week one include:

- Adzuki beans
- Black beans
- Kidney beans
- Lima beans
- Navy beans
- Pinto beans
- Split peas
- Tofu (organic only, no more than once a week)
- White beans (cannellini or northern)

Grains

Grains are a controversial food item these days, but may be especially important if you're in SOS or have Hashimoto's. For some women, a very low-carb diet triggers the brain's "danger signals," triggering SOS, and may lower the thyroid's production of T_3 because your body thinks it's in energy conservation mode.

A slow-carb versus low-carb diet is the answer. Legumes, whole grains, and cooked potatoes are examples of foods that contain high amounts of resistance starches, indigestible fibers that increase healthy and decrease unhealthy gut flora, and improve blood sugar balance and insulin sensitivity. Eating legumes several times weekly, if you tolerate them, actively promotes weight loss. And winter squashes and sweet potatoes are excellent starch-containing "energy vegetables" (see page 149).

Eating slow-burning carbs from grains or energy vegetables about four hours before bed increases your natural production of melatonin, which helps you to fall asleep more easily. This increases the amount of time you get deep sleep, and as a result, improves your cortisol curve and hormonal balance. It also improves fat burning. Having your grain or energy vegetables at your dinner meal will not cause you to gain weight as long as you're not filling up on carbs all day, too.

During the first week, you're going to kick it off grain-free and legume-light, however, because one week of going grain-free has been shown to help restore the microbiome to a more favorable colonization of beneficial organisms. If eating grains causes you to feel tired, chances are that you are not digesting them well due to gut dysbiosis. In this case, you can keep them out of your plan until after the 4R Program for Gut Health (chapter 6), substituting energy vegetable dishes into your menu in place of grain sides. You can reintroduce the grains after week two when you've been on the 4R Program for Gut Health for a week.

I recommend never having a predominantly grain- or legume-based meal for breakfast; they leave you tired and hungry by midmorning. A protein food, ideally animal protein-based (eggs, for example), is optimal for steady blood sugar and lasting morning energy, balanced mood, and focus.

While you will be avoiding grains for the first week, quinoa, buckwheat, wild rice, and red, pink, and black rice are not technically grains; they are a different form of seeds, and you can eat them even during week one.

Examples of whole grains and grain-like seeds:

- Brown rice,
  brown rice noodles
- Buckwheat (kasha)
- Millet
- Oats
- Quinoa
- Wild rice; red, pink, or
  black rice

Nuts and Seeds

Nuts and seeds, particularly almonds and walnuts, may be one of the most important common denominators in the health benefits of the Mediterranean diet. Even just a handful each day (about an ounce) can prevent heart disease in conjunction with an otherwise healthy diet. Because they are high in fat and protein, they are the perfect energy package, making them an excellent addition to meals and a great snack.

Seeds are also rich in healthful oils and are rich protein sources. They are rich in vitamin E, an important antioxidant. You can use them in any form: raw, dry-roasted (not oil-roasted), and in nut and seed butters. Some companies include palm oil and sugar in nut butters, so read labels. While most are good options, the healthiest Reboot choices are almonds, walnuts, and any of the seeds. During week one we'll be eliminating nuts because they are inflammatory for some individuals.

Examples of healthy nuts and seeds include:

- Almonds
- Brazil nuts
- Cashews
- Coconut
- Flaxseed
- Hempseed
- Pecans
- Pine nuts
- Pumpkin seeds
- Sesame seeds
- Sunflower seeds
- Walnuts

Energy Vegetables

These vegetables provide you with energy and also allow you to pass on the grains if you don't tolerate them. They are also loaded with vitamin A, which supports your immune system and helps to heal the lining of your digestive tract. The starch serves as great food for healthy microflora, which also means they are great for keeping your bowels healthy and regular. Because they are relatively high in sugar, you should have only one to two portion sizes per day, as recommended in the menus.

Examples of starchy vegetables include:

- Beets
- Parsnips
- Sweet potatoes
- White, yellow, and purple potatoes (note these are nightshades)
- Winter squashes (delicata, pumpkin, acorn, spaghetti, butternut, etc.)

Leafy Green Vegetables

Leafy greens are particularly important in the Reboot and Replenish Plans. They are rich in powerfully detoxifying and antioxidant nutrients, essential for the ability of your liver to detoxify environmental toxins and hormones, support methylation, and provide some of the most important fiber you can get to encourage a healthy microbiome and proper elimination. I recommend including about four cups of total leafy greens in your

Greens and Your Thyroid

If you have Hashimoto's, you may have heard that you need to avoid veggies in the *Brassicaceae* family: broccoli, cabbages, kale, Brussels sprouts, cauliflower, and collards. These veggies contain a thyroid-suppressing compound, as do millet, soy, and cassava, to name a few foods. However, the risk due to green veggies in this family appears to be associated with eating them raw in large quantities, or if you have Hashimoto's *and* iodine deficiency. Daily intake of moderate amounts of these vegetables cooked does not appear to present a problem at all, and has protective effects on most aspects of health. If you have a slow-functioning thyroid, avoid large amounts of raw *Brassicaceae* vegetables. Fermenting these vegetables (for example, eating cabbage as sauerkraut rather than raw) may also inhibit their ability to slow thyroid function.

diet daily, two at lunch and two at dinner. See "Greens and Your Thyroid," above.

Examples of leafy greens include:

- Arugula
- Bok choy
- Broccoli and rapini
- Brussels sprouts
- Cabbage (red, green, Chinese)
- Cauliflower
- Chard / Swiss chard
- Collard greens
- Dandelion greens
- Kale
- Lettuces and salad greens (all varieties except iceberg)
- Mustard greens
- Spinach

Rainbow Vegetables

The rainbow-colored vegetables are nutrient warehouses filled with phyto-chemicals that your body uses for detoxification, squelching inflammation, and literally thousands of enzymatic, metabolic, and immune reactions around the clock. These can be eaten in abundance, although if these are a trigger for you, you'll eliminate the nightshades for the three weeks of the Reboot. They are marked as such (NS) in the recipes; if you see them as a vegetable addition, simply omit; if you see canned or crushed tomatoes, swap with vegetable or organic chicken broth; if you see tomato paste, omit except in tagines or curries—and then swap with coconut cream to thicken.

Examples of "rainbow vegetables" include:

- Asparagus
- Carrots
- Celery
- Green beans, snow peas
- Onions (yellow, red)
- Purple broccoli (also a "green")
- Red cabbage (also a "green")
- Red, yellow, and green peppers, tomatoes, eggplant (note that these are nightshades)
- Yellow summer squash
- Zucchini

Does Organic Matter?

Organic does matter. Toxins in your food (herbicides, pesticides, hormones, antibiotics) accumulate in your body and can cause obesity, hormone disruption, and cellular damage, and alter your immune responses. Going organic clears these toxins out of your system in just days. Organic meats, eggs, and dairy are a priority; the price you pay now will save you in health problems and misery later. For produce, I recommend following the Environmental Working Group's Clean Fifteen and Dirty Dozen guidelines. The Clean Fifteen are those conventionally farmed foods that you can eat without worrying about toxins; the Dirty Dozen are the foods most heavily exposed to pesticides and herbicides. Eat these organic only or avoid them. See ewg.org.

Oils and Fats

Oils (liquid at room temperature) and fats (solid at room temperature) are our most energy-dense forms of nutrition, and contrary to thirty years of misinformation on low-fat diets, we now know that it takes healthy fats to burn fat and to protect us from disease. Good-quality fats are also mainstays for keeping your blood sugar steady and to support brain and nervous system health, and mood. Every meal should include a serving of healthy fat.

The Replenish Super Foods

Nutrient-rich foods are the leading ladies in your body's ability to detoxify and fight inflammation. You won't be disappointed as you read the list of foods that also act essentially as healing medicines! They help your brain to learn and remember; they rev up your detoxification support, cool inflammation, normalize blood pressure and cholesterol, and boost your mood—naturally.

Leafy green vegetables in the *Brassicaceae* family (broccoli, kale, collards, Brussels sprouts, cabbages, and bok choy) contain a host of naturally occurring chemicals called glucosinolates, which break into chemicals that bump up the volume on liver detox while giving your gut flora the best nutrition possible (yes, gut flora need good nutrition to flourish, too!). They also contain fiber that promotes a good daily BM—which not only keeps you feeling peppy and makes you drop pounds, but also clears out environmental toxins and prevents estrogen excess.

Berries. Talk about awesome medicine for the body and deliciousness in life! All the berries are fantastic for you. Blueberries, red raspberries, strawberries (organic for these, please!) and blackberries are my top go-tos. They contain proanthocyanidins, ellagic acid, and polyphenols in the most delicious package ever!

Pomegranate has three times the antioxidant effects of green tea and red wine. It improves detoxification in the liver and helps keep cholesterol and blood sugar balanced. Take two ounces of unsweetened pomegranate juice concentrate in eight ounces of still or sparkling water daily for a lovely natural "spritzer" that is safe even for diabetics because it reduces insulin resistance!

Olive and coconut oils. Olive oil, 2 to 4 tablespoons daily, will not only help you lose your weight and improve your cholesterol, it will also decrease isoprostanes, nasty little inflammatory chemicals that your body makes. Rich in naturally healthy phenols, olive oil gives a power boost to your body's production of naturally occurring detox chemicals such as glutathione. Olive oil, like the other foods and herbs listed here (for herbs, see page 155), can also help mitigate damage to your DNA because they create chemicals that scavenge free radicals, harmful little inflammatory forms of oxygen that get loose in our bodies as a result of toxins and detox problems.

Flaxseeds help you to feel full, eat less, lose weight, and improve your bowel health and regularity because they feed good gut flora, act as a gentle bulk laxative, and help to balance your hormones. In supporting good gut flora, flaxseeds help your body eliminate harmful estrogens you may have produced or picked up from the environment, which not only keeps you in better hormonal health but also may prevent breast cancer. They also improve blood sugar, reduce inflammation, and bring down cholesterol. Add 1 to 2 tablespoons of freshly ground flaxseeds daily to a smoothie/shake, or toss them into your salad or onto grains (don't heat the flaxseeds).

Herbs and spices. Rosemary, a powerful anti-inflammatory and antioxidant, is perhaps the queen of detox seasonings, and can also be taken in capsules and extracts for its ability to help the liver do its job of getting rid of toxins; but any of the herbs and spices I mention on page 155 can boost your health. See my Olive Oil Lemon Salad Dressing (page 343) and Lemon-Rosemary Chicken (page 367) for two ways to start incorporating fresh or dried rosemary into your daily diet.

Dark chocolate. I wouldn't be "The Women's Natural M.D." if I didn't include dark chocolate, now would I? But I'm not including it just to make you like me. Dark chocolate really is good for you. It's rich in magnesium, supports healthy brain function, reduces blood pressure, and makes people happy because it's a natural mood booster. It keeps cholesterol in check and is a powerful antioxidant. If you're struggling with cravings or blood sugar problems and "can't eat just one," then wait until after the 21-Day Reboot to enjoy dark chocolate, or use unsweetened cacao nibs or powder in your shakes to get the benefits without the sugar (it's a bit bitter—be forewarned); otherwise, you can enjoy a couple of ounces of dark chocolate (two to four squares) daily, but it has to be 72 percent dark or higher and contain no soy lecithin, carrageenan, or emulsifiers.

Don't worry—you will not gain weight from good-quality fats and oils. All oils should be cold-pressed, organic, non-GMO, and ideally sold in dark bottles or opaque packaging to protect them from oxidation due to light exposure.

My favorite healthy fat choices are:

- Avocado
- Coconut oil and unsweetened coconut milk
- Extra-virgin olive oil
- Ghee (clarified butter)
- Olives, black or green
- Sesame oil
- Sunflower oil
- Walnut oil

Fruits

Fruits are an incredible source of vitamins and phytochemicals important for preventing inflammation and oxidative stress; they are also high in sugar, so during the Reboot, I recommend the lowest-sugar-containing fruits, in limited amounts. Omit or keep to one serving daily if you struggle with chronic yeast or fungal infections, gas and bloating, or metabolic syndrome. All berries should be organic, fresh or frozen.

The Reboot-friendly fruits include:

- Apples
- Blackberries
- Blueberries
- Cherries
- Kiwi
- Raspberries
- Strawberries

Half of a ripe banana may be included in your smoothie, or citrus juice added to salads and dressings in small amounts. Lemon and lime juice may be used in water or salad dressings.

Microbiome-Friendly Fermented Foods

Naturally fermented vegetables are important parts of rebuilding a healthy microbiome, and are parts of most traditional diets around the world. Since you'll be dairy- and soy-free during the Reboot, I recommend including a small amount of unpasteurized (look on the bottle) fermented vegetables with at least one meal daily, for example:

- Coconut yogurt or kefir (unsweetened)
- Kimchi
- Sauerkraut

If you don't enjoy fermented foods, taking a probiotic once daily, as described in the next chapter, will help keep your microbiome healthy.

Spice It Up for Health and Weight Loss

Cooking spices are nature's delicious herbal pharmacy. Studies show that including even small pinches of fresh or dried herbs such as rosemary, thyme, or oregano in a salad, for example, increases weight loss, reduces inflammation, and boosts detoxification. They may be one of the "secret" ingredients in Blue Zone diets—diets that lead to the greatest health and longevity in the world. Here are some of my favorites; you'll find more in the shopping list on page 314.

- Basil
- Cardamom
- Cayenne
- Cilantro (fresh)
- Cinnamon
- Cumin
- Curry blends
- Dill
- Garlic
- Ginger
- Mint
- Oregano
- Parsley
- Rosemary
- Turmeric

Beverages

The healthiest drink is filtered water. Consider a charcoal countertop water filter (a Brita, for example), an under-the-sink reverse osmosis filter (you or a plumber can install this, and over time it's a cost savings over purchasing water), or delivery of five-gallon glass containers (plastic may contain BPA or BPS). When you're out, you can drink still or sparkling water from glass bottles, or carry your own glass or stainless steel water bottle with you. I love the Life Factory bottles—they last forever and are dishwasher-safe. Here are the healthiest Reboot beverages:

Coffee Break or Coffee Breakup?

If your mind is already fighting against giving up the coffee—it's the one item that usually provokes a protest—I understand. You're exhausted and this is what gets you through your days. It's delicious and part of "you time."

Coffee has some great science showing that it can keep our minds sharp well into our senior years and reduce the risks of dementia, Parkinson's disease, diabetes, and stroke. But here's the thing: You're reading this book because you have SOS. And if you're sensitive to caffeine, it can keep you jumpy and irritable during the day and jacked well into the night. Many women find that coffee causes plummeting blood sugar, PMS, and monthly painful breasts, and worsens their hot flashes. That's because it causes the release of stress hormones.

My recommendation is to let it go for the three weeks of the Reboot. I promise that you can do it, and it's much less painful than you think; if there are any withdrawal symptoms, they usually last only three days. I'll help you ease off carefully in the plan, and if you start the Reboot on a Friday, you'll be cruising without it by midweek. If you're thinking, "There's no way I can do that because I *have* to have my morning coffee," or "Yeah, I'm not addicted, but I like my coffee ritual and I don't want to give it up," then you're addicted and absolutely should break up with your coffee for a week to reclaim your addicted brain and reset your stress hormones. It will also give you a chance to see how severe your fatigue is without it.

Fatigue and headache are the most common coffee withdrawal symptoms, and if you rely on coffee to get your bowels going in the morning, they might slow down a bit (take 300 to 800 mg of magnesium citrate, or a little senna and peppermint tea, before bed to fix this problem). Withdrawal symptoms usually clear in two to three days. Drinking a lot of water and keeping your energy up with balanced blood sugar and a high protein diet will get you through.

Coffee alternatives are water (hot or room temperature) with lemon, herbal tea (caffeine-free), a morning shake (see recipes), caffeine-free chai (see recipes), or turmeric Chai Golden Milk without the black tea (see page 157). If you just can't deal with the no-caffeine transition and still function, try green tea instead. It's got less caffeine and it's loaded with antioxidants.

Here is a delicious chai tea recipe that you can try today to start incorporating as a coffee alternative or simply a delicious tea.

Chai Golden Milk

- 1 tbsp. fresh grated turmeric root or 1 heaping tsp. turmeric powder
- 1 tsp. fresh grated ginger
- 1 cinnamon stick
- 1 green tea bag or 2 tsp. green tea leaves
- Coconut milk (or almond milk)

To prepare: Bring 1 cup of water to a boil and turn off. Add the spices, keeping the green tea aside, and steep for 10 minutes. Add the green tea or tea bag to the water and steep 5 minutes more. Strain, and if you'd like it hot, add the liquid back to the pot, bringing it to a simmer. Pour into a cup and add coconut milk or almond milk in the amount you like in your tea. Alternatively, you can use coconut milk or almond milk instead of the water, lightly simmering the spices in it for 10 minutes, turning off the heat, and adding the green tea, straining all and enjoying after another 5 minutes of steeping.
Drink 1 to 2 cups daily as a beverage. One cup now and again is also safe during pregnancy and breast-feeding.

If you'd prefer a simpler route, use one tea bag of any good-quality chai tea and combine with one heaping teaspoon of Gaia Herbs Golden Milk powder, and prepare as directed on the package.

Herbal Medicine 101

- Turmeric, which you'll see throughout this book, is profoundly anti-inflammatory and helps to reset cortisol, especially when elevated due to chronic stress.
- Ginger is also anti-inflammatory, and both ginger and turmeric heal the gut lining, symptomatically relieve gas and bloating, and are helpful for pain.
- Cinnamon not only tastes great and benefits digestion, it also helps lower high blood sugar and improves insulin resistance.
- Green tea is a powerful anti-inflammatory with compounds that improve natural detoxification while supporting healthy metabolism.

- Water
- Carbonated water
- Water with lemon
- Green tea
- Herbal teas

Don't Count Calories; Eat Healthy Portion Sizes

Calories don't tell you anything about the quality or healthfulness of foods, and counting them contributes to food neurosis—which I want you to completely get free of. Eating only healthful foods that support optimal metabolism and healing SOS will naturally lead to weight loss as a side effect.

Knowing what to eat is one part of the story; how much is another. Large portion sizes are very much a U.S. phenomenon that goes hand in hand with our obesity problem—and most of us were taught to put too much on our plates. It gets particularly complicated because if you're in SOS or are struggling with being overweight, your brain's chemical messages that are supposed to tell you when you're hungry and full may be a little wonky until you get reset, which can take a few weeks or so. But since you're not there yet, the list below shows you what to include at each meal during the Reboot and is followed by what's considered a healthy portion size.

Portion sizes per serving are roughly as follows:

- Meats: 4 ounces red meat (the size of the palm of your hand or a deck of cards), 4 to 6 ounces for poultry and fish (the size of your hand or a checkbook)

- Grains, beans, and legumes: ½ cup cooked (or how much would fill a cupcake wrapper or ½ tennis ball)

- Veggies: 1 to 2 cups (1 cup is about the size of your fist) of raw or cooked leafy greens and ½ cup raw or cooked rainbow veggies

- Energy veggies: ½ to 1 sweet potato, ½ to 1 cup equivalent of winter squash

- Nuts and seeds: 1 handful

- Nut butter: 1 tablespoon is about the size of your thumb tip

- Oils and fats: 1 to 2 tablespoons olive oil, 1 tablespoon solid fat (e.g., coconut oil), and ½ avocado; 2 tablespoons salad dressing (would fill up a Ping-Pong ball)

- Fruits: ½ cup berries, 1 piece single-serving fruit (e.g., an apple, an orange, a kiwi)

- Fermented vegetables: 2 tablespoons

There are several strategies that can also help you to eat "the right" amount.

- Serve and store: serve your plate, then immediately store away the remaining food for leftovers before you eat. This simple technique reduces food intake by 14 percent over serving a small portion and then coming back for more.

- Eat from smaller packages, bowls, and plates: this reduces the amount you eat (see page 160 for healthy snack recommendations).

- Eat more slowly: it takes about twenty minutes for your brain chemistry to catch up with what's going on in your stomach; if you eat too fast, you override these messages and risk overeating.

HARA HACHI BU
AND THE ART OF MINDFUL EATING

Have you ever eaten a whole meal and not remembered what you just ate or realized you inhaled your food so fast you never tasted it? This is the opposite of mindfulness and usually happens when we've been eating and multitasking. Watching television, talking on the phone, working on your computer, and driving your car while you're eating, for example, all increase the likelihood of overeating. Watching TV increases food intake by at least 50 percent, whereas paying attention to your meal is linked to eating less—both now and later. Mindful eating means giving your meal your full attention.

Hara hachi bu, the Japanese tradition of eating until you're 80 percent full or satisfied rather than stuffed, is another way to eat the amount your body needs without overdoing it, and it reharmonizes your brain-gut communication. Here are a few food mindfulness practices to get you started:

- Set your kitchen timer to twenty-five minutes, and take that entire time to savor your meal. More relaxed eating has been shown to improve digestion.

- Start each meal with one minute of silence and gratitude.
- Slow down by eating with your nondominant hand, or try eating with chopsticks if you don't usually do so (studies show this trick helps with weight loss).
- Take small bites and chew well.

The No-Crash Emergency Stash and Replenish Snack Recommendations

Keeping an emergency Snack Stash with you is important if you tend to get low blood sugar. Here are my no-crash emergency stash and Replenish snack recommendations:

- Keep a small container of almonds or walnuts, or individual nut butter packets on hand.

- If you eat meat, keep some organic beef or turkey jerky with you.

- Make hard-boiled eggs, and carry them in a small paper or plastic bag, or container; one or two make a great snack.

- Have Hippie Mix (see page 372) with lots of nuts on hand to keep your energy steady.

- Pack hummus and veggies or gluten-free crackers in a small cooler, or keep them in the fridge at home or work.

- Make quick turkey roll-ups or another type of lettuce wrap (see page 346).

- Have a small container of unsweetened coconut yogurt with some nuts and seeds, or a handful of Hippie Mix or fresh berries tossed in.

You want to stay prepared so you never find yourself at the airport or driving home from a workout or standing in front of your colleague's M&M bowl, starving. You may not be famished, but you don't want your brain to feel like it's starving. I don't use the word "starving" lightly, but from a primitive perspective; that's what your brain thinks it's doing.

MAKE TIME FOR REST AND REPAIR

Traditional cultures around the world have periods of time built into the annual calendar for fasting—either a day or a week periodically of omitting certain foods from the diet (for example, meat and dairy), or even a month of eating nothing before sunset, followed by breaking the fast; or a week or month of excluding certain foods. These practices likely originally coincided with times of natural food scarcity, and some evolved into religious practices.

Fasting for short periods of time has been shown to improve energy, reduce inflammation, boost metabolism, and prevent oxidative stress. However, for women with SOS, eating regularly and preventing blood sugar drops is critical, so fasting is generally not recommended. Still, there is a way to get the benefits of fasting while resetting your natural cortisol rhythm without tanking your blood sugar: stop eating each evening no later than 7:30 P.M., and don't eat again for at least ten hours. This simple "whole ten rule" can give you a major reset while supporting the normal repair and detoxification that are traditionally meant to happen overnight when we're living in harmony with natural circadian rhythms.

MAKE SURE YOU'RE GOING TO THE BATHROOM DAILY

Elimination isn't just about what you're taking out of your kitchen or diet; your digestive elimination is equally important. Having a daily bowel movement will allow your body to eliminate toxins while you're Rebooting. Your response to the Reboot could be that you naturally start to have more regular BMs, but if you are usually constipated or become constipated when you start the program, because of new dietary changes, here's what you can do:

- Increase your fiber; your fiber goal should ideally be 30 to 35 g daily regardless. Fiber helps you to lose weight; it fills you up, decreases unhealthy cholesterol, and improves the elimination of broken down hormones from your digestive system. Good-quality fiber from vegetables and resistant starches also nourishes healthy gut flora. To get this much fiber in your daily diet you can increase your vegetable intake to about a pound of veggies per day, and also add supplements such as flaxseed and psyllium, available at your local pharmacy or health food store, to your foods and smoothies.

- If you're not having a bowel movement at least once daily, add 400 to 800 mg of magnesium citrate before bed.

- Take a probiotic containing *Lactobacillus* and *Bifidobacterium* strains (it will say this on the label) each morning.

- If your bowels are still sluggish or if you tend to get indigestion when you eat fats, this bitters support blend, or one with similar herbs that you can purchase, can help bring relief. Mix ¼ teaspoon each of the following herbal tinctures (extracts) in ¼ cup water or in ½ to 1 cup sparkling water before or after each meal:
  - Artichoke
  - Burdock root
  - Dandelion root
  - Gingerroot

See "Resources" (page 393) for companies that sell herbal products.

BLOOD SUGAR SOLUTION

If you've been on a chronic blood sugar roller coaster, it could be because you're often running on low energy, not putting enough of the right fuel or too much of the wrong fuel (fast-burning sugar, refined foods, empty carbs) in your tank, or you're not filling your tank often enough. Blood sugar balance is key to staying out of SOS and reversing the problems that keep you inflamed, your hormones and detox systems out of whack, and your mind and mood in a rut. Willpower is no match for biochemistry, but you can also eat your way back to willpower by keeping your blood sugar balanced.

There are a few simple "must follow" rules for keeping your blood sugar balanced all the time.

Power start your day, every day: Eat breakfast within an hour of waking to keep your energy steady through the morning, maintain your focus and clarity, and avoid blood sugar crashes that send you heading for a sugar fix. Breakfast should always be high-protein and have healthy fat; I recommend no grain other than an occasional piece of toast or wrap with eggs or your other protein source (gluten-free while on the Reboot); absolutely no sweets at breakfast (not even orange juice); fruit at breakfast only if in a morning smoothie; and if you refuse to kick the coffee habit, make sure you're having it *with* your breakfast, not before or instead of breakfast.

Eat only high-nutrient foods: High-nutrient foods pack in a lot of nutrition in every serving. This is in comparison to processed foods that offer practically no nutrition or have "empty calories," meaning they're high in calories but devoid of nutrients. Don't bother eating foods that don't pack a whole lot of nutrients into a portion. They're a waste of your time—and your health.

Don't go hungry: A wee bit of hunger or an appetite by the time you're ready for your meal is not unhealthy, but don't ever let yourself get *overly* hungry to the point of having low blood sugar symptoms (page 65). If you're a high-octane woman like me, you've got to put the best fuel in your tank, probably about every three hours. Protein and fats are blood sugar's best friends: protein helps you feel satisfied and provides sustainable energy for about two hours after you eat it, fats for up to four hours. They keep your blood sugar steady and prevent insulin and leptin resistance, as well as weight from coming back after you lose it. You may be afraid of eating fat, but it takes fat to burn fat, so avoiding it may be preventing you from burning calories, and a low-fat diet could lead you to binge on less-healthy, quick-burning fuels—such as sugar and empty carbs.

Rest and digest: It's important for your body to have clear times for eating and clear times for digestion. Don't eat *more* often than every three hours, and don't nosh all day long. Additionally, don't eat within three hours of going to bed, to maintain your healthy evening cortisol rhythm. That said, by the time you get home from work, feed the kids, get the kids to bed, etc., it can be late, and if you haven't eaten, it's better to eat something healthy than nothing because you don't want to wake up ravenous and blow your plan or have a cortisol spike because of low blood sugar stress. Also, pregnancy and breast-feeding are exceptions—eat as your body dictates, but keep it 100 percent nutrient dense and natural.

If you're prediabetic, insulin-resistant, or have type 2 diabetes (DM2), maintaining healthy blood sugar with your diet is mission-critical for you, even if you're on blood sugar medications. Reversing high blood sugar even if you have DM2 is possible, and often happens as a result of following this plan. If you notice that you're feeling like you have low blood sugar on this plan, or if you check your sugars and they are running low, talk with your doctor; you may be able to lower your medication—or come off of it altogether—if you've reversed the problem. This can happen in as short as a few weeks on the plan, so pay close attention. Additionally, if you are struggling with elevated blood sugar, a number of supplements have been shown to be helpful in making your cells more sensitive to insulin, including vitamin D and magnesium, which are already in your Daily Dose Supplements. See "SOS Rx: Daily Dose Supplements" on pages 166-67.

BRIDGE YOUR PHYTONUTRIENT GAP

Food is your most important source of nutrition, and supplements are just that—supplements to real food. But the reality is, most of us are just not getting the nutrients we need from our food to maintain optimal health in the setting of the added demands placed on us by twenty-first-century living—higher stress levels, as well as the additional nutritional needs we have for detoxification of the environmental toxins we're exposed to.

Here's just a short list of the nutrients most American women are commonly low in according to 2009 statistics from the U.S. Department of Agriculture:

- Vitamin E: 86 percent
- Folate: 75 percent
- Calcium: 73 percent
- Magnesium: 68 percent
- Zinc: 42 percent
- Vitamin B_6: 35 percent
- Iron: 34 percent
- Vitamin B_{12}: 30 percent

We are also chronically and often severely low in essential fatty acids, critical for the health of our cells, including our nerve cells, and necessary for keeping inflammation at bay, and vitamin D, more accurately a hormone than a vitamin, involved in hundreds if not more critical functions for health, including immunity, blood sugar metabolism, bone health, and mood. A 2016 study by the American Psychiatric Association, not notoriously the most nutrition- or supplement-forward-thinking group, found that many of the above are among the nutrients also critical for brain health and for healthy emotional lives, including depression prevention and reversal. In addition were found to be fiber and vitamins B_1, B_9, and E.

In addition to following the Reboot meal plan and making sure to get a variety of the Replenish Super Foods in your diet regularly, I recommend that everyone following the SOS Solution include the Daily Dose Supplements each day, starting as soon as you can get them, and indefinitely for your long-term wellness.

STOCK UP

Now it's time to stock your pantry and fridge with the real foods and ingredients you'll want to have on hand as you go through the Reboot. Select the recipes you'll follow for this week from the Sample Daily Menus, page 171, and use the Replenish Shopping List on page 314 as a checklist to take to the store. You can find additional copies at avivaromm.com /adrenal-thyroid-revolution.

READY, SET, REBOOT

Now that you've done your prep and know which foods to eliminate and which to include, what supplements to take, and how to keep your blood sugar steady, it's time to Reboot. If you're wondering how to put all of this together, here's a blueprint for an inspired day. The inspired day is an ideal—not meant to overwhelm, just to use as a guide to pick and choose from. Visit my website, avivaromm.com/adrenal-thyroid-revolution, for a free gift of the Replenish Lifestyle Planner to record how you feel, and inspired daily exercises to support you as you go through the program.

Also, while it's important to track your food-related symptoms, don't feel obligated to write down everything every time you eat, but do pay attention to when you're feeling especially energized and well, or when you're feeling tired or have other symptoms—this can give you huge clues that you can then use to identify food triggers.

SOS Rx: Daily Dose Supplements		
Herb/ Supplement	**Uses and Cautions**	**Dose**
EPA/DHA (fish oil, cod liver oil, or algae-derived)	Protects cells from oxidative stress, reduces inflammation, protects nervous system, boosts mind and mood. See resources for brands known to be safe from environmental toxins.	850 EPA / 200 DHA 1 to 2x/day
Magnesium (glycinate is the preferred daily dose form)	Called "the calming mineral," yet one that most of us are deficient in, magnesium is an important daily supplement for hundreds of important reactions in our bodies, including blood sugar and insulin regulation (it appears to improve insulin sensitivity and aid pancreatic function, helping to counter hyperglycemia), bone health, mood, detoxification in the liver, muscle relaxation—including keeping your heart muscle in a regular rhythm—and blood pressure, to name a few.	300 to 1,200 mg/ day total (If you need to take magnesium glycinate for constipation, you can combine the different forms of magnesium toward the maximum total daily dose.)

Herb/ Supplement	Uses and Cautions	Dose
Multivitamin	Provides a general baseline for bridging the phytonutrient gap. Look for a multivitamin that doesn't contain sugar, artificial dyes, or additives and that contains B-complex with methylfolate and methyl B_{12}, zinc, selenium, and iodine. B-complex with methyl-B vitamins supports a healthy nervous system and liver detoxification; zinc provides a boost to your immune system, keeping you resilient and resistant to infections; selenium boosts liver detoxification by increasing glutathione, one of your body's most important detoxification compounds (more in the next chapter), reduces anxiety and depression, supports healthy thyroid function, and may reduce thyroid antibodies. Many women are low in iodine, which is needed in low amounts for healthy thyroid hormone production.	As directed; a one-a-day is usually easiest to keep up with
Vitamin D_3	Supports immunity, boosts mind and mood, especially for depression; it is also essential for optimizing blood sugar when elevated, healthy functioning of your immune system, thyroid, and the health of your intestinal lining, among hundreds of functions essential for your wellness. Improves insulin levels by protecting the pancreas and increasing insulin resistance.	2,000 units/day; up to 4,000 units/day for 3 months if your testing shows that your blood level is low or you have elevated blood sugar or insulin resistance

INSPIRED DAY BLUEPRINT

Morning

- Ideally, wake up an hour before you have to leave for work, get your family in gear, or get started on your day so you have breathing room.

- Before you get out of bed, give yourself two to five minutes for a Quickie (see page 199—it's not what you think!), deep breathing, or another meditation that you enjoy.

- When you rise, drink a glass of room-temperature water with a squeeze of fresh lemon.

- If time allows, even if you have only five minutes, do some movement (yoga or stretching, or if you have more time, a brisk walk) or try a seven-minute workout (app).

- Eat breakfast within an hour of waking, and do not skip. Take your supplements with breakfast. If you haven't packed a lunch and your emergency Snack Stash, do.

- Make time to go to the restroom before you get too busy with your day.

- Midmorning: Have a healthy snack if you need one and make sure to hydrate. Take some bathroom time if you haven't already.

Noon to Late Afternoon

- Take a mindful lunch break for at least thirty minutes, an hour if you can, off the computer, at least a few times each week. Try to eat within three hours of breakfast. Hydrate.

- Take five to fifteen minutes to stretch, walk, and go to the restroom during your lunch break or at midafternoon.

- Late afternoon: Have a healthy snack and take two to ten minutes to do a brief meditation, visualization, or breathing exercise. Hydrate.

Evening

- Take fifteen minutes to decompress after your workday (see page 201) to set yourself for a healthy evening cortisol rhythm.

- Plan your dinner prep so you're making leftovers for tomorrow's lunch if you can, and have some fun making dinner—this can become a relaxing, pleasant time for you. Take the remainder of your supplements with dinner. Try to finish dinner by 7:30 P.M. if you can.

- After your evening responsibilities, make time, even if just ten minutes, for a Replenish Self-Care.

- Power down about an hour before you head to bed. Try to get to bed by 11:00 P.M., or whatever time will give you at least seven hours of sleep. Take sleep supplements at bedtime if needed (see page 203).

- For extra inspiration, head over to avivaromm.com/adrenal -thyroid-revolution, where I walk you through the Inspired Day Visualization.

Troubleshoot the Reboot

Take Back Your Kitchen

You'll probably be amazed to find that eating at home, even healthy and organic, is often less expensive than eating out. It's also satisfying to prepare and eat a delicious meal, and if you plan ahead, you'll have leftovers to make the next day's lunch easy and healthy.

When you cook at home, you have control over what's in your food, allowing you to avoid added sugar, excess salt, and other ingredients that make you pack on pounds and can be hidden food triggers. Many of my patients, for example, report flares of symptoms after "getting glutened" by "gluten-free" foods in restaurants (see avivaromm.com, "Gluten Free? What to Do If You 'Get Glutened'"). Eating at home is a sure way to drop some unwanted pounds. Just one meal out each week translates to a two-pound weight gain each year; and get this—the average American adult eats out five times per week. Restaurants know that we love to get a big bang for our buck, and increasing portion size doesn't add much to a restaurant's overhead, so we get served supersize portions. The Good Girls in us feel obligated to finish what we're served. Our waistlines—and our health—pay the price.

At my website, avivaromm.com/adrenal-thyroid-revolution, you can find tips on how to order healthy when you inevitably do eat out.

Watch Out for Weekends and Weak Spots

As a rule, Americans tend to binge out on weekends—we eat more calories, junk, drink more alcohol, and overdo the bad fats between Friday and Sunday. Why? Because by the time the weekend comes we're willpower fatigued from following the rules and toeing the line all week. So we say screw it and go for the quick fix relaxation, even if we know that by Monday we're going to feel awful and regret it. The same thing happens when we're overtired, overworked, over-hungry, and show up at a birthday party or holiday event. A healthier strategy is to try to stop bottling up your stress all week by making self-care a daily part of your life, and having a plan for when you do get to the weekend (or party or holiday) so you can enjoy it without making yourself feel awful. Here are a few weekend and weak spot rescue tips:

- In general try to stay out of SOS heading into the weekend; stay replenished so you're not setting yourself up for food benders.

- Have a healthy snack before you go out, and keep an emergency Snack Stash item in your bag so you don't end up somewhere over-hungry with your only menu choice being a pizza, heart-attack burger, or 600-calorie piña colada.

- Eat before you drink alcohol—or at least while you're drinking; otherwise you'll end up smashed and famished, with no control over what you eventually scarf down to sop up the alcohol and set yourself straight.

- Sip slowly and sip smart: Order simple drinks that are gluten-free, cut with still or sparkling water, and ask that they have no simple sugar added. Wine coolers, vodka with lemon and sparkling water, or gin and tonic are examples. Or stick to red wine, no more than two glasses, and sip slowly.

- Try to stick to your weekday eating habits as much as possible on the weekends and before parties and social events. If you usually eat at 7:00 A.M., noon, and 6:00 P.M., do that on the weekends, too.

WEEK 1: REBOOT, DAY BY DAY

Week 1 Sample Daily Meal Plan

Breakfast Example

8–12-oz. Smoothie (Shake)
or
Breakfast protein + good-quality fat (+ optional veggie)

Lunch Example

Protein entrée + green veggie + rainbow veggie
+ energy veggie + good-quality fat

Dinner Example

Protein entrée + green veggie + rainbow veggie + energy veggie
+ good-quality fat + small amount of fermented veggie (if tolerated)

Week 1
Sample Daily Menus and Lifestyle

	Day 1	Day 2	Day 3
Morning practice	The Quickie meditation (page 199)	Dry brush (page 232) in morning shower	5 minutes of deep breathing (page 191) and stretch
Fresh Start	Drink a glass of room-temperature or warm water with a squeeze of lemon.		
Breakfast + Daily Dose Supplements	Smoothie Bar (Green Dream) (If fruit is a food that you're omitting, swap in one of the egg-based breakfasts for smoothies this week.)	East Meets West Frittata + mixed greens with Olive Oil Lemon Dressing	Smoothie Bar (Omega Brain Power)
Mid-morning	Jump Start Detox Nutrient Broth	Jump Start Detox Nutrient Broth	Jump Start Detox Nutrient Broth
Mindful lunch + SOS Solution Supplements (if you've personalized your plan ahead)	Salmon Caper Board (skip the potatoes and crackers)	It's a Wrap option (use lettuce) or Make Your Own Salad + a soup	Leftover frittata + mixed greens with Olive Oil Lemon Dressing
Mid-afternoon	Jump Start Detox Nutrient Broth	Jump Start Detox Nutrient Broth	Jump Start Detox Nutrient Broth

Day 4	Day 5	Day 6	Day 7
The Quickie	Dry brush in morning shower	5 minutes of deep breathing and stretch	Day off from as much social media and electronics as possible
Asparagus & Onion Breakfast Scramble (omit the starch) + mixed greens with Olive Oil Lemon Dressing	Smoothie Bar (Choco Cherry Greeny)	Breakfast Scramble or Omelet of choice + mixed greens with Olive Oil Lemon Dressing	Smoothie Bar (Hot Mama Super Smoothie)
Coconut yogurt with raw cacao nibs or hemp seeds	Hardboiled egg with Himalayan sea salt sprinkle	Coconut yogurt with raw cacao nibs or hemp seeds	Hardboiled egg with Himalayan sea salt sprinkle
The Middle East Board (make with last night's dinner leftovers; omit crackers and nuts)	Green Tara Lentil Bowl (use wild rice or quinoa) or, if you're skipping legumes this week, swap in Rosemary Roasted Chicken + a Green Salad and use this for leftover lunch or dinner tomorrow	Nappy Raw Citrus Salad	The Middle East Board (omit crackers and nuts)
Hardboiled egg with Himalayan sea salt sprinkle	Jump Start Detox Nutrient Broth	Hardboiled egg with Himalayan sea salt sprinkle	Coconut yogurt with raw cacao nibs or hemp seeds

Week 1
Sample Daily Menus and Lifestyle

	Day 1	Day 2	Day 3
Cortisol Reset	Reset your cortisol for the evening with 15 minutes of any Replenish Repair Kit practice		
Dinner + SOS Solution Supplements (if you've personalized your plan ahead)	Sweet Potato and Kale Salad (omit the corn) + Lemon Rosemary Chicken and/ or Chickpeas as a vegan option	Grilled Tangy Chicken with spinach (or vegan option) + Roasted Root Veggies	Satay Chicken + roasted cauliflower with curry powder
Replenish Self-Care	Replenish Bath	Gratitude or Worry Journal	Digital Detox and read

Day 4	Day 5	Day 6	Day 7
Satay Chicken or Beef with quinoa or wild rice	Nappy Raw Citrus Salad	Fiesta Fish Tacos + Ginger Lime Kale + Guacamole + roasted root vegetables	You're a Dahl Buddha Bowl
Gratitude or Worry Journal	Digital Detox and read	Replenish Bath	Gratitude or Worry Journal

REFRAME

Calm Your Mind and Mood

| Reboot: Remove Food Triggers | Reframe: Chronic Emotional and Mental Stress | Repair: Root Causes and SOS Damage | Recharge: Your Adrenals and Thyroid | Replenish: No More Running on Empty |

Our key to transforming anything lies in our ability to reframe it.

—MARIANNE WILLIAMSON

WELCOME TO THE second part of week one, the Reframe.

A flight attendant truism: you've got to put your own oxygen mask on first if you're going to be able to save anyone else. It's also true that if you don't take care of your need for time in Repair mode, it's harder to reclaim your energy and get out of SOS. Why? Being burned out is not just a metaphor for feeling crispy and tired, it also means burned—as in inflammation. When you're fried, you also inevitably find ways to soothe yourself that are less than healthy (think ice cream, too many glasses of wine, or a shopping spree that was beyond your budget). If you've found yourself wondering where the pause button is or wishing you had the superpower to stop the world for a minute so you could sit down and catch up on your massive to-do list or just take a breather, or if you scored high on the stress Root Cause questionnaire, this chapter is for you. If you feel you've been living like you're stuck in the ON position, you're in the right place.

This chapter is going to give you Permission to Pause. It's an Rx for self-care.

It starts with Reframing our belief that we don't have time for self-care or deserve it.

Most women think we have to push and push, give and give, until we have nothing left. Overwhelm and overwork are so common that most working parents perpetually feel they're not getting enough done, and fewer than 20 percent feel that they are truly flourishing. The first and most important Reframe is that you do have the right—and deserve—to take care of yourself. Not to make you a better mom, or better at anything else. Just simply because you deserve to, because *you are worth taking care of.* You can—and have to—learn to live and give from a place of feeling replenished, not depleted and constantly trying to stay afloat. I'm going to share tools you can use to navigate away from constantly feeling exhausted, overwhelmed, and running on empty, and instead put you in the driver's seat of your life.

You're also going to refresh your relationship with sleep, because without good sleep, everything else suffers.

HOW DO YOU FEEL?
(YOUR BODY DOESN'T LIE)

Your body is your barometer, your personal gauge that tells you when the pressure is getting too high. The symptoms you get may be physical (headaches, disrupted sleep, digestive symptoms, aches and pains, worsening hot flashes) or emotional (anxiety, depression, irritability, frustration, overwhelm). For me, it's overwhelm combined with disaster thinking; I get anxious that everything is going to fall apart if I "stop," and I overcompensate by working more. Remember, the stress response is your body's way of protecting you from harm, so when you feel these symptoms, listen to what your body is trying to tell you. This is your "body-speak."

Yet, too many of us ignore our bodies. *We actually forget to feel how we feel.*

Listen to Your Body Intelligence

- Set a timer for three minutes.
- Sit upright in a chair, or lie on a comfortable surface.
- Close your eyes and breathe regularly at first, then more slowly and deeply for eight breaths.
- Now deepen your breath. Let your breath wander throughout your body to anywhere that feels tight, blocked, or "stuck." Use your breath to imagine massaging out that tension or releasing the blockage. *Is there anything in your life that you associate with the tension you're holding?* Let the answer rise to the surface and just listen.
- Now ask your body if there's anything you need to know.
- Listen for the answer, and if you're inspired, jot it down to return to in the future as a "note to self."

It starts young, ignoring when we need to pee, for example, because we don't want to raise our hands in class for permission to use the bathroom. And we pay the price when we ignore little messages because eventually those can turn into louder messages, and eventually symptoms and conditions.

The body doesn't lie. You may have noticed this in the past—for example, when things were going on in your life that were hard to handle head-on, or when you took a path that was inconsistent with your gut feelings, physical or emotional symptoms manifested. Take my patient who, in her early thirties, developed severe eczema only under her wedding ring when she began to wonder if her husband was having an affair (he was and she left him). That's a very dramatic and specific, but telling, example. Pay attention to that pit in your stomach (it's exactly what trusting your gut really means) or the tightness in your throat when you're not speaking your truth—for example, you're saying yes when you want to say no. Your body and brain are one. Valuable information can come to you in the form of a thought or a physical sensation that may arise from your organs or nervous system, a phenomenon known as *interoception.*

PERMISSION TO PAUSE

Women in particular . . . need to do a better job of
putting ourselves higher on our own "to do" list.

—MICHELLE OBAMA

Recently, one of my best friends was pushing herself so hard at her work that she hit a wall. She was irritable and cranky, and instead of honoring her need to push her own pause button, she just ended up getting stressed out, picking a fight with her husband, feeling miserable, and ultimately not getting anything done on her to-do list. Sound familiar? She texted me late in her day, saying that she finally "just had to cave." So she literally created a cave. She crawled into bed, pulled the covers over her head, tuned out the pressure to constantly do more and be more, and decompressed for an hour, after which she felt like a new woman.

I texted back saying, "That's brilliant. Caving—I'm going to write that up. It's the perfect metaphor."

How often do we push when we know we really need to cave? We feel the crash or emotional explosion coming, but we push. Yet, just by stopping for a short time and replenishing ourselves, giving ourselves what I call *Permission to Pause*, we can prevent the breakdown. Permission to Pause is a big philosophy in my life and medical practice. It also makes good physiological sense. For example, we are all guided by not just our circadian rhythm, the daily rhythm that creates, for example, your diurnal cortisol rhythm, but also our shorter cycles called *ultradian rhythm*—90- to 120-minute bursts of focus. If we pause at the end of or throughout our day, for even just 15 minutes of self-care, deep breathing, walking, or anything to reset us for the next ultradian cycle, we are naturally more focused and productive.

But getting more focused and productive isn't the only game in town.

Getting good at giving yourself Permission to Pause in a bigger life way is the secret sauce to overcoming overwhelm, for living life with your gas tank full, rather than constantly hovering at or below empty. High-performance athletes, top musicians, and successful entrepreneurs all know this secret: making time for repairing, recharging, and rejuvenating yourself is key for success in anything—including health success.

So why do most of us find it so hard to make time for ourselves? Why are we riddled with guilt and anxiety when it comes to stopping and replenishing? It's true: the demands of external life—just what it takes for most of us to make a living and keep up with our responsibilities—can feel relentless and put a lot of pressure on us. But there's more. Somewhere along the line we got the idea that self-care is self-indulgent. We have also internalized patterns that keep us feeling like we always have to do more, give more, push harder. These come with names such as *Perfectionism, FOMO* (Fear of Missing Out), and *Good-Girl Syndrome* and cause enormous physical and emotional strain. Before we dive into how to pause, let's look at some of the common patterns that add unnecessary pressure to our lives.

THE STORIES WE BELIEVE

Step out of the history that is holding you back.
Step into the new story you are willing to create.
—OPRAH WINFREY

There's more than one way that we get stressed, and everyone reacts to stress differently. For me, it's perfectionism, big time. It drives me to take on too much at one time and then overdeliver in the attempt to make it all perfect—all the while worrying it won't be good enough or as good as everyone else's. The amazing thing, though, is that once I learned *how* my SOS and stress pathways show up in my life, I could name them and tame them.

If you continually find yourself with too much on your plate, chronically stressed out, and with no time for self-care, it's worth exploring whether there are patterns and personal stories you're self-perpetuating that are putting you there, too. I didn't become fully aware of my own perfectionist pattern that was driving me until I met Marni. Her story changed my life.

At fifty-eight, Marni was a powerhouse. A successful career and marriage, and five grown children, all high-powered earners; she had it all.

Except for energy. She was exhausted, yet working out for two hours a day, keeping up with research in her field, and traveling to teach at conferences and visit her children. When she came to me, she was underweight, had Hashimoto's, and couldn't sleep. Listening to her story, I discovered that she grew up the child of immigrants who had to scrape together every dime to feed their kids and had a lot of anxiety about basic survival. She started working at a young age to help support the family, and became determined to escape poverty. She pushed herself to be the best at everything—and succeeded. But what was once an adaptive survival pattern that got her out of rough beginnings, by her early forties became maladaptive. She went into overdrive; although she'd achieved financial security, her brain never got the memo that she could slow down. I looked at her—well dressed, perfect makeup, and a body like Madonna, and said, "Marni, you're feeding hungry ghosts that aren't actually chasing you anymore. You can give yourself Permission to Pause." Several years later she told me that conversation was the turning point in finally being able to relax and enjoy her life.

Meanwhile, I realized that I, too, had used high achievement to escape a vulnerable childhood situation. But as an adult, I was still living as if poverty were always a step away, saying yes to every opportunity even when my gut said no, worried that if I wasn't always working, there wouldn't be enough money. True confession: I was such an overachiever that I actually felt that something was wrong or I wasn't doing something I should be doing if I felt relaxed or something felt too easy. It took becoming aware of how my past was driving me, deciding how I wanted to feel, then practicing staying in tune with that to make choices that kept me feeling that way. I had to learn that success doesn't require stress. Before long, that old pattern began to take a backseat to a healthier and more empowered life. It also wasn't until after I used the term "hungry ghosts" with Marni that I discovered it was a Buddhist term for being perpetually driven by unmet inner needs—which was uncannily close to how I'd used the term, and how so many women live.

Addiction to overwork is an example from my own life. In my childhood, getting high grades and "performing well" not only "bought" me love from my mom, but also won approval from teachers. I became savvy at using my intellect for self-protection and parlayed that same approval into a scholarship out of my rough neighborhood and into college at age fifteen.

That was amazing. But the thing is, even well into a happy, secure adult life, I felt that I had to work hard and achieve *all the time* to "survive." If I wasn't stressed out and working, I truly felt that something was wrong. SOS was driving me to achieve out of survival fear. Because I continued to be rewarded for my behavior professionally and socially, I became addicted to a self-perpetuating cycle of overwork and reward. Marni's story was a cautionary tale of burnout, and like she now does, I continue to learn to enjoy my drive without being *driven* by SOS.

As I began to talk with women (and men) about how perfectionism, addiction to stress, and FOMO were hungry ghosts, the response was unanimous: "I'm feeding those, too." Fatigue, stress, overwhelm, anxiety, depression, and many of the physical symptoms we experience go beyond physical causes. SOS happens when our brains don't register that we're safe, and we can't feel safe if we think ghosts are after us. That's the stuff a pill can't fix, but the insights you get from this chapter, and bring forward into the SOS Solution four-week plan, can. You're going to learn to kiss that self-perpetuated, maladaptive stress good-bye.

Addiction to behaviors causes the same feel-good chemical responses that happen in your brain as other addictions. The difference is that unlike drug or gambling addictions, overachievement, overwork, and perfectionism are socially and professionally rewarded, temporarily filling a primal human survival need to belong, be recognized, and feel economically secure or validated. It's why when we don't feel like we fit in or belong, we feel terribly afraid, alone, and vulnerable. It's also why we strive so hard to fit in.

These behaviors themselves aren't inherently harmful—high achievement, volunteering, working hard, being focused, and making money are all wonderful, and there's no need to change the beautiful you that you are. Becoming driven by fear (SOS), rather than motivated by passion, self-love, and enjoyment, however, can cost you your health, happiness, downtime, relationship time, and personal sanity.

Enter the term *neuroplasticity*. Until recently, our brain patterns were considered fixed. This is far from the truth. The world of neuroscience is exploding with studies showing that you can change the pathways in your brain that have been shaped by life circumstances and dictate how we think and behave—by creating new thought and behavior patterns. Once you understand that you no longer need certain patterns, you're able to retrain your brain so that you're living and thinking intentionally, not reactively. You can ask yourself if you're living in a way that allows you to feel how you want to feel, and correct your course when you are not. I still have to work at it, but life is so much easier now that my own brain has received the message that I don't have to strive all the time for life to be great. Marni has had the same experience, as have many other women I've worked with. It takes practice and commitment, but it's completely within your reach.

Ready to look at a few of the most common patterns dogging women? I'm sure you'll recognize at least one.

PERFECTIONISM

At a swank yoga retreat where I was teaching, I asked a roomful of more than a hundred fit "yogini" students to raise their hand if at any time in the past six weeks they'd passed a mirror and criticized their bodies. Immediately, every woman in the room shot her hand up in the air. Every time I ask that question to groups of women, the same thing happens. It's not surprising given that 91 percent of women are dissatisfied with their bodies and that 97 percent of us have at least one "I hate my body" thought every day. During our waking hours we're barraged with images "proving" to us that we're not enough—thin enough, perfect enough, detoxed enough, good enough mothers; you name it. If there's anything we women have in common, it's the feeling that we're never enough. Perfectionism is a survival pattern that most women struggle with—some even more than others, particularly if love and achievement were tied together when you were young.

While aspects of perfectionism might have brought you some mighty benefits, there may be an exhausting shadow side you're ready to kiss goodbye—a relentless pressure to be better that keeps you striving more than thriving, the "imposter syndrome" that leads you to fear you're going to be found out to not be as good at something as people think you are, or the inability to rest and relax because you always have to do more. These feelings not only make you feel awful, they also drive you into SOS. Your cortisol goes up just like with any chronic toxic stress. Pretty soon the acclaim

Overexercising? Get Off the Treadmill

I've worked with numerous women whose symptoms of SOS began after months of training for an athletic event or after years of being an athlete, or whose perfectionism shows up in the form of overexercise to have "the perfect body" (which, don't kid yourself, can show up as wanting to have "the perfect yoga body," too!).

In moderation, running, or any aerobic training, has a positive effect on health. However, the physical stress of overtraining can cause overtraining syndrome, which is adrenal depletion with symptoms including chronic fatigue and burnout, particularly if the overtraining is accompanied by a triggering stressful event, and without adequate recovery time, that pushes you beyond your coping level into SOS. Conversely, low-intensity exercise lowers cortisol levels and is much more in keeping with a plan to leave SOS. If you're in SOS, or notice that you crash and burn after a major workout, it might be time to cut back on your training plan, get more restorative for a while, and replenish yourself.

and success you receive are overshadowed by the exhaustion you feel or the symptoms you develop, and you really want to crawl into a hammock and sleep for six months.

Symptoms of perfectionism include:

- Feeling there's always something more you *should* be doing or *should* have accomplished by now
- Always feeling unprepared or underprepared before a test, presentation, or paper, even if you've been working hard on it
- Frequently comparing yourself to others
- Always feeling like you could "do it better"
- Black-and-white thinking—you're either successful or you're a failure

That brings us to the next pattern, which nearly always accompanies perfectionism.

STRESS ADDICTION

Many of us grew up in stressful environments and unwittingly re-create feeling stressed out for ourselves, because as uncomfortable as it is, it's a familiar emotional default. There are many ways by which we can create drama in our lives to perpetuate comfortable misery. Here I'm going to focus on a highly acceptable form—addiction to stress, overwork, and overwhelm.

Symptoms of stress and overwork addiction include:

- Being chronically stressed out or overwhelmed
- Chronic overscheduling
- Feeling there's never enough time to get things done,
  yet taking on more
- Going from one pressure cooker to the next

Being chronically overwhelmed and overscheduled are, in and of themselves, sources of anxiety. So to change your inner experience, you've got to shift the patterns. That leads us to the next pattern, a natural cousin to perfectionism and overwork—the need for approval, which often drives us to these first two patterns.

GOOD-GIRL SYNDROME
(APPROVAL ADDICTION)

"Be a good girl" is one of the earliest rules we're taught, and it holds many women back from speaking up, taking risks, and stepping out. From our earliest years we're told to be polite, to be good, not to interrupt, to say "thank you" and fake appreciation even when we don't like something, to be pleasant, not to make waves, to be seen and not heard, not to question authority, not to stand up for our rights, not to be bossy—the list of how we're taught to "be good" is endless. Good-Girl Syndrome also often arises from a home life where you were the peacemaker (sometimes in an unstable situation), where you needed to fly under the radar to avoid getting noticed or into trouble, or in which your security (being loved, being taken care of, noticed) depended on "good behavior."

But being a Good Girl can get in the way of reaching for your dreams. It can make you say yes to taking on things even when you want to say no, and being a Good Girl isn't necessarily good for your health when it translates into being a good patient. Good patients don't question authority. They don't challenge the need for the test, the diagnosis, or the treatment. Doctors and nurses, just like parents and teachers, favor the Good-Girl patients, and they dread those who are known in common medical parlance as "difficult patients." "Compliant" is the word used to describe cooperative patients who do what the doctor tells them. But many Good Girls have suffered for months, even years, with symptoms of depression, weight gain, hair loss, dry skin, constipation, postpartum problems, or other symptoms because they didn't know they could insist on further testing or another opinion or a different medication that might reveal or improve a thyroid problem. Learning to insist on something you feel you need (for example, the right thyroid tests) isn't easy for everyone, especially for women, but your life really could depend on it. To read more about this, see avivaromm .com, "How Being a Good Girl Can Be Hazardous to Your Health."

Symptoms of Good-Girl Syndrome include:

- Exhausting yourself trying to please others
- Keeping the peace (conflict may cause you anxiety)
- Difficulty telling the truth if it might hurt someone's feelings
- Always being the "Good Samaritan" or the volunteer; taking on projects even when you don't have time so you don't disappoint anyone
- Fearing that if you say no to something someone asks you to do, you won't be liked or loved

That leads us to the next pattern.

WORRY, FOMO, AND OTHER SCARCITY THINKING

FOMO (Fear of Missing Out) and scarcity thinking (fear that there's not enough—usually money, time, or love) are rooted in "what if?" thinking. This type of thinking often arises from a history of loss, trauma, or inadequate resources, which then formed a neural pathway that hardwired your brain to anticipate danger in even the slightest risk, and that keeps you hypervigilant—always on the lookout for catastrophe. The problem is that if you think this way, no amount of external security usually changes the inner reality—so you'll always strive for more security, and never feel you have enough.

Symptoms of worry, FOMO, and other scarcity thinking include:

- Fear there's not enough time, money, love, "room at the top"
- Catastrophe living—always worrying that the other shoe is about to drop
- Overworking to make sure there's enough
- Saying yes to going to an event or joining a group when you really want to say no

Now let's look at some of my favorite strategies for consciously breaking free of these (and other) patterns so you can enjoy your life a lot more and be free of SOS triggers that you don't need anymore.

HOW TO HIT THE PAUSE BUTTON

*In any moment, no matter how lost we feel . . . we need
only pause, breathe, and open to the experience of aliveness
within us. In that wakeful openness, we come home
to the peace and freedom of our natural awareness.*

—TARA BRACH

Stopping is a spiritual practice. It serves you. It serves everyone. It creates a ripple effect and is a gift that keeps on giving. Running on empty doesn't benefit you or anyone else. It makes you less effective in your work, less kind in your relationships, and less happy. Running on empty leads most of us to feel conflicted, victimized, resentful, angry, exhausted, and irritable. There's overwhelming evidence that if you are happier and more relaxed, you are better for everyone and at everything you do. And besides that, you deserve to take care of you. You deserve Permission to Pause, regularly.

What we crave when we want to hit the pause button is the exact opposite of the feelings we have when we're in SOS. We crave the quiet and inner calm we get when we're relaxing at the beach, soaking in a hot bath, getting a deep massage, in meditation, or in *shavasana* at the end of yoga class. This feeling is called the *relaxation response*. Physiologically, it is the mirror image of the stress response. It's the OFF to SOS's ON. It's the parasympathetic nervous system talking, instead of the sympathetic response, and it supports rest, digestion, and tissue healing. It's also accompanied by relaxed heart and respiratory rates, normal blood pressure, and a calm mind. The health benefits of spending time in this state for even thirty minutes several times a week are vast and are well documented in hundreds of medical studies on meditation, yoga, and other relaxation practices.

SLEEP WELL

Sleep is the ultimate pause you need at the end of the day. It's almost impossible to stay out of SOS without good-quality and enough sleep, let alone avoid cravings, caffeine, and brain fog. Here's the magic number: You need at least seven hours of good sleep every night to reset your natural clock and cortisol rhythm, to dump the chemical toxins that accumulate in your brain and body all day, and for your brain to do the work of sorting and filing new information from that day.

TOP SEVEN TIPS FOR GREAT ZZZS

Here are my top seven tips for great zzzs. Doing them all will bring you the best results. Note that many sleep medications can backfire and interrupt your sleep. I've provided my favorite natural sleep remedies below. These can generally be taken before you take your sleep medication, so you can still take the appropriate amount of them if you need to, and they can replace sleep medications if they do the trick for you. If you're on a benzodiazepine drug, it's essential to work with your doctor on a safe taper and not try this on your own.

1. **Get a head start** by setting the stage for a good night's sleep:

   - Avoid caffeine after 2:00 P.M., including chocolate if you're sensitive
   - Skip daytime naps
   - Exercise for at least twenty minutes daily, but not within three hours of bedtime (with the exception of restorative yoga)
   - Avoid alcohol within three hours of bedtime (even red wine keeps a lot of women awake)
   - Avoid eating within three hours of bedtime, and skip the reflux triggers (citrus, tomatoes, peppers, coffee, spicy foods, chocolate) if heartburn keeps you up
   - Skip fluids within two hours of bedtime if you typically wake up for a bathroom trip

2. **Make your bedroom a sleep sanctuary.** Insomnia can make your bedroom feel like a nightmare. To turn it into your sleep sanctuary:

   - Use your bed for sleep, sex, and inspirational reading only
   - Keep it cool; most people sleep better at about 68°F
   - Reduce ambient noise and light; use an eye pillow or mask and earplugs
   - Invest in comfy bedding
   - If you're having trouble falling asleep, don't lay there tossing; get up and read something relaxing until you're ready to try to sleep again

3. **Power down** from all electronics, stimulating conversation, and activities one hour before bed, and keep your bedroom electronic devices turned off. Instead, read a book—something inspirational or relaxing; practice deep breathing or yoga; or listen to relaxation or guided visualization recordings (the exception for electronics).

4. **Do your worrying *before* bed.** Create a Worry Journal. About forty-five minutes before you get into bed, sit anywhere in your house—but not in your bedroom—and pour your worries into a notebook. Write down anything that could remotely be keeping you up or weighing on your mind or spirit. Then, on the flip side

of the page, brainstorm your next day's to-do list so that nothing pops into your mind with an "Oh, shoot, I've got to remember to . . ." and makes you jump up to write or text yourself a last-minute note. You'll sleep with a clearer head. My patients *love* this practice.

5. **Soak it up.** Take a hot bath before bed to relax your mind and muscles. See the Replenish Bath under "Soak It Up" on page 200. Soak away your day's troubles. This is perfect to do after you write in your Worry Journal. If you feel uncomfortable in your bathtub, you can simply soak your feet or place a warm cloth over your eyes.

6. **Breathe deeply.** Staring at the ceiling doesn't help anyone fall asleep. Deep breathing does. Lay on your back or side, close your eyes, place one hand on your belly, and feel the rise and fall of your abdomen with each deep breath. When distracting thoughts slip in, return to following your breath. You will soon fall into a restful sleep.

7. **Reset your circadian rhythm** by getting up at the same time daily, preferably no later than 7:00 A.M., and getting to sleep at the same time each evening, preferably by 11:00 P.M. If you have severe insomnia, try sunlight exposure (sit in front of the window, even if cloudy, while you're having breakfast) or use a light box for thirty minutes each morning to help reset your cortisol awakening response.

How do you know when you need to get into the relaxation response? If you find yourself irritable, short-tempered, with your shoulders up to your ears, overwhelmed, impatient, overly hard on yourself, unable to unwind, unable to sleep, having a hard time focusing—pretty much any symptoms of emotional and mental SOS—you need it. Actually, you needed it before you got to that point, so pay attention to how you're feeling and try to recalibrate before you cross from the You Zone into overwhelm. Most of us need to practice relaxation several times every day, but think of it this way: Your energy and emotional resilience levels are the gauges on your fuel tank. Are you full? Three-quarters full? That's pretty good! But if you feel you're heading toward empty, or worse, are living off of your reserve tank or on fumes, it's time to replenish. The cool thing

If You Have to Work Nights

This is a tough situation—because working nights is inherently harder on your stress response system and does tend to cause problems. But there are things you can do to protect yourself:

- **Get extra sleep *before* your shift.** I know that sounds wonky, but a phenomenon called sleep banking—sleeping ahead to store up on rest—really is scientifically proven to help prevent exhaustion and physiological consequences from missed sleep.

- **Eat well on the job.** It's so tempting to nosh out at night, especially on junk and liquid calories (soda, "Mochachocalattatios" and other high-calorie coffee drinks, juice), but keeping to nutrient-dense foods only overnight can keep your cortisol sane and the unhealthy calories off.

- **Take adaptogens** (see page 248). Eleuthero has been especially useful for offsetting the stress on body and brain of night shift work.

- **Decompress when you get home,** just as you would after any job, and rest up in your downtime.

is that you can get into the relaxation response in just minutes, as you'll see with one of my favorite activities, the Quickie (on page 199, and not what it sounds like!), and the more you practice, the easier it becomes. My patients tell me these practices not only make them happier people, but also allow them to tap into their true potential as moms, wives, partners, and professionals.

Here's the thing, though. You have to value yourself enough to make it nonnegotiable. This means getting clear on your life priorities and boundaries, not letting your inner guilt gremlin talk you out of your time to yourself, and checking in with yourself regularly on whether you're prioritizing self-care. Taking "me time" isn't selfish; it is self-respecting and healthy. If you're just not good at creating downtime for yourself, feel you can't, or just don't have the time, I can personally tell you, as an incredibly busy woman myself, that you're making excuses and you have to get over that. There is time, and getting into this space more often actually makes you feel that you have more time and space in your life. How awesome is that?

But still, if you think you have no time to relax, please answer these questions:

- How can you fit in nonnegotiable "self-nourishing time" a few times over the next two weeks?
- What are you going to do during it?
- What are your obstacles, and how are you going to overcome them?
- If you took some time for yourself, what would be the best thing that could happen?
- The worst thing?
- How, specifically, are you going to create this time, for how long, and when?

Now schedule it!

REWRITE YOUR STORY, REWIRE YOUR BRAIN

Remember, the entrance door to the sanctuary is inside you.

—RUMI

We weren't born having negative thoughts about ourselves and our lives. These evolved as we encountered people and situations in our lives that fed us negative, doubting, inhibiting messages and beliefs. These same thoughts—and the patterns they lead us to—can be some of the most powerful toxins we swallow each day. And each thought we have becomes the narrative by which we create and live our lives. Changing thought patterns and behaviors—and with them your personal story—takes some practice, especially when they've been around for a long time. Imagine walking on a well-worn hiking trail. The path is carved out for you—you don't have to work hard to get where you're going. If you've been walking on the same thought path for a long time, your brain is naturally going to gravitate toward it because it's easy—your brain has an actual neural circuit for it.

Now think about the work of walking through the woods with no path. You'd practically have to swing a machete in front of you to clear the underbrush. But once you walk on the new path over and over, it, too, gets easier, until taking the new one is as easy as the old one. This is what forming new thoughts—and with them new neural pathways—is like. Once the path is clear, it's much easier to live in inner peace, confidence, and optimism more of the time, the perfect antidotes to living in anxiety, stress, self-doubt, and fear. Brené Brown says, "Owning our story can be hard but not nearly as difficult as spending our lives running from it."

Here are my top seven strategies for creating new thought pathways.

1. Stay Present

Staying present is one of the fastest ways to get over fear, worry, and FOMO. When you're in the present you aren't regretting the past or worrying about the future. Here are simple practices to get you present-minded:

- Sit quietly, and for one minute, simply notice all the sounds around you.

- When you wash the dishes, focus only on the sound and feel of the water and the dish you're holding. Practice this with other chores as well.

- Savor the aroma and taste of your food for one minute of your next meal.

If your attention wanders, bring it back. It's that easy. Stay present.

2. Get Rid of ANTs (Automatic Negative Thoughts)

Can you imagine walking up to your best girlfriend and saying, "Honey, what is wrong with you, your ass has gotten so big?" Or "What, you broke up with your boyfriend? It's definitely because you're not good enough." Or "Yeah, you're never going to get that job—you're too much of a loser."

None of us would ever talk to our best friends the way we do to ourselves. But this is how we talk to ourselves—every day! These are called ANTs—or *automatic negative thoughts*. And they can invade your life. Here are some of the common underlying beliefs, or ANTs, women have that hold us back:

- I don't deserve to put time (or money) into myself.
- There's not enough time to do this.
- I'll never be able to get what I want.
- Actually, I really am fat and lazy.
- Everything I try fails.
- I never stick to anything, so why bother?
- My mom and grandmother were like this, so I probably will be, too.
- Does this stuff *really* work, or am I deluding myself into false hope?
- I already "cheated" on the plan, so what's the point of continuing?

Start paying attention and you'll notice your own. Here's how to get rid of those pesky ANTs:

Be your own best friend: Being your own best friend is a powerful way to retrain your thought patterns to speak to yourself the way you would to someone you really love. It can spare your adrenals from being in overdrive and help you to resolve many adrenal-fatigue-related symptoms as side effects! Here's a quick trick I use: Imagine your best friend talking to those critical thoughts on your behalf. What would she say? My guess is she'd tell them to get lost and then she'd tell you something awesome about yourself. Try it—you have permission to crush your inner critic.

Watch them like a cloud: ANTs are habit thoughts that can make you take action—such as indulge in a pint of Ben & Jerry's. But they aren't true and don't have to control you. My favorite technique is the same one I use for any emotional impulses, including food cravings (see page 142), which is to feel what arises when I have a thought or impulse, and just watch it pass by like a cloud on a breezy spring day. Watch. Watch. Watch. Don't react. Just feel it. And it passes.

Talk back: If you have a particularly persistent self-critical thought pattern, you can also challenge and disprove the thought with a contradictory one. For example, if you think you'll never be successful, recall a time when you did have success at something. When I have an unhelpful "old thought" pop up, I thank it for coming from my past to try to help me, and I tell it, "I have it from here, sister. Thank you, but you can go, and you don't have to come back." Takes practice but works like a charm.

Welcome in the new: Here are examples of positive reframes of negative thoughts you can use to replace the ANTs. Over time, these can become second nature, or at least intentional thought substitutes when you notice ANTs popping up:

- I can relax. The universe has my back. I am provided for and have all I need.

- I know how I want to feel and am taking steps right now to feel that way.

- I love and approve of myself exactly the way I am.

- My body is beautiful and perfectly designed for wellness.

- It's okay if the laundry sits or the dishes aren't done. It's more important to nourish myself right now.

3. Quit "Shoulding" on Yourself

The word "should" is a harsh taskmaster—an especially sneaky ANT telling you you're not enough, you're not doing enough, and that you don't deserve to push pause. It often sounds like, "I should be more successful than I am," "I should be thinner than I am," "I should be married by now," "I should be working harder than I am," "I should say yes (or no)."

Pay attention to how many times a day you "should" on yourself, and about what; you might be shocked. And you might learn a lot about what's driving you. After a few days of noticing the word "should" in your life, practice removing it from your vocabulary and see what happens. It can be transformative.

4. Quit Comparing

As a perfectionist-in-recovery I'm familiar with the comparison gremlin who loves to remind me that everyone else is more successful, accomplished, and smarter than I. It's an extension of "shoulding" on yourself.

Having role models you admire and learn from is powerful, and it can motivate and inspire you; comparing is toxic. You can never be someone else, so comparing is a losing battle that is sure to leave you exhausted from trying to keep up or be better, while fighting inadequacy feelings. The antidote? Love YOU for who YOU are. Also, try this little trick: Next time you catch yourself comparing, send a little mental love note to the person you're comparing yourself against. Wish them success in your mind, go to their Facebook page and "like" something, drop an appreciation email—and remind yourself that the world needs us all. Focus on bringing *your* gifts to the world, rather than being distracted by someone else's, and appreciate them for theirs. It's healing and it's generous.

5. Count Your Wins

Make it a practice each evening before dinner or before you go to bed to recount at least one thing you did that day that made you feel good about yourself—whether that was holding a door open for an elderly person at a grocery store, saying something kind to someone, or checking some things off of your to-do list that have been nagging at you. We all deserve praise, and who better to get it from than your own best friend—you! Plus, optimism and gratitude release hormones that counteract the stress response and rewire your brain so you don't get stuck in SOS, and weirdly, there's scientific evidence that optimism can help you to attract more wealth and success into your life.

6. Tend and Befriend

While many of us instinctively reach out to others for support when we're under a lot of pressure, when we get too busy, it's easy to neglect a basic need: girlfriend time. Sometimes we don't reach out because pride gets in the way of admitting we need help. But being connected to each other powerfully reduces SOS. Stanford researcher Shelley Taylor has identified this as the "tend and befriend" response, a unique way that women naturally antidote the stress response. This works because connecting leads to release of the antistress, confidence-building hormone oxytocin.

Known as the "love hormone" because it's released when a new mother bonds with her baby, when we have orgasms, and when we connect with a friend, oxytocin counterbalances the stress response. It decreases fear, anxiety, and being stressed out, while increasing confidence, trust, courage, generosity, and empathy—not just for you, but also in the person you're reaching out to. Do something social—anything that allows you to bond with others. You don't need to discuss problems to get the benefit of social bonding, though studies do show that when we verbalize what's going on with us it automatically reduces the stress response. Next time you're feeling stressed out, anxious, or blue and want a hit of the love hormone, phone a friend. It'll be good for both of you.

7. Reframe Stress: Excite and Delight

You don't *have* to cave when you feel pressure. Try another approach: the "excite and delight" response. When you feel burdened by the "I have tos," reframe your thinking to "I get to" and get curious. This can switch the negative effects of stress to the positive effects because you're shifting into the You Zone I showed you on page 32. Positive psychology researcher Carol Dweck calls this switching into a "growth mindset." It's the opposite of a "fixed mindset," in which stressful situations cause us to make quick judgments about ourselves, or interpret or internalize the situation as "hard" or "bad" rather than as a challenge to be welcomed. This fixed mindset is the default of the fight-or-flight response, in which hormones limit our perception of the bigger picture. If you adopt a growth mindset, a challenging situation can become an exciting opportunity to learn or experience something new. Curiosity expands your options for how to solve problems, and usually helps you to solve them more quickly and easily.

THE REPLENISH REPAIR KIT

Volumes have been written about relaxation, meditation, and mindfulness, and it's absolutely essential to bring some form of relaxation response into your daily life to stay out of SOS. Below I am going to give you suggestions for my favorites in the Replenish Repair Kit—pick one or several to make your own. You'll also find suggestions in your day-by-day plans.

Cave Proactively

You've earned it and don't have to make everything fall apart to get the rest you need. When you've hit the wall of overwhelm, stop everything. Unplug. Step away from your cell phone, stay off of the Internet, turn off alarms and notifications, and take some time to be a human being—not a "human doing." It takes downtime to get out of SOS and for productivity to blossom, clarity to return, and your mood to smooth out. For how long? Depends on how overwhelmed you are. Could be a minute, an hour, or a vacation! But when you need it: cave.

Grab a Quickie
(Not What You Think, but It's Really Good)

Meditation, one of the techniques that bring you into the relaxation response, also reverses SOS. It even rebuilds the thickness of your brain's cortex, and along with it, improves memory and emotional regulation, and renews willpower. It prevents shortening of your telomeres, the protective end caps on your DNA sequences, whose greater length is associated with longevity. Even if you've never meditated or tried intentionally focusing your breathing before, try this. The Quickie is the best meditation I've ever learned. It can be done anytime, anywhere, and immediately shifts your mindset and relieves tension. It takes just two minutes, but it can be repeated for a longer meditation.

- Sit or stand comfortably, becoming aware of your feet on the floor. If you're in a place where you can, close your eyes.
- Take a few normal breaths in through your nose, out through your mouth.
- On your next inhale, breathe in deeply through your nose for a count of four while saying to yourself, "I am."
- Now exhale deeply through your mouth for a count of six while saying to yourself, "at peace."
- Repeat four to eight times, then open your eyes.
- Take a few seconds to note how you feel.

If you love the Quickie and other mind-body practices you're find-ing in this book and want more, you can visit my website, avivaromm .com, and look for Mind and Mood. As you see here, meditation doesn't have to mean sitting on a mat with your eyes closed and saying "Om" for an hour, though it can be that, too, which is powerful. But it can also be quick techniques like this one that bring you inner calm and reset your stress response, really fast.

Practice Yoga—or Find Your Move Groove

Regular physical movement of pretty much any kind, in moderation (see page 185), improves your health, relaxes your mind, and does good things for your cortisol curve. Yoga, in particular, releases deep tension and sets tissue healing in motion, while calming the mind and helping you to be in the present—all of which powerfully invite the benefits of the relaxation response. Restorative yoga is particularly effective at bringing you into deep relaxation fairly quickly, without stress and strain on your muscles. You can even be a total yoga newbie and do it. I highly recommend it if you scored high on the mental-emotional stress questionnaire. Most yoga studios offer restorative yoga classes, or you can stream videos online for guidance (see "Resources" on page 393).

Soak It Up

I call this the Replenish Bath, because that's how you feel when you get out, replenished—like you've had a long moment of *Ahhhh*. Before you go to bed, or anytime you need to soak up some relaxation response, fill your tub with water as warm as you can tolerate and enjoy; add one cup of Epsom salts and seven drops of lavender (or other relaxing) essential oil. If you have candles, light them, and soak away your troubles, practicing a few minutes of deep breathing while you're in the tub, too.

Have a Daily Ritual

A daily ritual can be as simple as a cup of tea or coffee, sipped in peace and quiet for fifteen minutes, a regular thirty-minute walk alone or with a friend, a five-minute meditation, or a hot bath (see above)—all of which can reset your HPA axis. Pick one ritual that you make your own. Daily is too much to fit in? Pick one evening or one weekend morning a week for self-care, mark it off on the calendar, and make it happen. Religiously. You have to show up for yourself.

Journaling

Journaling does not require great writing skills; simply grab a pen and a notebook and write what comes to you. Here are two journaling techniques:

Worry Journal: Thirty minutes before bed, write out your fears, worries, and troublesome experiences. This has been demonstrated to reduce cortisol, alleviate anxiety, and help to overcome PTSD. It has also been shown to reduce the frequency of visits to the doctor and reduce chronic illness and inflammation. Fifteen minutes a day of journaling for just four days in a row, one time, can lead to benefits lasting up to eight months.

Gratitude Journal: Several times each week, simply write down three things you're grateful for. Practicing gratitude has also been shown to have numerous health benefits and improves quality of life.

The After-Work Reset

Women who take time to relax and Reboot mentally and emotionally after a workday, especially a stressful workday, enjoy healthier evening cortisol levels and sleep better than women who don't take this rest and repair time. Make it a daily end-of-work habit to decompress for fifteen minutes with any of the relaxation response practices in this book when you get home, to keep your cortisol from being jacked in the evenings. My favorite end-of-day practice is a *solo dance party*. I play loud music and dance like no one is watching—even if someone is watching. I don't care. I sing really loud, too. Also, give yourself one evening a week completely off from work and chores. This simple act can work wonders to keep you feeling like you're a human being, not just a "human doing."

Digital Detox

Information overload is a new kind of toxin that is addling our brains and making us feel that we never know enough, do enough, or are happy enough (especially if you believe everyone else's perfect happy life pictures on Facebook). Additionally, staying on the computer and other electronic devices too close to bedtime not only introduces other people's agendas and a whole lot of social concerns into your awareness, but also the blue light itself emanated from these devices keeps your cortisol elevated and inhibits melatonin production, interfering with sleep. So I dare you. Unplug yourself from your digital habit every evening by nine o'clock, and for one full day each week be Internet- and device-free. No cell phone. No email. No Facebook. No computer. It's a game changer. I promise.

Get Some Fresh Air

Ancients have always known what science now proves—that nature heals your brain, reduces cortisol, reduces inflammation, and shifts you to a calm, happy mindset. The caveat is that you unplug while you're enjoying it. You don't have to buy a farm or a vacation home in the country; walking in a park for thirty minutes a couple of times a week can make a difference. Or try standing outside in the sunshine, bare feet on the ground, and breathe consciously, even if just for three minutes, directing your breath to wherever you feel discomfort or tension in your body, and for a moment, clear your mind.

Play

Play is as necessary for health and happiness as exercise, and laughter puts you straight into the relaxation response. Make some time to play with friends, with your kids, or with your neighbors' kids if you don't have any, or pick up a hobby that you used to love but haven't let yourself enjoy in years. Do it with no pressure, no self-judgment—just for pure pleasure. Fun is good. What do you miss doing? Roller-skating? Riding a bicycle? Pottery-making? Hula-hooping? (I have one!) Just do it.

Have Sex

In a book on women and stress, a whole chapter on sex probably wouldn't be too much for some readers. Stressful relationships can sap our moods, motivation, and diet. Research shows that even our sleep is interrupted when sleeping next to a partner who's stressing us out (and like so many stress statistics, men's sleep is not as affected). On the other hand, sleeping next to, and having sex with, someone you love is an SOS antidote that improves sleep quality, reduces cortisol overdrive, and boosts your mood. Good relationships with intimacy can offset daily tensions, improve your immunity, and increase your longevity. That said, having orgasms is good for you even if you're the only one involved. It's still a stress buster and oxytocin releaser. So you don't have to wait for someone else to get your mojo going. Hint: if your sex drive isn't quite what you want it to be, the Hot Mama Super Smoothie on page 319 can work wonders to help you get back in the groove.

NATURAL SUPPORT FOR SLEEP, MIND, AND MOOD

In addition to your Daily Dose Supplements, the following herbs and nutrients can nourish your nervous system, restore balance in your autonomic nervous system (ANS), support neurotransmitter production, and give you extra help in relieving anxiety and depression and improving mood. They are safe, nonaddictive, and nonsedating. These gentle supplements can help you rest soundly without sleep medications. You can safely combine any of these or try any solo, experimenting with which work for you. You can expect to see results within five days of starting any of these.

For sleep, take the herbal extracts diluted in two ounces of water within thirty minutes of going to bed. If sleep is really tough for you, you can take a dose one hour before bed, then again at bedtime. Unless specified, these are *not* recommended during pregnancy, though they may be taken while breast-feeding.

In chapter 7 you'll also learn about "adaptogens," herbs that relieve SOS and have a specific affinity for boosting immunity, energy, and mental clarity.

SOS Rx: Natural Support for Sleep, Mind, and Mood (Also see "SOS Rx: Adaptogens," page 248)		
Herb/ Supplement	**Uses and Cautions**	**Dose**
L-theanine©	A calming amino acid found almost exclusively in green tea, L-theanine, much like meditation, increases relaxation yet supports focus and alertness by increasing alpha brain waves. It compares favorably to antianxiety medication in the prevention of anxiety, even under stress, within one hour of taking a dose. It also enhances the production of neurotransmitters, including serotonin, dopamine, and GABA, producing a state of well-being. It may also help to reduce blood pressure.	100 to 200 mg/day
Lavender©	Deepens sleep, reduces anxiety. Scientific studies support the use of lavender for the relief of tension, whether used as a tea or herbal extract, or even inhaling the essential oil (aromatherapy). My preferred form for reducing anxiety and sleep disruption due to frequent waking is oral lavender oil. I've had patients who have successfully tapered off of long-term use of antianxiety medications after starting on just 60 mg of lavender oil (in capsules) daily. It can be taken before bed, or in the morning. It's shown equal effectiveness to antianxiety sleep medications such as benzodiazepines with none of the risks. It is also especially helpful for performance anxiety—for example, regarding test taking. While at this dose, I do not have concerns about the very mild potential estrogen effects of lavender oil; don't use if you personally have had estrogen-receptor-positive cancer or are at high risk due to immediate family history (your mother or sister has had estrogen-receptor-positive cancer). Aromatherapy use acceptable in pregnancy.	One lavender oil capsule (60 mg) before bed

Herb/Supplement	Uses and Cautions	Dose
Magnesium	Promotes relaxation, relieves anxiety and depression. Can be taken before bed to promote mental and muscular relaxation. Magnesium also helps if restless leg syndrome or muscle cramps keep you awake.	400 to 800 mg/day
Melatonin◎	Helps initiate sleep and may also improve menopausal night sweats. Numerous studies support effectiveness and safety.	0.5 to 3 mg in the hour before bed
Passion-flower	Promotes sleep and improves sleep quality; helps you feel more rested when you wake; also useful for anxiety.	40 to 60 drops of the tincture (or 320 mg in a capsule)
Probiotics	Should contain *Lactobacillus* and *Bifidobacterium* species; reduces stimulation of the HPA axis. Exciting research on the gut-brain connection has yielded a whole new field of study: psychobiotics—looking at the use of probiotics to improve mood and cognitive function—and studies are not disappointing. We now know that enhancing the presence of beneficial gut flora relieves anxiety, alleviates depression, reduces inflammatory cytokines, and reduces HPA axis overstimulation. *Bifidobacterium infantis* and *B. longum* are among the strains of probiotics that have been found to be particularly beneficial, leading to reductions in depression, irritability, and anxiety, and improving stress-coping abilities.	1 to 2 capsules/day, with a minimum of 10 billion CFUs (colony forming units) daily
Relora◎	Sleep, anxiety, energy. A combination of magnolia and phellodendron, reduces SOS and anxiety, improves sleep and energy, reduces cortisol, and may help to safely raise DHEA.	500 mg at bedtime

SOS Rx: Natural Support for Sleep, Mind, and Mood (Also see "SOS Rx: Adaptogens," page 248)		
Herb/ Supplement	**Uses and Cautions**	**Dose**
SAMe (S-adenosyl methionine)⊘	This amino acid, important for methylation, appears to be as potent as some pharmaceutical options for depression. Also helpful in the treatment of anxiety, pain and inflammation in osteoarthritis, and muscle soreness with fibromyalgia.	400 to 1,600 mg/day; may take 1 to 2 months to notice effects because it has to build up in your system
St. John's wort	In more than eighteen studies with nearly six thousand individuals, St. John's wort has been found to be as effective as or more effective than antidepressant medications, with none of the side effects.	300 to 600 mg/day of products standardized to 0.3% hypericin and/ or 3 to 5% hyperforin
Turmeric	Because of its overall anti-inflammatory effects, turmeric, as well as one of its main active constituents, curcumin, is an important herbal supplement to consider if you're struggling with brain fog, anxiety, or depression.	1 to 3 mg powdered turmeric or 1,200 to 2,400 mg curcumin daily
Vitamin B$_6$	Taken before bed specifically to relieve night waking by reducing nocturnal cortisol spikes.	50 to 100 mg
Vitamin B$_{12}$ (methylcobalamin)	Plays an especially important role in allowing your body to reset its circadian rhythm, possibly due to its effects on melatonin production, and improves quality of sleep, leading to feeling refreshed when you wake up.	1,000 mcg taken sublingually

Key: ⊘ = Not safe for use in pregnancy.

DREAM BIG, LIVE ON PURPOSE

And the day came when the risk to remain tight in a bud
was more painful than the risk it took to blossom.

—ANAÏS NIN

Look back at that You Curve (page 32). There's a boredom end and it's where you find lack of fulfillment and quashed desire leading to lower function and performance. This can also translate into irritability, depression, anxiety, anger, disappointment, resentment, and a whole host of other emotions, while at the same time translating into physical health symptoms. This is because satisfaction, fulfilled desires, and the ability and space to develop and express your talents are all ingredients in the recipe for human health and happiness.

If you're living a life out of harmony with fundamentally feeling happy and enjoying your day, your SOS risk goes up. I've had so many women come into my practice and write to me expressing the challenges they feel in fulfilling their hopes and dreams. I know it can take a tremendous effort to leave an unfulfilling job, to end an unhappy relationship, or to shift careers. It's also very scary sometimes. I'm not telling you to do any of those things hastily, or at all if you just can't. But I can tell you that your health does depend on life satisfaction and a feeling of safety. Believing you "can't," whether it's healing your body and mind, changing your career, or trying something new, is an old story. You are a fabulous, mature, strong, smart woman who can now recognize that those are just false stories and old beliefs—and that you can write a new script for yourself. You can be the author of your life. Be a witness to your automatic negative thoughts—understand where they came from, thank them, and send them on their way. Make it a daily practice to replace automatic negative thoughts with new, positive ones based on your ability to design your life. Consider the possibility that you could start to intentionally doubt your fears, and believe in your dreams. The ability to make change rests on the belief that we can reinvent ourselves. Often we get stuck in the belief that we can't change our lives; the reality is that your health may depend on making change. One of the greatest known risk factors to health is lacking a feeling of control over your time, work, and life.

Too often we've gotten comfortable with habits, lifestyles, and symp-toms that actually aren't comfortable at all. We confuse familiar with safe and easier. Taking the risk to change, to fulfill your dreams, is a powerful self-rescue from SOS. The poet Mary Oliver asks, in "The Summer Day," "Tell me, what is it you plan to do with your one wild and precious life?"

It is a question I believe every woman deserves to ask herself. I hope you will, too.

Who looks outside, dreams; who looks inside, awakes.

—CARL JUNG

REPAIR

Heal Your Gut, Boost Immunity, Support Detoxification, and Balance Your Hormones

Reboot: Remove Food Triggers

Reframe: Chronic Emotional and Mental Stress

Repair: Root Causes and SOS Damage

Recharge: Your Adrenals and Thyroid

Replenish: No More Running on Empty

*As soon as something breaks, tears, or malfunctions within us,
the instructions in our cells begin to supervise repairs.*

—KATE WHEELING, *YALE MEDICINE* (AUTUMN 2014)

WELCOME TO WEEK TWO of the SOS Solution. Congratulations! You're already well on your way to vibrant health with the dietary changes you've made and adding in practices to unstress your life.

This week you'll continue on your 21-Day Reboot with the menus and recipes provided and now you'll explore the nutrients, herbs, and solutions that will allow your intrinsic repair mechanisms to do their jobs to reverse

the Root Causes of SOS—gut imbalances, toxic overload, immune disruption, and stealth infections—while boosting immunity and reducing overall
inflammation. Because your body is an intricate web, if you heal one area,
the whole benefits.

How to Approach the Repair Work

- If you scored 3 points or above on the gut health questionnaire,
  start with that section, adding in the supplements and approaches
  that you see are recommended for your symptom picture.

- If you did not score more than 3 points on the gut health
  questionnaire, start with the area you scored highest in on the
  Root Cause questionnaires, focusing on the recommendations
  in the corresponding section below, and then, after three days,
  add in recommendations from the next-highest-scoring section,
  and so on.

- If you scored high in several categories, start at the beginning
  of this chapter and work your way through the chapter in order,
  giving a few days for each section before you add in supplements
  from the subsequent section.

- Continue to stay on the plan for each section as you add in the next
  section, throughout the four weeks, or as directed.

Remember, this is a lifestyle, not a "quick fix plan." Feeling pressured and
rushed is old SOS thinking. Try your best to let go of the rush, and enjoy
the path and the process. You're already on your way, learning a new way
of life, new tools you can turn to for healing, and a new way of eating that
will transform your health for your whole lifetime.

Also recall that you will see redundancies in supplements across sections. Herbs and nutrients work by activating various self-healing mechanisms and address Root Causes of inflammation and other underlying
imbalances triggered by and causing SOS. Don't add in *more* of the same
supplement if it appears more than once; the dose you take for one imbalance will cover you for all.

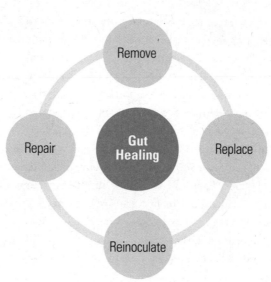

THE 4R PROGRAM FOR GUT HEALTH

Healing your gut is not hard to do, and it is the most important step in treating most chronic conditions, in addition to the dietary changes you're making. Gut health is central to nutrient absorption, immune system regulation, and detoxification. Inflammation in your gut, as you've learned, is also a major Root Cause of general systemic inflammation, weight gain, insulin resistance, brain fog, hormone imbalances, depression, and anxiety. Gut dysbiosis, celiac disease, and gluten intolerance are also associated with higher levels of Hashimoto's and other autoimmune diseases, and determine the reactivity of your stress hormone. Hashimoto's, in turn, leads to decreased peristalsis, and as a result, constipation, which can then lead to gas, bloating, and bacterial overgrowth that may result in diarrhea.

The 4R Program for Gut Health is a very effective four-step process to reverse leaky gut, get rid of the "bad bugs" that cause SIBO, yeast overgrowth, weight gain, and even anxiety, and replace them with healthy flora, heal inflammation in your intestinal lining, and replace important digestive enzymes and stomach acid if these are low. Depending on the severity of your symptoms, it can take from about four to six weeks, and sometimes even as much as six months to *fully* heal your gut. Here are the steps, which can be done consecutively, or concurrently if you prefer, or you can select from the parts of the 4R that are most relevant to the results of your gut imbalances questionnaire on page 111.

1) **REMOVE** the inflammatory and disruptive triggers to your gut lining that are damaging your microbiome and causing bacterial or yeast overgrowth, 2) **REPLACE** missing digestive enzymes and improve stomach acid to aid in digestion, 3) **REINOCULATE** your microbiome with healthy flora and good-quality fiber, and 4) **REPAIR** and **HEAL** your gut lining with appropriate herbs and supplements. The exciting news is you're already well on your way. The first step involves removing all triggering foods—and you've already been doing that for a week now, so you'll keep going with your Reboot food plan, and progress now to add in specifics for gut healing.

REMOVE

Now that you've removed food triggers, we're going to work on reducing the overgrowth of unhelpful and even harmful bacterial and yeasts in the gut, as well as doing our best to remove potentially gut-damaging medications when possible.

Remove Triggers and Stop Bacterial Overgrowth

Remove the "Big Four" Gut-Disrupting Medications: Antibiotics, NSAIDs, Tylenol, and PPIs

Most medications have unintended consequences, and when it comes to antibiotics, proton pump inhibitors, NSAIDs, and acetaminophen, the consequences are damage to your gut ecosystem and infrastructure. To protect both our health and our planet, we have to reduce the number of pharmaceuticals we use. The best way to do this, of course, is by staying healthy and needing fewer medications. But we also need to begin "thinking beyond drugs," and return to more natural approaches to healing. The good news here is that this program is designed to significantly help boost immunity. Each day on the SOS Solution improves your overall health by removing the key stressors and allowing the body's natural ability to heal take center stage. You will be amazed to find that you get sick much less frequently than in the past, and get well much more quickly when you do. However, please check with your doctor before going off of doctor-prescribed medications—these may be important for your health and safety.

Antibiotics: Antibiotics are gut enemy number one. More than 70 percent of those prescribed in the United States are medically unnecessary, yet by the time the average American is thirty years old, he or she has had thirty courses of antibiotics. On top of this, over half of all antibiotics produced in the United States are fed to cattle to make them grow fatter, faster—meaning you're getting an extra dose with every (nonorganic) chicken or steak dinner. While the gut microbiome has amazing resilience, it can take only so much. Even just one round of antibiotics can wipe out an entire species of your gut flora—permanently. Hand sanitizers are a related problem. *Antimicrobial products* not only contain triclosan and other endocrine disrupters, but they, too, can breed antibiotic resistance. A lot of household products, including dish and body soaps, contain them as well. Nix them. Use companies such as Seventh Generation and Ecover in the kitchen, and wash your hands with plain soap and water. To learn how to avoid unnecessary antibiotic exposure for your health and safety, see page 214.

Nonsteroidal anti-inflammatory drugs (NSAIDs): Medications in this category include ibuprofen, Aleve, Motrin, and many of those familiar to women with menstrual cramps, headaches, migraines, and chronic pain. Their ubiquitous use makes them seem benign, but they aren't. Even five continuous days of use can lead to gastrointestinal (GI) bleeding, and many chronic users develop chronic inflammation of the GI tract—a major cause of leaky gut and, potentially, autoimmune disease.

Proton pump inhibitors (PPIs): These medications, including Prilosec, Prevacid, and Nexium, to name a few, are used for the treatment of acid reflux (GERD or, commonly, heartburn). In addition to interfering with vitamin B_{12} absorption, which increases risks of depression,

Natural Alternatives to Common Pain Medications

Below you'll find my "green medicine cabinet" must-haves—the top herbs to use singly or in combination to help you avoid unnecessary or excessive use of acetaminophen and NSAIDs for pain and inflammation—so you can protect your gut and detox system. To avoid unnecessary antibiotic use, eat eight to ten servings of a rainbow of veggies and berries every day, take your Daily Dose Supplements, and use herbs and supplements on pages 166-67 to keep your immune system optimized.

Herb/ Supplement	Comment	Dose
Boswellia⊘	Reduces inflammation and pain of osteoarthritis and inflammatory bowel disease supplements	350 mg three times daily
Bromelain⊘	An enzyme from pineapple, can be taken daily to reduce chronic inflammation and also helps with digestive symptoms	200 to 320 mg twice daily
Capsaicin	Derived from hot peppers, highly effective for reliving chronic nerve pain when applied topically	Apply to the affected area three times daily. Wash hands after applying, and do not touch your eyes!
Curcumin⊘	Relieves inflammation and pain	1,200 to 2,400 mg daily
Devil's claw⊘	Shown to be better than conventional medications for low back pain	50 to 100 mg harpagoside, the active chemical in the herb, daily

Herb/ Supplement	Comment	Dose
Ginger	Shown to be as effective as NSAIDs for relieving pain and inflammation in menstrual cramps, headaches, and arthritic joints	500 to 1,000 mg one to two times daily
Lavender or peppermint essential oil	Alleviates headaches when applied topically	One to two drops applied to the temples for headache, or seven to ten drops in a hot bath
SAMe⊘	Specifically beneficial for osteoarthritis knee pain	200 to 400 mg three times daily

Key: ⊘ = Not safe for use in pregnancy.

detoxification problems (due to interference with methylation—see page 235), and neurologic problems. PPIs can increase the growth of bacteria in the small intestine, causing small intestinal bacterial overgrowth (SIBO), which can contribute to food intolerances and thus chronic inflammation.

Tylenol: Acetaminophen damages the delicate lining of the stomach and can lead to gastrointestinal bleeding and problems with the absorption of nutrients needed for gut health. It is one of the leading causes of liver damage in the United States annually. It depletes the most important detoxifier we have in our bodies—glutathione.

Get Rid of the "Bad Bugs"

If you have gas, bloating, frequent loose stools, dysbiosis, or SIBO symptoms on your gut imbalances questionnaire, then it's time to get rid of the "bad bugs." Herbal remedies are very effective at eliminating the overgrowth of less friendly gut bugs, including for the treatment of SIBO. The most effective of these include goldenseal (or other berberine-containing herbs), garlic, and essential oils of oregano, thyme, and sage,⁹ all of which can be found in combination products readily available from major herbal supplement companies (see "Resources" on page 393). Follow the instructions for the product you choose, and take for at least four, and up to eight, weeks. These products are not appropriate for use during pregnancy, and check with your midwife or doctor before using while breast-feeding.

Sometimes people feel a little worse when they start to kill off the bad bugs, especially Candida, a yeast, because as these organisms die, they release chemicals into your gut and bloodstream that can cause what are called "die-off" symptoms. These most commonly include:

- Achiness
- Brain Fog
- Constipation
- Diarrhea
- Fatigue
- Gas, bloating
- Headaches

If these are mild, you can just drink extra water and ride it out. It usually lasts at most a few days. If symptoms are more intense, drink at least eight glasses of water each day, make sure you are having a BM every day, and take NAC (see below), 300 mg three times daily, for detoxification support. If any of these symptoms lasts more than three days, or is accompanied by other concerning symptoms or those not on the list above, this is not likely a die-off reaction and is more likely an illness, such as flu or other infection; get appropriate medical evaluation as needed.

REPLACE

Here we'll add in supplements to support what your body tries to do naturally with each meal but is sometimes struggling to do adequately: produce and release digestive enzymes and stomach acid.

Replace Digestive Enzymes and Boost Stomach Acid

Digestive enzymes are helpful if you have undigested food in your stool, gas, or bloating after meals. These are taken at the start of each meal to coincide with when your body would naturally start to pump out these enzymes.

Boost stomach acid with any of the following:

- *Digestive bitters*◎ at the start of your meal are one of my practice go-tos, *or* one to two tablespoonfuls of *apple cider vinegar* in water at the beginning of your meal at one or two meals daily, *or*

- *Betaine HCl*, starting with one pill (they usually contain 650 mg), and increase by one at each meal, to a max of three if needed, at the start of your meals (do not take if you are on an antacid or without talking with your primary provider if you have ulcers). If you get any burning sensation in your stomach, the dose should be decreased by one pill. As your body starts to produce more stomach acid, you'll be able to decrease the dose. Take for one to two months.

If you suffer from GERD (reflux), consider DGL licorice,◎ one to three chewable tablets or capsules between meals, and before bed if needed. Zinc carnosine, 30 mg daily, can help heal gastric inflammation.

REINOCULATE

It's not enough to just get rid of the "bad bugs"; we have to add in the healthy ones, which you'll do with lacto-fermented foods, probiotics, and healthy fiber.

Restore Your Gut Flora

Please feed your good flora:

- Eat *dark leafy greens* (page 149), at least two cups at two meals each day, and one serving of *fermented vegetables* (page 154) once daily with your meal to repopulate your gut with the good guys. This is something that should be done daily for your lifetime for optimal gut health, but at least stick with it throughout the entire SOS Solution.

- *Healthy fiber* from a variety of plant sources serves as the best food for a healthy microbiome. Most of us get less than half of the daily

SOS Rx: Gut-Healing Herbs and Supplements at a Glance		
Herb/ Supplement	**Uses and Cautions**	**Dose**
Apple cider vinegar	Boosts stomach acid, improves digestive secretions	1 to 2 tbsp. in water at the beginning of meal, once or twice daily
Betaine HCl	Boosts stomach acid	Start with 1 tablet and work up to 3 if needed
DGL licorice[○]	Relieves GERD (reflux)	1 to 3 chewable tablets or capsules between meals
Digestive enzymes	Undigested food in stool, gas, or bloating after meals	1 or 2 at the beginning of each meal
Fiber	Decreases unhealthy cholesterol, improves detox of hormones from digestive system, nourishes healthy gut flora	Ideally 30 to 35 g/day
Flaxseed	Adds fiber	2 tbsp. freshly ground seed/day
Herbal bitters[○]	Take any of a combination of: Dandelion root Burdock root Artichoke	¼ tsp. each of the herbal tinctures (extracts) in ¼ cup of water or in ½ to 1 cup of sparkling water before or after each meal. Add ¼ tsp. gingerroot as well for taste and gut-healing effects
L-glutamine[○]	Nourishes and heals the intestinal lining	5 to 10 g powder 2x/day for at least one month
Magnesium citrate	Helpful with constipation	400 to 800 mg before bed

Herb/ Supplement	Uses and Cautions	Dose
Marshmallow root	Heals gut lining	2 to 6 capsules/day, or 1 to 2 cups of tea/day made by steeping 2 tbsp. in 2 cups of boiling water for 30 minutes
Probiotic	Should contain *Lactobacillus* and *Bifidobacterium;* restores normal balance of flora and repairs gut barrier	1 to 2 capsules/day
Turmeric	Heals gut lining	2 to 10 g of powdered turmeric/ day
Zinc carnosine	Heals gastric inflammation	30 mg/day

Key: ⃠ = Not safe for use in pregnancy.

recommended 25 to 38 grams of fiber. If gut flora don't get fed, they begin to eat away at the important protective mucosal layer of the intestines, causing inflammation and eventually leaky gut. Add fiber in the form of two cups of veggies with at least two meals each day, and add two tablespoons of freshly ground flaxseed to your daily diet.

- Take a *probiotic* that contains ten billion CFUs and a variety of *Lactobacillus* and *Bifidobacterium* species to help restore the normal balance of flora in your gut and repair your gut barrier function. I recommend taking them daily for a couple of months, then back down to a few days each week if you feel you're continuing to find them helpful. Sometimes if you have significant dysbiosis, or SIBO, taking a probiotic can cause gassiness or bloating. If this happens, discontinue the probiotic, follow the recommendations under "Get Rid of the 'Bad Bugs'" above for four to six weeks, and reintroduce the probiotic two weeks after you start that treatment, at which time you'll likely tolerate it without a problem. If it still causes you trouble, try another product at the lowest possible dose, or reintroduce the product you have four weeks after starting the "Get Rid of the 'Bad Bugs'" plan.

- *Prebiotics* are starches, including fructooligosaccharides (FOS), found in garlic, onions, asparagus, Jerusalem artichokes, oats, and arabinogalactans from larch trees (used in supplements) that are food for your gut flora. Dose: 4 to 10 grams daily. They are commonly found in combination gut-healing products.

REPAIR

Now you'll learn to repair the digestive system lining to reduce leaky gut and heal gut tissue to reduce inflammation, optimize nutrient absorption, and create a healthy terrain on which your healthy microbiome can flourish.

Repair Your Gut Lining and Heal Leaky Gut

Your intestinal lining is renewed approximately every five days. These supplements and herbs can help with the healing process and reverse leaky gut:

- *Turmeric root, marshmallow root, and DGL licorice* are some of the most effective herbs for healing the gut lining. The dose of turmeric is 2 to 10 grams of the powdered herb per day, or fresh root can be added to smoothies.
- *Zinc* is an integral mineral in maintaining the intestinal tight junctions and halting inflammation in the intestinal lining and also healing stomach ulcers. A form called *zinc carnosine* is optimal, but any form can be used. Dose: 30 mg daily.
- *L-glutamine* powder is an amino acid that nourishes and heals the intestinal lining. Dose: 5 to 10 g of powder twice daily for up to 3 months.
- *Antioxidant vitamins A, C, E, and the mineral selenium* are necessary for a healthy intestinal lining and are in most good-quality multivitamins (see "Resources" on page 393). Make sure to also get plenty of antioxidant-rich vegetables, nuts, and seeds in your diet.

COOL INFLAMMATION, BOOST IMMUNITY, AND FIGHT STEALTH INFECTIONS

Your immune system is responsible for the massive job of sorting out what's you from what's not, in order to protect you from invading bacteria, viruses, and other microorganisms. When you're in SOS, your immune system is unable to properly process messages—you can be turning on inflammatory signals excessively, or be unable to turn them off. Regulating immunity is at the heart of healing from SOS and is essential for maintaining resilience to stealth infections, those viruses, especially Epstein-Barr virus (EBV), that can lie dormant in your body but become problematic if you are under stress, and that can cause fatigue, aching, and brain fog, and have been associated with autoimmune disease. Getting your cortisol rhythms back on track will also help your immune system to reset itself so it can properly differentiate between self and other, and respond appropriately to signaling messages.

If you're in SOS, you, by definition, have some rogue inflammation, so I recommend taking *curcumin*,⊚ *green tea extract*,⊚ *N-acetylcysteine (NAC)*,⊚ or a combination of these (see "SOS Rx: Anti-inflammatory Herbs and Supplements," page 222) for at least the next few weeks while you're doing the SOS Solution—and if you notice improvements, continue for three to six months longer.

Remember that Hashimoto's is a problem of immune dysregulation affecting the thyroid, rather than inherently a thyroid problem itself. So cooling the flames of inflammation and regulating immunity is one of the strategies for healing Hashimoto's—and removing its underlying causes so they don't lead to further autoimmunity or other conditions for you to deal with later.

If you scored high on any of your immune system or inflammation questionnaires, see the sections that relate to your needs, and make sure to take the following daily in the doses listed in "SOS Rx: Herbs and Supplements to Boost Immunity" (page 225), and add in additional relevant herbs from "SOS Rx: Anti-inflammatory Herbs and Supplements."

- A probiotic with *Lactobacillus* strains
- Zinc
- Vitamin D

SOS Rx: Anti-inflammatory Herbs and Supplements

Herb/ Supplement	Uses and Cautions	Dose
Curcumin◎	An extract from turmeric, a spice that has been used in Indian cooking for thousands of years, is a natural anti-inflammatory. It is specifically effective in treating major depression resulting from SOS-related inflammation and oxidative stress. Curcumin helps with arthritis pain, helps with pain and gut inflammation in Crohn's disease and ulcerative colitis, reduces brain fog, and reduces DNA damage from oxidative stress.	1,200 to 2,400 mg/day of extract
Essential fatty acids	Omega-3 fatty acids (DHA/EPA) have been shown in numerous studies to protect against and reverse inflammation and oxidative stress, and with that, protect against heart disease, depression, dementia, and other inflammation-related conditions.	850 EPA/200 DHA 1 to 2x/ day. If you don't eat fish, algae-based vegetarian sources are available.
Ginger	Relieves pain and inflammation. Ginger has been shown to be as effective as NSAIDs for relieving pain and inflammation, including pain due to osteoarthritis, and also menstrual cramps.	500 to 1,000 mg, 1 to 2x/ day
Green tea extract◎	Green tea boosts liver detoxification, helping you to break down and get rid of toxins while acting as an antioxidant and putting out the fires of inflammation around your body, promotes healthy flora, and supports estrogen detoxification. It can be taken as a tea, but in extract form it is a potent supplement for weight loss, hormonal balance, and detox.	200 mg/day of green tea catechins

Herb/ Supplement	Uses and Cautions	Dose
N-acetylcyste-ine (NAC)⊘	Boosts detoxification by building up gluta-thione, one of your body's chief detoxi-fiers. Glutathione is depleted by inflam-mation, oxidative stress—the damage to your cells caused by the smoldering fire of chronic inflammation—and infections. Low levels are associated with autoim-mune conditions and chronic fatigue.	300 mg 3x/day
Quercetin⊘	A flavonoid from foods, including onions and apples, quercetin is an immune-supporting anti-inflammatory that is also particularly effective if you suffer from food intolerances, seasonal allergies, eczema, hives, or histamine intolerance.	250 mg 3x/day

Key: ⊘ = Not safe for use in pregnancy.

Herbs and Supplements to Cool Inflammation

If you're in SOS, you're likely experiencing mild to significant chronic inflammation. So, too, if you are experiencing depression or fatigue; have painful, red, or swollen joints; have memory problems, chronic pain, PMS, or menstrual cramps; feel achy a lot; are overweight; are struggling with insulin resistance, prediabetes, metabolic syndrome, high cholesterol, or high blood pressure; always feel like you're coming down with something; get hives or chronic rashes; have PCOS; have chronic fatigue syndrome, leaky gut, or food intolerances; spend most of your day sitting; have eaten an American diet for a long time; work a night shift—or have many of the symptoms or conditions in this book.

Select one or several of the herbs and supplements in the table on page 222 to add to your daily plan. Within weeks you'll notice that many downstream symptoms, from joint aches and pains to menstrual cramps to depression, start to improve. Additionally, if you have chronic

Connecting the Dots: Healthy Boundaries, Better Immunity?

When we aren't honoring our boundaries emotionally—when we let too much in because we can't say no—not only do we run the risk of overwhelming ourselves mentally and emotionally, but this burnout also can impact our immune boundaries. Immunity is also your body's barometer for resilience. When you find your immune resilience low, look at the whole picture— are you overwhelming your resilience by not giving yourself time to replenish and rest in your life?

pain due to inflammation, see page 222 for safe and natural pain relief alternatives.

Herbs to Boost Immunity

If you tend to get sick often or seasonally, try these immune-boosting herbs, especially just prior to the onset of seasonal changes, cold and flu season, or times of increased stress, and continue throughout. Also see adaptogens in the next chapter (page 245).

Herbs to Fight Stealth Infections

In addition to the herbs and supplements to boost immunity, the following herbs are specifically effective at preventing viral infections, and may help keep latent viruses quiet. Remember that chronic stress has a significant impact on recurrent HSV and EBV, so managing stress with relaxation response practices and herbs and supplements for stress (page 192) is particularly important. The herbs in the table below can be taken preventatively or to clear infection for up to three months at a time. Please discuss treatment of viral infections with your primary care provider, and if you are positive for infections and are immune-compromised or pregnant, work with your doctor or midwife to decide on the best treatment for you. In chapter 7

SOS Rx: Herbs and Supplements to Boost Immunity		
Herb/ Supplement	**Uses and Cautions**	**Dose**
Andrographis◎	Used traditionally as an anti-inflammatory, antiviral, antioxidant, and immune-enhancing herbal medicine, also preventative for colds and flu.	2,000 to 6,000 mg daily; or if a concentrated product, 200 mg daily
Probiotic	*Lactobacillus* species have been shown to boost immunity and reduce the incidence of respiratory infections and inflammatory reactions.	1 to 2 capsules/day
Reishi mushroom◎	This medicinal mushroom is a powerful immune-system tonic in a category of herbs called *adaptogens* that nourish the adrenals and specifically address the impact of SOS on your immune system, as you will learn in chapter 7. Reishi is especially effective for chronically recurring infections and prevents against viral infections.	3 to 9 g dried mushroom in capsules or tablets/ day or 2 to 4 mL tincture in water 2 to 3x/day
Vitamin D$_3$	Important immune-system and mood benefits, with thousands of research studies.	2,000 units/day of vitamin D$_3$. You may need as much as up to 4,000 IU of vitamin D$_3$ a day in the winter, or to bring yourself up to the optimal range if your vitamin D is low (see page 382).

SOS Rx: Herbs and Supplements to Boost Immunity		
Herb/ Supplement	**Uses and Cautions**	**Dose**
Zinc	Reduces inflammation in the intestinal lining. Has been shown not only to boost immunity, but also to be specifically effective at fighting infections in the herpesvirus family, which includes Epstein-Barr virus. Food sources rich in zinc include beef, lamb, turkey, pumpkin seeds, sesame tahini, lentils, garbanzo beans, cashews, and quinoa.	30 mg/day; take with meals to avoid nausea

Key: ⃠ = Not safe for use in pregnancy.

you're going to learn about an amazing group of herbs called *adaptogens* that are also powerful immune boosters.

SUPPORT DETOXIFICATION

The environmental toxic burden we're facing, along with diets insufficient in the nutrients we need for optimal detoxification functioning, has been overwhelming our intrinsic detoxification processes.

The biggest player in "detox" is your liver, which breaks down harmful chemicals and then packages them up for elimination (primarily through your bowels, and also your kidneys). Detoxification imbalances are at play in numerous conditions, including acne, allergies, hormonal problems (PMS, endometriosis, uterine fibroids, cyclic breast tenderness, and fertility problems, for example), chemical sensitivities, chronic fatigue, stubborn weight, headaches, autoimmune conditions, chronic inflammation, and much more. The liver is also a major site of conversion of inactive thyroid hormone (T_4) to the active form (T_3), so liver health is crucial for preventing symptoms of hypothyroidism.

SOS Rx: Natural Approaches to Stealth Infection		
Herb/ Supplement	**Uses and Cautions**	**Dose**
Echinacea	A gentle yet effective antiviral and immune tonic. I often include echinacea into a seasonal plan for a woman getting "every cold that goes around." It is safe enough for use in pregnancy and can be taken if you have an autoimmune condition, though check with your doctor first if you're on immunosuppressive medication.	300 to 500 mg up to 3 times daily
Lemon balm	Antiviral, relieves stress and anxiety. Research conducted over the past decade has demonstrated impressive results using lemon balm as an antiviral herb for the HSV.	300 to 1,200 mg daily in tea or capsules, 40 to 60 drops of tincture 1 to 3 times daily
Licorice⊘	Numerous studies have shown licorice preparations to have antiviral, anti-inflammatory, and a wide variety of immunomodulating effects. It should not be taken if you have high blood pressure.	150 to 300 mg daily
St. John's wort	St. John's wort has combined benefits on the nervous system. It works as an effective antidepressant, and as an antiviral, making it particularly appropriate when stress is an issue in viral reactivation or frequent viral infections.	300 to 600 mg daily

Key: ⊘ = Not safe for use in pregnancy.

Do the Detox Two-Step

1. Remove "the bad stuff" by reducing toxin exposure.

2. Add in "the good"—the right foods and supplements to support detoxification.

SOS Rx: Herbs and Supplements to Boost Detoxification		
Herb/ Supplement	**Uses and Cautions**	**Dose**
Artichoke leaf extract◎	Supports liver detoxification; is an antioxidant; and boosts detox compounds produced in the liver.	320 to 640 mg/day
Curcumin◎	Boosts glutathione production, and naturally supports detoxification.	1,200 to 2,400 mg/ day of extract
Green tea or green tea extract◎ **(decaffeinated)**	Boosts liver detoxification. It can be taken as a tea, but in extract form it is a potent supplement for weight loss, hormonal balance, and detox.	200 mg/day of green tea catechins or 4 to 8 cups of tea/day
Methylfolate	If you scored high on the detoxification questionnaire (page 114), have elevated homocysteine (page 384), or know you have one of the MTHFR gene mutations (page 384), make sure to get at least 800 mcg of methylfolate in a daily supplement.	800 mcg/day
N-acetylcysteine	Discussed on page 223, boosts detoxification by building up glutathione, one of your body's chief detoxifiers.	300 mg 3x/ day

Remove the Bad Stuff with Low-Toxin Living

"Rules" for low-toxin living:

Eat a wide variety of vital natural foods. Not junk. It's that simple. By doing this you avoid most of the agricultural and added chemicals that act as toxins in your body.

Eat only organic meats and dairy.

Follow the Environmental Working Group's Clean Fifteen and Dirty Dozen (page 151) for fruits and vegetables.

Herb/ Supplement	Uses and Cautions	Dose
Pycnogenol⊘	An extract of maritime pine bark, pycnogenol reduces inflammation, oxidative stress, cellular membrane and DNA damage, and damage due to the impact of chronically elevated blood sugar on the cells. It contains the same compounds, procyanidins, that make cacao, green tea extract, grapeseed extract, and berries so health-promoting and protective. Benefits include improved cognition and focus, reduction in harmful cholesterol, increased sense of well-being, reduction in inflammatory cytokines (after just five days of use), lasting reduction of symptoms with endometriosis, reduced menopausal symptoms, reduction in wrinkles, and reduced osteoarthritis pain. It may also reduce fat accumulation that happens as a result of inflammation, and improve insulin sensitivity.	100 to 200 mg/day
Schizandra⊘	Schizandra, which you'll learn more about on page 254, is a liver tonic that appears to protect the liver, and acts as an antioxidant. Its effects on the liver may be due to anxiety and stress reduction that lessen the adverse effects of stress on the liver. It also increases glutathione production and appears to have protective effects against damage from environmental toxins, medications, and heavy metals. Consider taking this if you have Hashimoto's and poor T_4 to T_3 conversion (see page 227).	20 to 30 drops of extract 1 or 2x/ day or 2 to 4 capsules/ day

Key: ⊘ = Not safe for use in pregnancy.

Use natural household cleaners, cosmetics, and body products, as well as organic lawn and garden care products, household paints, and building materials and furnishings to the extent you're able.

Avoid unnecessary medications. In addition to those I mentioned that impact your digestion system, many medications are metabolized (broken down) and processed by your liver, and as such, many can overload your body's own natural detoxification systems. For example, Tylenol uses up your natural stores of glutathione (that's why giving NAC is our primary treatment when patients come into the hospital for Tylenol poisoning). I am not suggesting you go off of any of your currently prescribed medications—in fact, please don't without discussing this with the practitioner who prescribed them—but to the extent that you can going forward, learn to use natural remedies whenever possible for common symptoms.

My website, avivaromm.com, has an entire section, Natural MD Library, devoted to helping you do this. For a start, you can use the recommendations on page 214 under "Natural Alternatives to Common Pain Medications" next time you have a headache or menstrual cramps, instead of automatically first reaching for Tylenol or Motrin. You'd be amazed at how effective many natural remedies can be for run-of-the-mill symptoms, from colds to fevers to aches and pains.

Add in the Good

The foods you're eating on the Reboot are exactly what your body needs to support detoxification. You'll find that within days to weeks your energy, health, and mood are picking up! Additionally, take a probiotic, make sure to emphasize leafy greens and a rainbow of fresh veggies and berries, and add several of the super-detox botanicals and supplements on page 228 for an extra boost, for example, curcumin, though you may be on one or more of these by now.

HEAVY METAL DETOXIFICATION

The most common heavy metal burden is mercury, almost all of which is coming from fish intake; taking fish out of the diet (switch to an omega-3 supplement) is often enough to normalize mercury levels, which can happen in just a few months. Chlorella, buffered ascorbic acid, and fiber are safe supplements commonly used to bind and excrete (chelate) heavy metals. Your body uses NAC to manufacture glutathione, which also helps to clean up heavy metals, as well as other environmental toxins. One lesser-known aspect of probiotics is their ability, through your digestive tract, to bind heavy metals. A number of environmental microorganisms have long been known for their ability to bind metals, but less well appreciated are human gastrointestinal bacteria. Species of *Lactobacillus*, present in the mouth, gut, and vagina and available in fermented foods and from probiotic supplements, have the ability to bind and detoxify some of these substances.

If you suspect you have been exposed to a high level of heavy metals, and by the end of the SOS Solution are having resistant symptoms, work with a functional or integrative medicine doctor who can help you to obtain appropriate testing and treatment to reduce your heavy metal body burden. You should not intentionally try to do a heavy metal detox within three months of getting pregnant, during pregnancy, or while breast-feeding, as this can send a toxic download to your baby.

HOME AND PERSONAL CARE DETOX

You've been making big changes in your diet to eliminate toxic food triggers. You'll want to support that good work with clearing out the cosmetics and household cleaning products that can be harming your health.

Green Up Your House: It's Easier Than You Think

A rule in environmental science called the *precautionary principle* nicely boils down to something I've been saying to patients for thirty years: *When in doubt, leave it out.* When you're unsure about the safety of a food, household cleaner, or body product, find an alternative. It's clear that even small amounts of endocrine disrupters can lead your hormonal symphony (including your thyroid hormones) into confusion and chaos. Pretty much any product these days can be replaced with a healthier alternative, and it's amazing what vinegar, baking soda, and a little lemon can do, but if that's too "crunchy" for you, there's no shortage of natural cleaning products on the market.

Dry Brush for Detox Support

Your skin is your largest detoxification organ, eliminating 30 percent of your body's waste each day. Dry brushing takes five minutes, is free beyond the cost of the brush, and can do wonders for stimulating your skin and removing toxins.

Here's how you do it:

1. Purchase a natural (not synthetic) bristle dry brush. A very long handle gives you the best reach to your whole body.

2. Stand naked in the shower, with the water off.

3. Start by brushing your neck and shoulders, working your way over your arms, down your back and belly, buttocks, thighs, legs, all the way down to your feet, going in a gently clockwise overlapping circular motion several times, over as much of your body's surface as you can, slowly. Be gentle but firm and take care with sensitive areas (breasts, thighs).

4. When you're done, turn on the shower and rinse off, starting with warm water and ending with a brisk, cool rinse. Pat dry and apply a gentle natural moisturizer.

Dirty Looks

Your body products go way more than skin deep. From the time she's a teen, the average woman applies literally dozens of chemicals before she even leaves home in the morning for school or work, hidden in hair and body products, cosmetics, and perfume. We absorb these chemicals into our circulation, where, like the other endocrine disrupters I've talked about, they do their dirty work of increasing our estrogen exposure. What can you do? Lower your exposure to toxins absorbed through your skin with a "beauty products makeover." I personally like the approach that is often attributed to French women: less is more. Still, if you like to do it up, there are some great cosmetic companies with products that will dazzle. (See "Resources" on page 393.)

Genetics, Mood, and Detoxification

There are two common inherited genetic mutations: MTHFR, discussed on page 384, and one called COMT, which determines the ease with which you detoxify environmental toxins, hormones, and adrenaline. When you don't detoxify well, you are more susceptible to chemical sensitivities and related illnesses (for example, chronic fatigue syndrome, fibromyalgia, endometriosis), and also anxiety and depression.

If you scored high on the detoxification questionnaire, if you have a history of miscarriage or complications, or a strong family history of heart disease (suggestive of the MTHFR gene), or if coffee, thrill rides, or scary movies leave you feeling like your heart is beating out of your chest and you're on red alert (suggestive of COMT), then consider daily supplementation with methylfolate (800 mcg daily), vitamin B-complex, and SAMe (400 mg daily) to help circumvent the impact of these mutations.

The Dirty Truth About Feminine Hygiene Products

In 1982, reports first started being published about the presence of dioxin, pesticides, and other toxins in sanitary pads and tampons that act as carcinogens and endocrine disrupters. Other chemicals are also found in douches, feminine wipes, and lubes, all products that do not have to be regulated the same way that foods and pharmaceuticals do, so it's basically open season on the ingredients—which increases risks of early puberty, endometriosis, and cancer, to name a few problems. I recommend switching to organic products. This can make a difference in your health, particularly if you're struggling with endometriosis, PMS, fibroids, or fertility problems.

SOS Rx: Herbs for Hormone Balance		
Herb/ Supplement	**Uses and Cautions**	**Dose**
Chaste berry (Vitex) The women's hormone-balancing herb	Chaste berry, or Vitex, is nature's hormonal balancer and one of my favorite herbal medicines for women in all stages of life. While it doesn't contain any hormones, it improves estrogen and progesterone balance, kicks PMS's butt, easing depression and irritability, bloating, breast tenderness, and cravings, and helps to regulate menstrual cycles. Vitex reduces environmentally induced inflammation that contributes to endometriosis, promotes fertility, and is used to prevent miscarriage, possibly due to effects on progesterone. Vitex relieves vaginal dryness, sleep problems, and hot flashes associated with menopause. Try for a minimum of three months for best results; you can continue to take it as long as you are benefiting. Discontinue if it makes your mood low; this is a rare but possible side effect.	500 mg in capsule 1 to 2x/ day or 40 to 60 drops of tincture up to 3x/ day
Maca⊘	This is a gentle, safe herb for restoring cortisol balance and as a result balances female hormones, and can be taken medicinally or added to your smoothies (see page 318). See discussion on page 251.	

Key: ⊘ = Not safe for use in pregnancy.

FROM HORMONAL CHAOS TO HORMONAL HARMONY

The Root Causes of SOS and the downstream effects, including "cortisol steal," microbiome disruptions, excess weight, insulin resistance, inflammation, environmental toxins, and overwhelmed detoxification systems all lead down the same road: hormonal imbalances.

So what's a girl to do? The SOS Solution! The beauty is that you're already doing all of the right things proven to balance hormones, resolve infertility, heal endometriosis, break the cycle of monthly breast tenderness, irregular periods, and PMS, and boost libido. You're taking the very steps needed to bring your hormones from chaos back to harmony—and you'll learn even more about how nourishing your adrenals and supporting your thyroid can help, in the next chapter, along with how to use some of my favorite herbs, the adaptogens. For extra support to naturally balance your hormones, you can also use "SOS Rx: Herbs for Hormone Balance" and see articles on specific hormonal problems at my website, avivaromm.com.

WEEK 2: REPAIR, DAY BY DAY

Week 2 Sample Daily Meal Plan

Breakfast Example

8–12-oz. Smoothie (Shake)
or
Breakfast protein + good-quality fat

Lunch Example

Protein entrée + green veggie + rainbow veggie + energy veggie + ¼ cup cooked grain (if tolerated) + good-quality fat

Dinner Example

Protein entrée + green veggie + rainbow veggie + energy veggie + ½ cup cooked grain (if tolerated) + good-quality fat + small amount of fermented veggie (if tolerated)

Week 2.
Sample Daily Menus and Lifestyle

	Day 8	Day 9	Day 10
Morning practice	The Quickie meditation (page 199)	Dry brush (page 232) in morning shower	5 minutes of deep breathing (page 191) and stretch
Fresh Start	Drink a glass of room-temperature or warm water with a squeeze of lemon.		
Breakfast + Daily Dose Supplements	Smoothie Bar	Frittata + mixed greens with Olive Oil Lemon Dressing	Smoothie Bar
Mid-morning	Snack Stash option	Rise and Shine muffin or Power Balls	Snack Stack option
Mindful lunch + SOS Solution Supplements (if you've personalized your plan ahead)	Fresh Turkey "Russian" Wrap or Vegan Nori Wrap	The Middle East Board	It's a Wrap option
Mid-afternoon	Coconut yogurt with raw cacao nibs and berries or Olive Oil Granola	Snack Stash option	Snack Stash option

Day 11	Day 12	Day 13	Day 14
The Quickie meditation	Dry brush in morning shower	5 minutes of deep breathing and stretch	Day off
Breakfast Scramble or Omelet + optional mixed greens with Olive Oil Lemon Dressing	Smoothie Bar	Breakfast Scramble or Omelet + optional mixed greens with Olive Oil Lemon Dressing	Power Parfait with optional Olive Oil Granola
Jump Start Detox Nutrient Broth	½ apple sliced with 1 tbsp. almond butter	Coconut yogurt with raw cacao nibs and berries or Olive Oil Granola	Snack Stash option
Spicy Sushi Buddha Bowl with leftover Salmon from dinner	Leftover frittata	Cajun Lime Fish "Taco" + Not Your Mother's Slaw + Guacamole (vegan option is to use Mexican Black Beans) (Leftovers)	Make Your Own Salad option
½ size any It's a Wrap	Snack Stash option	Jump Start Detox Nutrient Broth	Snack Stash option

Week 2
Sample Daily Menus and Lifestyle

	Day 8	Day 9	Day 10
Cortisol Reset	Reset your cortisol for the evening with 15 minutes of any Replenish Repair Kit practice		
Dinner + SOS Solution Supplements (if you've personalized your plan ahead)	Thai Steak Salad (make extra steak for next day; also chicken or vegan option) + ½ cup cooked grain of your choice	Basil Coconut Curry Tagine + Sautéed Spinach (or Dandelion Greens) and Pine Nuts or Curried "Popcorn" Cauliflower + ½ cup cooked grain (brown basmati rice)	Miso-Glazed Salmon + Sautéed Orange Ginger Carrots + Roasted Brussels Sprouts + ½ cup cooked grain of your choice
Replenish Self-Care	Replenish Bath	Gratitude or Worry Journal	Digital Detox and read

Day 11	Day 12	Day 13	Day 14
Green Tara Lentil Bowl + "Popcorn" Cauliflower + sautéed spinach	Cajun Lime Fish "Taco" + Not Your Mother's Slaw + Guacamole (vegan option is to use Mexican Black Beans)	Broccoli Sesame or Eastern Wisdom Buddha Bowl	Butternut Squash Curry Coconut Soup + Moroccan Spinach, Coconut, and Chickpeas + ½ cup cooked basmati rice
Gratitude or Worry Journal	Digital Detox and read	Replenish Bath	Gratitude or Worry Journal

I choose to make the rest of my life the best of my life.

—LOUISE HAY

RECHARGE

Nourish Your Adrenals and Thyroid

Reboot: Remove Food Triggers

Reframe: Chronic Emotional and Mental Stress

Repair: Root Causes and SOS Damage

Recharge: Your Adrenals and Thyroid

Replenish: No More Running on Empty

The part can never be well unless the whole is well.

—PLATO

WELCOME TO WEEK THREE of the SOS Solution. At this point you've done the heavy lifting needed to get your self-repair mechanisms into high gear. I hope you're already noticing more energy when you wake up in the morning and throughout the day, no 4:00 P.M. energy crash or sugar cravings, regular and better digestion, and more and deeper sleep. Ideally, you feel less puffy and swollen, and it feels like someone's turned the windshield wipers on in your brain! But even if you haven't started to notice gigantic changes, do pay attention to the little wins, because your body is in the process of healing, which is a process that can take time.

This week you'll be Recharging your energy glands—your adrenals and thyroid—with the exact nourishment they need. Why did I wait to talk about these important organs when they got top billing on the book cover? Because starting directly with the branches often misses the roots. While herbs and supplements for your adrenals and supplements and hormone replacement for your thyroid can make a world of difference in your energy, metabolism, mood, mind, hormones, and weight, they don't address the deeper causes that got you to where you were when you picked up this book. In the long run, you'd still be at the mercy of Root Cause imbalances, which could show up in any area of your health. Taking a thyroid medication, for example, replaces low or missing thyroid hormones, but it doesn't reverse autoimmunity—which could then strike another organ or system— nor does it reverse inflammation, fight stealth infections, or reduce environmental toxins that can be at the heart of the problem.

You have to heal the Root Causes. And that's exactly what you've been doing. Now you'll top that off with some targeted support.

The first part of this chapter, "Nourish Your Adrenals," is for every woman— because we all need it. And I don't want you to learn to protect your energy the hard way—when it's really late in the game. This section is especially important for you if you scored high on the SOS questionnaires (page 97). The second part of this chapter, "Heal Your Thyroid," will give you the answers you've been looking for regarding thyroid lab results, medications, and how to support your thyroid function with herbs and nutrients that can make all the difference. You'll also continue with the final week of your 21-Day Reboot. If your thyroid is calling out for help, make sure to also nourish your adrenals at the same time. They depend on each other.

As you move through this chapter, continue on the Reboot, and take your Daily Dose Supplements and any Root Cause-specific supplements you've added. Sprinkle in some Replenish Self-Care, and remember to track how you feel in relation to what you're eating.

NOURISH YOUR ADRENALS

When I'm tired, I rest. I say, "I can't be a superwoman today."

—Jada Pinkett Smith

At thirty-four, Wren, a long-distance runner and nutrition coach, had an "impeccable diet," as she noted in her health forms before her first appointment with me. She felt like she should be on top of the world.

But she wasn't.

She was working fourteen-hour days to manage her coaching practice, was training hard for marathons, and was exhausted all the time. After a marathon, she invariably got sick with a cold that would linger. "The other odd symptom I'm having," she told me, "is nighttime food binging. About an hour after I go to sleep, I wake up and feel truly famished. I down table-spoons of almond butter or coconut butter right off the spoon. Then I go back to sleep. I also wake up at about 6:00 A.M., and am especially exhausted in the morning—I feel groggy, like I've been drugged. It's not until I have one or two cups of coffee that I finally start to feel awake. I'm finding that my focus is off with my clients, and I'm just not recalling nutrition information like I should. Also my periods are completely irregular and my boobs hurt so badly I can't even put on my bra. My sex drive is in the toilet, and I'm a 'b-word' for a whole week before my period starts—and it's really impacting my relationship with my boyfriend."

Upon review of Wren's three-day food journal, something all of my patients bring for me to review at each visit (for a copy of my three-day food journal see avivaromm.com/adrenal-thyroid-revolution), I discovered that while her diet did consist of only high-quality foods, she wasn't eating nearly enough to meet her energy outputs. She subsisted largely on green juices for breakfast, a salad for lunch, and a handful of almonds in the afternoon, before her last meal at 4:00 P.M., usually another salad or a small amount of steamed vegetables and some gluten-free crackers. She was usu-ally awake until at least midnight, but didn't eat again before bed. She was completely carb-free. Sure enough, twenty-four-hour salivary cortisol test-ing (page 387) showed a highly elevated evening cortisol, a big stress-related cortisol spike at 1:00 A.M., exactly the time she was waking up each night with intense cravings for almond and coconut butter, which she'd binge out on before going back to sleep. A very low morning cortisol level was keep-ing her from getting going easily in the morning. Instead she felt "groggy" and "hungover."

I got Wren on the SOS Solution, including increasing her overall amount of food intake, increasing her dietary fat (what her body was craving at night!), and adding an evening meal that contained energy vegetables such as sweet potatoes, white potatoes, and winter squash, as well as a small amount of grains. Wren adopted a more gentle athletic training schedule

HPA Axis Quick Review

The HPA axis is the stress response system that starts in your brain, extends to your adrenal glands, and impacts pretty much every system and function in your body. When it's stuck in the ON position, you're wired, overstimulated, irritable, and living as if you're constantly on red alert—your blood sugar, blood pressure, and digestive, nervous, hormonal, and immune systems respond accordingly, and you end up with all of the problems associated with SOS-O. When your brain dials down the reaction to protect you from chronic overload, and with it, dials back your cortisol and adrenaline production, you end up in SOS-E, feeling exhausted, sometimes deeply, and your reactions are low—in everything from your metabolism, mood, and immunity to your mind, blood pressure, and hormones. Your thyroid function gets dialed down, too, so that you save energy, but hypothyroidism leaves you feeling sick and tired.

that added restorative yoga, and began taking a selection of the herbs and supplements from "SOS Rx: Adaptogens," and her life went from red alert to You Zone.

Wren's story might be different from yours—but most of us can relate to the constant pressures we're under to work more, be more, do more—and the price we're paying for our chronic overwhelm—exhaustion, brain fog, food cravings, frequent illness, stress and anxiety, poor sleep, the hormonal roller coaster, and more. These are all downstream effects of SOS—the impact of your stress response being stuck in survival mode and producing hormones and neurotransmitters that impact every system of your body, from the communication of your microbiome, belly fat cells, and brain influencing your appetite, food cravings, and weight storage as a protective mechanism against inadequate nutrition and the primitive response against famine, to ramping up your immune system so that you get sick too often, or worse, unwittingly sabotage your own cells with autoimmune disease. Also important to remember is that there are many kinds of overwhelm that can cause SOS—life stress is just one of these. Anything that overwhelms any of your body's systems—your digestive system, your detoxification system, or your immune system, can throw you into SOS.

The good news is that every SOS Solution step you've taken so far has been a vote in favor of supporting your adrenals and getting you out of overwhelm—and thus SOS.

- You've removed inflammatory triggers from your diet and environment.

- You're nourishing your body with the nutrients you need.

- You're hitting the pause button more often so you can take care of yourself and keep your energy replenished instead of depleted.

- You're working on getting better sleep.

- You're using tools from your Replenish Repair Kit to reset your cortisol each day and keep yourself out of SOS.

The next step is to add in a bit of extra help from nature's pharmacy: the adaptogens, a special group of herbs that will help you to take your healing efforts to the next level, and specific nutrients that help to restore and nourish your stress response system. If it's become overactivated, they'll help calm it down, and if it's gotten sluggish from wear and tear, you can restore it and enjoy more energy and resilience.

Adaptogens: Ancient Medicines for Modern Times

Adaptogens are a category of herbal medicines that are specifically restorative to the hypothalamic pituitary adrenal axis (see "HPA Axis Quick Review," on the facing page). Used for centuries in China and India, they are considered the "royalty" of herbs for helping you respond to stress, restore health, vitality, immunity, stamina, and sense of well-being. Adaptogens help your body to cope more easily with the demands of everyday life, providing a sense of calm and energy at a deep level. They also help you to establish a new stress set point—reprogramming your nervous system, boosting energy and relieving chronic fatigue, enhancing memory and mental stamina, improving mood, calming inflammation, regulating immunity, and helping to restore hormone balance. They are remarkable in that they normalize adrenal function whether you are in SOS-O or SOS-E.

Importantly, the goal isn't to use adaptogens to allow you to just keep going at a twenty-first-century pace—the goal is to hit the pause button more often, live at a healthier pace, and use adaptogens to help restore

Warning: Addison's, Conn's, and Other Adrenal Diseases

If you've been diagnosed with an adrenal disease such as Addison's or Conn's disease, while you can follow the SOS Solution, do not discontinue any adrenal medications you've been prescribed, and please discuss the use of adaptogens and adrenal support supplements with your practitioner *before* taking any.

you—and to help you get through when things do get hectic, which, of course, does inevitably happen at times in real life. The science behind adaptogens was pioneered by Soviet researchers, eager to find substances that could enable the increase of productivity and work hours of military and production forces. However, our goal isn't ramping up your "productivity" at the expense of your health. That is the opposite of the way we're using adaptogens here—our goal is to Repair and Replenish, not push harder and more.

In addition to everything you're already doing to heal SOS, the supplements in this section will specifically help you get to the root of your personal energy crisis: SOS. They regulate and heal your stress response by naturally dialing down your brain's perception that you're in survival mode, while dialing up your resilience and resistance to stress, and with that, normalizing your immune system's responses, resetting your hormones, improving your clarity of thinking, balancing your blood sugar, and more. You have to do your part to also remove the SOS triggers.

While it might seem a bold statement to say that a group of herbs can help to heal virtually every body system, based on what you now know of the far-ranging effects of SOS you might not be that surprised. The naturally occurring wealth of chemical compounds they contain heal, nourish, and reset the HPA axis from your brain's stress centers all the way to the downstream organs and systems—your immune system, endocrine system, and metabolism, for example, which are impacted by the stress response.

Here's what women have said to me after starting adaptogens:

JL: *My sympathetic nervous system's [fight-or-flight] "inner motor song" was the recurring theme music from* Run Lola Run—*cortisol pushing and racing and pushing me to mental exhaustion. However ... a recalculation of priorities, slowing down, and the use of adaptogenic botanicals (which you have beautifully suggested) have helped to shift my being into more of a parasympathetic mode [rest and digest]. Now my theme music is a lovely Brazilian samba—still good energy but smoother on the system.*

ML: *I just recently started taking ashwagandha and have noticed such major improvements! My anxiety has been cut in half, I'm not as hungry as often, and I just feel more energized! Can't wait to see how it helps as I continue to take it!*

Choosing Your Adaptogens

I've categorized the herbs in the following table as calming, stimulating, or nourishing and have given you symptoms and a "personality picture" to help you select the adaptogen or adaptogens that are right for you. I generally recommend starting with one of the more calming or nourishing adaptogens—for example, reishi mushroom, ashwagandha, and maca, then progressively adding additional herbs based on the descriptions that most relate to your symptoms and needs.

Select the adaptogen to start that seems the most specific to your needs based on the descriptions in the table below, and then, over the course of a couple of weeks, add additional choices to reach a combination of three or more. Individual responses vary. Starting slowly allows you to pay attention to how you respond. There's quite a bit of crossover in the effects of these herbs, so they can be used somewhat interchangeably, but each also has its own slightly unique "personality." You'll find variety combination products on the market that include several of these together, often combining the herbs and nutritional supplements.

Additional adaptogens you can also include are ginseng (stimulating, energizing, balances blood sugar), licorice (strong anti-inflammatory, very helpful for deep adrenal exhaustion with low blood pressure, dizziness, low cortisol—not for use if you have high blood pressure), and cordyceps (like other medicinal mushrooms, profoundly nourishes the immune system and calms the nervous system). Also see Relora on page 205 for reducing cortisol, improving DHEA, and improving sleep.

The SOS Rx: Adaptogens©—Women's Adrenal Support

Herb/ Supplement	Especially for You If You . . .	Uses and Cautions	Dose
Ashwagandha The mind, mood, and muscle soother Calming, nourishing	Are tired and wired Are nervous or anxious Are unable to fall asleep easily at night Experience chronic joint aches and pains, arthritis Struggle with memory and brain fog Have chronic fatigue syndrome, fibromyalgia, or chronic muscle tension	Ashwagandha is for deep exhaustion. It's known for gentle, soothing, calming effects, improving sleep, relieving anxiety, and alleviating nervous system exhaustion while improving memory and learning. It's also relaxing for muscles and reduces inflammation while acting as a mild pain reliever, so it's excellent if you're struggling with osteoarthritis or rheumatoid arthritis, chronic fatigue, or fibromyalgia. Ashwagandha has also been shown to improve blood glucose in diabetics and to improve cholesterol. Use cautiously or avoid if you are sensitive to plants in the nightshade family.	3 to 6 g dried herb in capsule/ day or 1 to 4 mL (20 to 80 drops) of tincture in water 3x/day

Start Low, Go Slow

Occasionally I get reports that an adaptogen increased anxiety, irritability, or worsened, rather than improved, a sleep or energy problem. The stimulating adaptogens rhodiola, eleuthero, or ginseng enhance mental and cognitive function and strongly boost physical stamina, so if you're already in SOS-O and overstimulated, they might be overstimulating to a small number of people. This could also happen if you're exceptionally exhausted in SOS-E and the adaptogen stimulation is a bit too much. The

Herb/ Supplement	Especially for You If You...	Uses and Cautions	Dose
Eleuthero The performance and focus enhancer Stimulating	Are struggling with brain fog or need more mental alertness and clarity Are getting sick a lot or have a stealth infection such as EBV Need detoxification support Work night shifts or very long hours that interfere with a normal sleep routine (this includes being a new mom!)	One of the best-researched adaptogens, eleuthero increases mental alertness and performance, increases energy and stamina, reduces stress and fatigue, reduces dream-disrupted sleep and insomnia, enhances immunity, especially against viral infections, and improves detoxification. It helps build muscle and prevents its breakdown as we age, and it relieves inflammation and pain in osteoarthritis. There have been rare cases of insomnia reported with eleuthero; if you have insomnia, select a different adaptogen or consider taking eleuthero before noon. Not if you have insomnia; not recommended for those with high blood pressure.	2 to 3 g dried root in capsule daily or 2 to 4 mL tincture in water 2 to 3x/ day

effects dissipate after the herb is discontinued but highlight the importance of finding the right adaptogen for *you*. I recommend starting at the lowest end of the dose range and frequency, staying at that dose if you're noticing improvement, and increasing slowly over a few weeks to reach the higher dose if you're not feeling optimized yet. Then simply adjust your dose down or up as needed. Admittedly, this can take some trial and error, so start low and go slow.

The SOS Rx: Adaptogens©—Women's Adrenal Support			
Herb/ Supplement	**Especially for You If You. . .**	**Uses and Cautions**	**Dose**
Holy basil The vitalizer Nourishing	Feel you need an overall gentle tonic for mind, mood, and immunity Are struggling with depression, anxiety, or low mood Have sleep problems Want help shifting to a new mindset and making healthy lifestyle changes Need more mental clarity Have chronic inflammation Have high blood sugar, cholesterol, or triglycerides	Holy or "sacred" basil calms the mind and spirit and promotes longevity. In Ayurvedic medicine it is called tulsi, which means "incomparable one." Holy basil improves energy and relieves fatigue, elevates mood, providing relief from anxiety and mild depression, and helps with nicotine withdrawal. It improves mental clarity, and increases motivation to make healthy lifestyle and mindset changes. Anti-inflammatory and antioxidant actions may protect the liver from stress and inflammation-related damage. It lowers blood glucose, triglycerides, and cholesterol, and improves immunity to common colds and bronchitis.	2 to 3 mL (40 to 60 drops) tincture in water 3x/day

What Should I Expect?

The amount of time it takes to see improvement with adaptogens is variable, and depends on the symptoms you're seeking to treat and finding the right herb for you at the proper dose. You should notice some improvement in your energy, sleep, mood, sense of well-being or inner calm, and mental

Herb/ Supplement	Especially for You If You . . .	Uses and Cautions	Dose
Maca[◎] The mother of hormone nourishers Nourishing	Want more vitality and feel you are missing deep nourishment Have low libido Have hormonal imbalances Want to improve your fertility Want to improve your mood, have anxiety or depression	A nourishing, restorative tonic. The Quechua Indians of Peru consider maca a food that promotes mental acuity, physical vitality, endurance, and stamina. It is also considered an aphrodisiac tonic that enhances sexual desire and performance, and is reputed to increase fertility, reduce anxiety and depression, and lower measures of sexual dysfunction in postmenopausal women. Dried maca root is rich in essential amino acids, iodine, iron, and magnesium, as well as sterols that may possess a wide range of activities that support adrenal and hormone function. It is used to treat menstrual and menopausal symptoms as well.	75 to 100 mg/ day

clarity and focus within a couple of weeks of starting. For the treatment of muscular relaxation, sleep improvement, and pain relief, you can see improvements in a few days. Expect it to take four to six weeks, up to several months, to experience improvements in PCOS and fertility problems, and for the blood pressure, blood sugar, and blood-lowering effects to be observable in lab tests.

While some research suggests that adaptogens work optimally in bursts of two to twelve weeks, traditionally they are used for extended periods

The SOS Rx: Adaptogens©—Women's Adrenal Support

Herb/ Supplement	Especially for You If You. . .	Uses and Cautions	Dose
Reishi mushroom© The immune nourisher Calming, nourishing	Want to improve your sleep quality and depth Want to boost your immunity Need help with detoxification Feel chronically overwhelmed and jangled	Reishi mushroom is highly regarded in Chinese medicine to nourish and support adrenal function. While best known for promoting immunity and reducing inflammation, reishi also helps support the body's abilities to detoxify from environmental exposures and calms the nervous system, and may be taken before bed to promote deeper, relaxing, and restorative sleep. Possibly avoid if you are allergic to mushrooms.	3 to 9 g dried mushroom in capsules or tablets daily or 2 to 4 mL tincture in water 2 to 3x/ day

of months at a time, and even up to a year. The bottom line is that you can take them for as long as you're getting benefit. If the benefits wane, take a two-week break and restart, or try a different adaptogen or blend. Of course, it's still important to focus on improved sleep practices and to get into your relaxation response at least once daily, rather than relying solely on adaptogens to reset your HPA axis response.

Can I Take These Supplements While Taking Other Supplements?

Yes, adaptogens can be taken with other supplements, and in fact I often recommend them in combination with those in "SOS Rx: Natural Support for Sleep, Mind, and Mood" (page 204). You can also take them with your thyroid hormone supplementation, and any of the other supplements in this book.

What About with Prescription Medications?

I always recommend checking with your primary care provider or specialist before starting herbs when taking prescription medications and working

Herb/ Supplement	Especially for You If You. . .	Uses and Cautions	Dose
Rhodiola The spirit calmer Stimulating	Struggle with anxiety Have mental fatigue or brain fog Want to heal from exercise-related inflammation, damage, or SOS Have anxiety or depression Feel irritable and burned out Struggle with fibromyalgia or chronic headaches Want to boost your libido or fertility	Rhodiola is perhaps the most important adaptogen for anxiety. It supports mental and physical performance and stamina and reduces mental and physical fatigue while repairing exercise-induced muscle damage and inflammation and improving exercise recovery. While it shouldn't be taken before bed because it's stimulating, its mood-regulating and nervous-system-supporting effects lead to improved sleep and reduced stress, irritability, and "burn-out." It also boosts the immune system, decreasing the frequency of colds and infections. It is used in the treatment of chronic fatigue syndrome as well as fibromyalgia and chronic stress headaches. Rhodiola boosts libido and fertility. It improves appetite and may be helpful in eating disorders, which often arise from SOS. Avoid if you have bipolar depression with manic behavior.	100 to 400 mg in capsules or tablets daily or 2 to 3 mL (40 to 60 drops) tincture in water 2 to 3x/ day Look for products labeled as standardized to 2 to 3% rosavin and 0.8 to 1% salidroside.

with an experienced integrative or functional medicine practitioner when starting an herbal plan if you're on medications, as interactions can occur. While this is thought to be rare with the adaptogens, they should not be taken if you are on blood pressure medications or immunosuppressive

The SOS Rx: Adaptogens©—Women's Adrenal Support			
Herb/ Supplement	**Especially for You If You...**	**Uses and Cautions**	**Dose**
Schizandra The detoxifier Stimulating	Have brain fog, memory, or focus problems Get tired out easily with physical exertion Have anxiety Need to support or boost your detoxification	Schizandra, revered as an elite tonic herb in traditional Chinese herbalism, is used to improve mental focus, while having calming, antianxiety effects. Schizandra is one of the primary herbs to protect the liver from damage, and appears to be effective at boosting both detoxification and clearance of toxins, especially environmental hormone disrupters. It's been widely used to enhance athletic performance and endurance, improving energy and stamina in general, and to relieve anxiety.	20 to 30 drops of extract 1 or 2x/ day or 2 to 4 capsules daily

drugs, and care should be taken if you are on medications for anxiety or depression.

Can I Take These Supplements While Trying to Conceive, During Pregnancy, or While Breast-Feeding?

Adaptogens can absolutely be taken while you are trying to conceive, and as you see in the chart above, several are used specifically to encourage fertility. Caveat: *discontinue as soon as you suspect you are pregnant.*

Good news for tired new moms, too: you can use adaptogens while you are breast-feeding. I recommend sticking with the more calming ones, and if your baby develops a rash or irritability, discontinue use and focus on the herbs and supplements in "SOS Rx: Natural Support for Sleep, Mind, and Mood" (page 204).

Herb/ Supplement	Especially for You If You . . .	Uses and Cautions	Dose
Shatavari The hormonal harmonizer, queen of women's adaptogens Nourishing	Feel you need rejuvenation, balance, and calm Have hormonal imbalances, including PMS, fertility, or menopausal problems	Shatavari is considered the "queen of herbs" in Ayurvedic medicine, where it is beloved as a rejuvenating tonic for women. It is nourishing and calming as well as hormonally balancing, and is used for irritability and many hormonal imbalances affecting the mood—for example, emotional symptoms of PMS and menopause. It is used as a fertility tonic and may be used for vaginal dryness, low libido, and sleep problems in perimenopause. Shatavari may improve insulin secretion and cholesterol levels. Avoid if you have a history of estrogen-receptor-positive cancer.	2 to 4 mL (40 to 80 drops) of tincture in water 2 to 3x/ day

Key: ⊘ = Not safe for use in pregnancy.

One of the more common questions I get about adaptogens is whether they can be taken in pregnancy. I understand how tired pregnancy can make you feel, but unfortunately I don't feel that there's enough safety data on the use of these herbs in pregnancy to recommend them at this time, and at least two, schizandra and licorice, are definitely not safe for use in pregnancy. Instead, see "SOS Rx: Natural Support for Sleep, Mind, and Mood" for safe, relaxing herbs you can take during pregnancy, and work with your midwife or doctor to determine whether there's an underlying reason for your pregnancy fatigue, particularly anemia or hypothyroidism.

SOS Rx: Women's Adrenal Support Nutrients		
Supplement	**Uses and Cautions**	**Dose**
Curcumin©	Unlike other adaptogens, which are based on whole plants, curcumin is an isolated plant compound, but early research suggests that it acts very much like an adaptogen, calming SOS-related stress, and is so important to every aspect of healing your Root Causes and SOS that I had to include it as one. Emerging research is confirming that curcumin reverses the effects of chronic stress and alleviates depression. Many of these effects are due to decreased inflammation with improved baseline cortisol levels, bringing them to nonstressed levels. It is a highly effective antioxidant, improves cholesterol (lowering "bad" LDL and increasing "good" HDL), improves adiponectin, a compound in VAT (visceral adipose tissue, or visceral abdominal fat) that protects against problems in hunger and fullness cross-talk, prevents against insulin resistance, improves intestinal motility, and may prevent cognitive decline.	1,200 to 2,400 mg/day of extract

Additional Adrenal Support

The supplements in the table above and on the next page provide important additional support for the adrenal glands and the stress response system. New data on curcumin show that many of its effects may be in part due to its ability to reset the stress response, while the additional supplements play a supportive role in rebalancing cortisol, and vitamin C restores what is used up by the adrenal glands in responding to stress.

Supplement	Uses and Cautions	Dose
Phosphatydil serine (PS)⊘	A compound similar to a dietary fat and found widely in the brain and nervous system, PS reduces excess cortisol and adrenaline release under stress. It has many adaptogen-like effects: improving mood, physical energy, and cognitive function, including enhancing memory, attention, and information processing speed, while also improving exercise capacity.	100 mg 3x/day
Vitamin B$_5$	Vitamin B$_5$ is included in many adaptogen blends for its purported ability to reduce high cortisol production under stress.	500 mg/day
Vitamin B$_6$	Important in the production of stress neurotransmitters as well as the production of relaxing neurotransmitters, including GABA and serotonin. Taken at bedtime, it rebalances overnight cortisol, preventing spikes that can cause night waking and morning fatigue.	50 to 100 mg before bed
Vitamin C	Found abundantly in the adrenal cortex, where it plays an important anti-inflammatory role protecting the adrenals, vitamin C is depleted by stress. Supplementation helps to normalize cortisol and replenishes the adrenal glands.	1,500 to 3,000 mg/day with bioflavonoids. Too much will cause loose stools; reduce your dose if that occurs. Do not exceed 2,000 mg/ day in pregnancy.

Key: ⊘ = Not safe for use in pregnancy.

HEAL YOUR THYROID

Claire, a cardiologist and the mother of two young girls, came to see me because she was sick and tired of feeling "fatigued, frumpy, and fat," as she put it. She completed a grueling medical residency in her last month of pregnancy, and only a few weeks later she was seeing thirty-five patients a day, juggling to keep up with paperwork, and trying to be "a perfect mom" when she got home from work. Three years and another baby later, Claire stepped onto her bathroom scale because she couldn't button her pants, and discovered she'd gained twenty pounds.

Sitting on the edge of her tub, she started sobbing and soon began taking stock of how she was really feeling. She felt tired all the time and unenthusiastic, had been ignoring pain in her wrist for months, had no sex drive, had high blood pressure when she checked herself at work, and was eating cookies like there was no tomorrow. She was bloated and constipated, which the cookies made worse, but she couldn't stop. Her usual glass of wine before bed had become two most nights, more on the weekends. The only saving graces were that she slept like a log and her lovely daughters were healthy.

I explained SOS to Claire. She got it. Teary, she took a deep breath and said, "Yup, that sounds like me. Let's get to work, Dr. Romm. I want to live a long life for my kids." I started Claire on the SOS Solution Reboot with an easy morning meditation practice, while we waited for lab results to return. When they did, I phoned Claire. She had low iron, low vitamin D, and severe Hashimoto's. I could hear her sigh. "I'm so relieved," she said. "All this time I'd been chalking my symptoms up to laziness—my willpower is gone." Still, she blamed herself for driving her thyroid into the ground. I gently reminded her that this was her body's wake-up call to her, and now that she heard it, she could make the changes she needed.

Claire was motivated. She took up the morning meditation practice, started going to yoga class once a week, learned to keep her blood sugar steady, and supplemented the nutrients she was low in. Her mood quickly improved, and with a low dose of natural thyroid replacement, she had fantastic energy and began to lose weight. Over time her joint pain disappeared, too. For the first time in years, she felt like she had the energy to take control of her food choices, and her life, too, making it her priority to set better boundaries for work, rest, and play.

Claire is just one of literally tens of millions of women who struggle with similar symptoms, as well as a host of others that can, in serious cases, devastate women's lives. Fortunately for Claire, she found the help she needed pretty quickly and got the treatment she needed to turn things around. Sadly, millions of women go for years without a proper diagnosis, experiencing infertility and miscarriages, depression and anxiety, embarrassing and confusing weight gain, and sometimes debilitating fatigue, too often dismissed because their labs seem to be normal, underdiagnosed because of lab test misinterpretation, or told by their doctors that they do not even need labs. Some have symptoms that are much less severe—but they live their lives just not feeling great. On page 389 you'll find insights into being an empowered health consumer so you *can* get what you need—and have a right to—in partnership with your health care provider.

The SOS Solution and Your Thyroid

Claire's story is a reminder of the connection between SOS and hypothyroidism. It's clear that her symptoms didn't come out of thin air. She was burned out, losing sleep, struggling with perfectionism, and deficient in several nutrients, probably for the entire three years leading up to the diagnosis. She had multiple Root Causes that could have brought her to her situation. It's also a reminder of the importance of taking care of ourselves, and not letting symptoms slide just because we're busy. Remember, we have to put on our oxygen masks, too.

Just to recap from earlier in this book, all of the five Root Causes that lead to SOS are also Root Causes of hypothyroidism. SOS itself puts the body into a state of overdrive and alert that signals the body to conserve energy. One of the main ways our bodies do this is by dialing down the heat on thyroid function—from production of thyroid hormone in the thyroid itself to peripheral conversion of T_4 to the active thyroid hormone T_3, to uptake of thyroid hormone at the level of your cells. So just like SOS can cause insulin, leptin, and cortisol resistance, it also can cause cellular thyroid hormone resistance. Additionally, chronic inflammation, toxins, leaky gut, and infection may play a role in hypothyroidism.

The entire SOS Solution has been created to prevent—and reverse—the Root Causes of SOS, *and hypothyroidism.* This next part of this chapter will help you take your thyroid health further into your own hands by telling you about the most thorough thyroid testing and how to interpret it, and discussing the targeted approaches to help you get the right treatment. It's imperative to stick with the SOS Solution even beyond just the four weeks to fully heal your thyroid function.

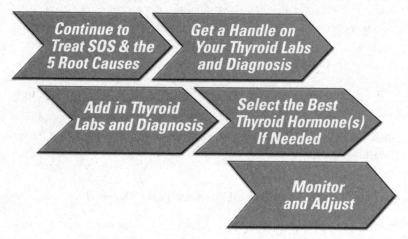

Hypothyroidism: "Test, Don't Guess"

First things first: when it comes to determining whether you have nonautoimmune hypothyroidism or the much more common Hashimoto's, testing is invaluable. It can help you to clarify your diagnosis, can point you toward the best solutions, and periodic retesting allows you to track improvement and to evaluate whether you're being optimally treated if you're on thyroid hormone supplementation. The *right* testing can make a huge difference in getting back in control of your health.

I absolutely recommend getting tested for hypothyroidism if:

- You scored greater than 3 points on the Hashimoto's pattern questionnaire.

- You're pregnant, even if you have no symptoms or history of a thyroid problem.

- You've previously been diagnosed with Hashimoto's or with hypothyroidism.

- You're currently on thyroid medication but still having symptoms.

I Don't Have a Thyroid— Can I Reverse My Hypothyroidism?

If your thyroid was removed or ablated, then you do need thyroid hormone supplementation to give you the hormones your body now can't produce. You don't have to have hypothyroid symptoms, however—the right doses of the right medication should keep you symptom-free as long as you're also taking care of your Root Causes and making sure that you don't have any problems with thyroid hormone conversion if you're only taking T₄, or have cellular resistance. You can also use the SOS Solution to heal the underlying Root Causes that still could be impacting other areas of your health.

The Key Thyroid Tests

Several standard lab tests evaluate the key players involved in thyroid production, conversion of inactive thyroid hormone to its active form, and thyroid immune health, and can unlock the mystery of whether you have Hashimoto's or nonautoimmune hypothyroidism.

Thyroid-stimulating hormone (TSH) is produced in a part of your brain called the pituitary gland. The job of TSH is to tell the thyroid gland that it's time to get busy producing more thyroid hormone. When the healthy thyroid gets this chemical message, it produces two main hormones: triiodothyronine (T_3) and thyroxine (T_4). In most cases, hypothyroidism occurs because the thyroid gland itself isn't functioning properly. In Hashimoto's this is usually due to antibodies that are attacking thyroid tissue and inflammation disrupting normal function. As a result the thyroid has trouble producing T_3 and T_4. TSH gets pumped out in an increasingly higher amount to try harder to stimulate the thyroid gland into action.

Think of it like this: You are TSH. Your best friend's house is the thyroid gland. When you go to visit your friend you knock on her front door. If she doesn't answer, what do you do? You knock louder to get a response. In just the same way, the TSH amps up to knock louder, hoping to get an answer. That's why an underfunctioning thyroid shows up as high TSH on lab tests. However, TSH can be normal in the presence of hypothyroidism in some cases, and you can still be having the symptoms of low thyroid when TSH is normal because of poor conversion of T_4 to T_3 (see page 277) or because of thyroid hormone resistance at the level of your cells. When stress is suppressing the pituitary gland enough to interfere with producing TSH, you might see low or normal TSH levels in the presence of low thyroid hormone production (T_3 or T_4), and hypothyroid symptoms.

Thyroid hormones (T_3 and T_4): Triiodothyronine (T_3) and thyroxine (T_4) are the hormones produced by your thyroid gland. T_4 is produced in a much larger amount and is then converted to T_3, the active form of the hormone. Free T_3 (FT_3) and free T_4 (FT_4) are called this because they aren't bound to proteins in your blood, making them free to perform their work in your cells—keeping your metabolism appropriately revved up for your optimal health. Measuring FT_3 and FT_4 tells you if you have enough active hormones in your circulation for the thyroid's important work.

Thyroid antibodies: Thyroid antibody testing is done to diagnose autoimmune thyroid disease and to distinguish it from other forms of thyroid dysfunction. The two thyroid antibody tests are *thyroid peroxidase antibody (TPOAb)* and *thyroglobulin antibody (TgAb)*.

The presence of TPO antibodies is definitive for Hashimoto's. If you have positive thyroid antibodies, but the rest of your thyroid testing is normal, it is very likely that autoimmune thyroid disease is brewing, though elevated levels of thyroid autoantibodies have been found in other autoimmune disorders as well, including systemic lupus erythematosus, rheumatoid arthritis, and type 1 diabetes, as well as fibromyalgia. Elevated TPOAb in pregnancy is very suggestive that you have subclinical hypothyroidism (see page 269), and this might need to be treated; it also suggests an increased risk of developing postpartum hypothyroidism. I discuss this more below.

Reverse T_3 (RT_3): When your body wants to conserve—rather than "burn"—energy, you divert the active T_3 into this inactive "reverse" form. This happens when you are acutely sick with fever, during infections, under prolonged stress, or undernourished (that is, if you're restricting calories), and with SOS. There is some controversy among conventional doctors about the utility of this test; I personally find it very useful for assessing thyroid function when lab tests are otherwise normal but there are hypothyroid symptoms.

Iodine: Your thyroid requires iodine to function the way a car requires fuel. It can't go without it, and women are commonly low in this element. About 90 percent or more of the iodine you get in your diet (or supplements) is eventually excreted through your urine, making a twenty-four-hour urine iodine test the most effective method to see if you're getting enough. A level of 100 to 199 mcg/L is considered optimal, and for pregnant women, urinary iodine concentrations of 150 to 249 mcg/L are considered adequate.

Additional testing: If your thyroid labs show hypothyroidism or Hashimoto's, I recommend testing for iron and vitamin D as well. As one woman wrote to me after following my blog, "My thyroid medication dose was constantly fluctuating. Then I found out that my vitamin D was also low. Once I got that back up, the weight started to come off! I am now a size six from a twelve!" Your body relies on these nutrients, as well as selenium, vitamin A, and others to properly produce, convert, and use thyroid hormones.

Clearing Up Thyroid Testing Confusion—and Controversy

Thyroid testing can be really confusing, and some doctors will give you pushback on ordering all of the above tests, since they've been trained to do only a TSH initially, and only if the TSH indicates it will they order additional tests. But TSH doesn't always tell the whole story. The TSH isn't always an accurate gauge of what's going on, and it's not the only gauge. For example, your thyroid can be functioning normally, producing ample amounts of free T_4, which gives your thyroid the message that everything's okay, yet all the while you aren't appropriately converting T_4 to active thyroid hormone, or you are, but your cells are resistant to it, both of which are discussed below (see "I'm Taking Thyroid Hormone Supplementation but I Still Don't Feel Better" on page 277). Or your labs could be normal *except* for high thyroid antibodies—which are a major harbinger that you're developing Hashimoto's. So your labs *look* normal, but you could have a problem that is undetected or brewing.

The matter of thyroid labs is hotly debated in the medical community, particularly the normal range for TSH. Most laboratories use values of 4.5 to 5.0 mU/L as the threshold needed for a diagnosis of hypothyroidism to be made. This is based on the fact that when a large population of the U.S. adults is tested for TSH, the typical range goes that high. However, when optimally healthy people who have no thyroid symptoms are selected out and tested, their range is actually much lower, which is why a paper published by the National Academy of Clinical Biochemistry argued that the range should be between 0.4 and 2.5 mU/L, based on the results of 95 percent of those thyroid-healthy people. This has been backed up by other studies, one of which shows, for example, that among those with the lowest levels of disease, the average TSH is 1.18.

While a narrower range like this could lead to overdiagnosis, which makes many doctors reluctant to accept it, one could equally say that the current range leads to underdiagnosis and unnecessary suffering for millions of women.

Further, even at the more conventionally used higher TSH range, most women with borderline tests do eventually develop hypothyroidism, so mildly elevated TSH levels shouldn't be ignored, though they usually are, with a woman told to come back in a year to retest.

So before assuming that your thyroid lab results are normal based on what your doctor said, look at the table "Key Thyroid Tests and Results" (page 266) to make sure you had the right tests ordered, and compare your results to the ranges in the table. Functional medicine practitioners, such as myself, have found that most patients feel best when their TSH is between 0.5 and 2.5 mU/L. Moreover, numerous studies have documented the medical benefits in treating according to lower TSH levels, whether or not individuals are symptomatic, including better long-term heart and cognitive health.

Having a clear plan before you go to your primary care provider's office can help. If you're getting pushback on getting the lab tests you need, see "Working with Your Health Care Practitioner—Or Finding Another" (page 389).

How I Order Thyroid Labs in My Practice

If symptoms are highly suggestive of hypothyroidism, I order all of the key thyroid labs right from the start. This provides the most comprehensive picture and means you only have to make one trip to the lab or doctor's office. You can then target the best treatment for your situation without delay.

If there are other diagnoses that are equally likely to explain your symptoms—for example, iron-deficiency anemia or Epstein-Barr virus infection—I order only the TSH, FT_3, and FT_4 initially, and test for other causes. If the thyroid labs come back borderline or positive, then I add in the remainder of the tests to see if it's Hashimoto's.

If symptoms are a dead ringer for Hashimoto's, but initial tests come back normal and other relevant tests are normal too, I recommend retesting for TSH and thyroid antibodies in four to six weeks, and again three to six months later. I also do this when only the antibodies come back abnormal on initial testing. Sometimes antibodies herald brewing Hashimoto's; they also can be positive in the presence of other autoimmune conditions. If the thyroid antibodies continue to go up, even though your other thyroid labs are normal, and you have symptoms of hypothyroidism, then you can reasonably treat for Hashimoto's.

There is an exception to thyroid labs in pregnancy: the TPO antibody test should also always be obtained.

Understanding Your Thyroid Labs

Whether you've been diagnosed with hypothyroidism in the past, or this is new territory for you, it's essential to understand your thyroid labs so you can proceed with the right diagnosis and proper treatment. I've provided a table below to help you make sense of what various sets of results might mean. This is not exhaustive, but it covers the main patterns.

My Doctor Said I Have Borderline Labs or Subclinical Hypothyroidism. What Does This Mean?

Anika came to see me because she was fatigued, moody, having heavy periods and no libido, and was bothered by constipation. She also wasn't sleeping well—waking up too early and unable to fall back to sleep, except

Key Thyroid Tests and Results			
Test Name	**What It Is**	**Optimal Range***	**Meaning If Out of Range**
TSH	A pituitary hormone that tells the thyroid to produce thyroid hormone	0.5 to 3.0 mU/L	If >2.5 mU/L with symptoms, suspect hypothyroidism
Free T_3 (FT_3)	The most active form of thyroid hormone	>3.2 mU/L (320 to 340 mcg/L)	If <3.2 mU/L (320 mcg/L) with symptoms, suspect hypothyroidism
Free T_4 (FT_4)	The precursor thyroid hormone to active thyroid hormone	>1.2 to 1.4 mU/L	If <1.2 mU/L with symptoms, suspect hypothyroidism
TPO	The most sensitive test for detecting autoimmune thyroid disease	Negative or <4 mU/L	If elevated with symptoms or other abnormalities, Hashimoto's
AntiTg Antibody	Thyroglobulin is a protein found in thyroid cells. This tests for antibodies to this protein.	Negative or <4 IU/mL	If elevated with symptoms or other abnormalities, Hashimoto's
Reverse T_3 (RT_3)	An inactive storage form of thyroid hormone	<10 ng/dL	If elevated, the body is conserving energy by storing active thyroid hormone as an inactive form
Iodine	A mineral necessary for the production of thyroid hormones	100 to 199 mcg/L 150 to 249 mcg/L in pregnancy	Iodine insufficiency or deficiency

* Based on standards discussed in this chapter.

If Your Labs Truly Are Normal and You Still Have Symptoms

If your labs truly are normal according to the information in the table "Key Thyroid Tests and Results" and you're still having symptoms that seem like hypothyroidism, it's possible that your symptoms are due to another cause. You could actually just be exhausted and needing more rest, for example, if you're a new mom or under extra stress. You could have remaining imbalances in any of the five roots—for example, food intolerances or gut dysbiosis causing fatigue. Hopefully by now in the program, though, these have been cleared up. It's also important to look into other possible causes of your symptoms. Diabetes, obesity, depression, sleep apnea, kidney disease, chronic fatigue, and congestive heart failure are some of the symptoms that can mimic hypothyroidism. Also, disease in the hypothalamus and pituitary can cause symptoms of hypothyroidism without classic lab findings; these are rare but, if the symptoms and the labs don't match, shouldn't be forgotten.

on weekends, when she could stay in bed, and then she felt she could sleep all day. She'd gained seven pounds in a couple of months even though she hadn't changed her eating habits. She was pretty sure something was wrong with her thyroid, so she asked her doctor to check her labs before coming to see me for a consultation. He tested her thyroid-stimulating hormone (TSH) only and told her that since it was in the normal range, though at the upper end of normal, she didn't have a thyroid problem. He suggested that maybe an antidepressant would be good to consider.

But her labs weren't normal. Her TSH was 4.4. One step over a thin line and she'd have had a slam-dunk diagnosis of the most common thyroid problem, hypothyroidism. In fact, this is what I diagnosed. She started the SOS Solution, customized to remove dairy, keep her blood sugar steady, and get more protein in her diet, along with thyroid treatment, and before long

What Do My Thyroid Labs Mean?					
TSH	FT$_4$	FT$_3$	Thyroid Antibodies Anti-TPO, AntiTgAb	Re-verse T$_3$ (RT$_3$)	What It Means
High	Low	Low	Normal	N/A	Nonautoimmune hypothyroidism or Hashimoto's but antibodies not yet elevated enough to detect
High	Normal	Normal	Normal or high	N/A	Subclinical hypothyroidism
High	Low	Low	Positive	N/A	Hashimoto's (autoimmune hypothyroidism)
Normal	Normal	Low	Normal	N/A	Hypothyroidism due to T$_4$ to T$_3$ conversion problem
Normal or high	Normal	High	Normal or high	N/A	Cellular resistance to FT$_3$
High, low, or normal	Low or normal	Low or normal	High	N/A	Hashimoto's likely in the process of emerging; high risk for developing Hashimoto's or another autoimmune condition; antibodies can be positive for seven years before symptoms appear or other lab abnormalities develop
Normal or high	Normal	Normal or low	Normal or high	High	Fatigue, stress, infection, SOS leading to "sick euthyroid," which is low thyroid hormone function due to storage of active thyroid hormone

she felt like a new woman. Her elimination improved, her periods stopped knocking her out, and she wondered why she'd been living with "the great flood" every month without anyone telling her it didn't have to be that way. She didn't need to sleep all weekend, and the irritable mood that made her wonder if she was just a grouchy person was gone. She actually felt cheerful!

Borderline thyroid labs mean that they are just a smidgen below the number needed for a diagnosis, and are usually stated in relation to the more conventionally used higher TSH, which, as I've established, should be revised.

If the TSH lower limit your doctor is using for hypothyroidism is 4.8, and your result is 4.7, you would be said to have borderline results.

Subclinical hypothyroidism is a term that gives doctors the latitude to not even diagnose hypothyroidism until the TSH is 10 mU/L or above, as long as the free T_3 and free T_4 are normal. It's estimated that as many as 10 percent of the population fits this bill. While endocrinologists and primary care doctors may not want to overdiagnose and overtreat, this has led to millions of women with hypothyroidism not receiving diagnosis and treatment.

The bottom line is that an elevated TSH means that your thyroid hormone levels are low. TSH is trying to drive the thyroid to produce more thyroid hormone. If it were responding, the TSH would quickly return to normal. Subclinical hypothyroidism is mild thyroid failure and should be treated. At least 30 percent of those with subclinical hypothyroidism have symptoms including depression, dry skin, poor memory, slowed thinking, muscle weakness or cramps, fatigue, cold intolerance, puffy eyes, and constipation. This mild dysfunction has been associated with higher rates of impaired cardiac function, including reduced exercise capacity, elevated cholesterol, atherosclerosis, peripheral vascular disease, and atrial fibrillation, which increases risk of stroke and increases risk for a heart attack 2.5 to 3 times. Every increase in TSH of 1 μL represents an increase in heart disease risk, which is worse if there's insulin resistance as well. Even only slightly low T_4 has been associated with an increased risk of insulin resistance and elevated cholesterol, and even mild thyroid dysfunction can cause metabolic syndrome.

Several large studies have shown that women who receive treatment with thyroid hormone, even when TSH is only marginally low, have improvement in cardiac and cognitive function. Treatment may even be appropriate if you don't have symptoms but have an elevated TSH. Keep in mind, too, as I explained above, that the lower limit most doctors are using for TSH is way too high, and accordingly, any TSH level above 2.5 to 3 would not be subclinical; it would be overt hypothyroidism.

Positive Thyroid Labs: What's a Girl to Do?

If you already knew or suspected that you have Hashimoto's, you might feel relieved to know that your symptoms have an explanation. If this is new territory to you, you might feel overwhelmed, frustrated, or sad, especially if you view yourself as an otherwise healthy gal and now see yourself with a future that includes dependence on medications. If you're feeling that way, it's totally normal. Anytime we have a change in self-perception, we might need to grieve for a minute. But having Hashimoto's doesn't mean you're not healthy, nor does it automatically relegate you to a life of medications.

Do I Have Increased Health Risks Now That I Have Hashimoto's?

When Hashimoto's is properly treated, it doesn't increase your health risks; you can live an absolutely healthy, happy, and normal life. Also, the risks accumulate over time, so you have time to try various interventions—supplements, herbs, dietary changes (the ones you're already doing)—and find the right medication for you, if needed.

Is It Possible to Reverse Hypothyroidism?

The answer is a resounding yes, it is possible for many women to reverse hypothyroidism. But not always.

If you have nonautoimmune hypothyroidism due to nutritional deficiency, then replacing missing nutrients can restore thyroid function. Similarly, if you have peripheral conversion problems or thyroid hormone resistance at the cellular level, removing the impediments can restore your thyroid hormone function.

Most women will recover from postpartum thyroid problems within six to twelve months after its onset, at which time medication, if you're on it, can be weaned by half for a couple of weeks, and then discontinued. If symptoms persist beyond eighteen months after onset, it is more likely that you've developed permanent hypothyroidism, and long-term thyroid hormone supplementation might be needed. About 30 percent of women who develop postpartum thyroiditis develop permanent thyroid problems. For women who have fully recovered from postpartum thyroiditis, repeat thyroid testing within five to ten years after the initial diagnosis is recommended as your risk of developing Hashimoto's later is elevated. Testing should also be obtained if you develop thyroid-related symptoms.

It is also possible to reverse Hashimoto's, though it doesn't happen for everyone. It is hard to predict who will have a reversal and how long it will take. My experience is that women with a clear trigger, for example, celiac disease, sometimes have a reversal after the trigger, for example, gluten, is removed from the diet.

As your inflammation goes down as a result of healing SOS and your Root Causes, so too will your thyroid antibody numbers, and with this, you can experience improved thyroid function, depending on how much of the thyroid has been left undamaged by the autoimmune attack. It takes at least several months and even a year to see a substantial change in antibody levels, but if you're getting to the root of the problem, you should see a change, and with it, your other thyroid labs return to normal. As inflammation resolves, you can also expect weight gain, brain fog, sleep problems, and other symptoms to improve. Thyroid medication can bring an enormous improvement in symptoms while you're working on healing the Root Causes, and does not make you dependent on it. You can wean off of it if and when your thyroid function is restored.

My Mom and Grandmother Have Hashimoto's. Am I Stuck with It?

A small percentage of individuals do have a genetic predisposition to Hashimoto's, either intrinsic to the thyroid or that interferes with thyroid hormone conversion. So if you have a first-degree family member with Hashimoto's (that is, your mom or sister), then you do have some increased risk, and if you have symptoms, should be tested. However, not everyone with the gene develops hypothyroidism, and not everyone with hypothyroidism has the gene. If you're at increased risk, practice a little extra TLC (thyroid loving care) by making sure you take thyroid-supportive nutrients, keep your inflammation low, and generally avoid the five Root Causes of SOS.

Do I Need Medication?

*Going up to the correct dose of thyroid medication
was a night and day difference in how I felt.*

—FROM AN EMAIL FROM M.S., WHO FOLLOWED THE
INSTRUCTIONS IN AN ARTICLE I WROTE

First of all, to clarify, I prefer to call thyroid medication *thyroid hormone supplementation*. It's more accurately what it is—supplying your body with the supplemental amount of hormone it is not able to make on its own, either currently or at all. Not everyone with hypothyroidism needs thyroid hormone supplementation, particularly if your thyroid labs aren't significantly out of the normal range or your symptoms aren't debilitating. With many patients, I spend at least six, and often up to twelve weeks helping them to identify reversible Root Causes.

However, if your TPO antibody numbers are far out of the normal range, if you've had long-standing Hashimoto's with prolonged highly elevated antibodies, and if your symptoms are seriously impacting your quality of life, thyroid hormone supplementation can be a game changer in how you feel, and starting one does not relegate you to a lifetime of it. But unless you have an identifiable and obviously reversible cause of hypothyroidism, there's a good chance that thyroid hormone supplementation is in your future. This can come as disappointing news, especially if you're trying to live as naturally as possible. But again, let me offer a word of reassurance: thyroid medication is not a medication that is doing something foreign to your body—it is thyroid hormone replacement therapy, giving your body what you'd naturally produce, but right now aren't because your thyroid function is suppressed. The goal of thyroid hormone supplementation is symptom resolution and normalization of thyroid labs; TSH, FT_3, and FT_4 will return to normal within six weeks; thyroid antibodies can take months to resolve. Once you've been feeling great for a number of months, you can work with your primary care provider to see if you can reduce the dose, and at some point you may decide to try to go off of the medication. This is done by slightly lowering the dose, and then testing your TSH, FT_3, and FT_4; if they are out of range off the thyroid hormone supplementation, you probably need to stay on it.

Finding the Right Thyroid Hormone
Supplementation for You

Historically, M.D.s have relied on a single treatment for hypothyroidism: levothyroxine (Synthroid), a synthetic form of T_4, making it one of the most widely prescribed medications in the world. While it is often effective, many women do not get relief from it. Unfortunately, doctors have been trained to use only levothyroxine, and are reluctant to offer options, leaving women inadequately treated, which can seriously impact quality of life and lead to long-term health consequences. Also, many women get started on a medication but never get their dose optimized, and have inadequate follow-up testing to keep their levels optimal.

Most M.D.s believe that the best and only necessary treatment for Hashimoto's is levothyroxine. However, there is a slowly growing recognition that many patients still have symptoms on T_4 alone, and that there may be a role for T_3 use in patients who don't improve on T_4 alone. The greatest concern is that T_3 can lead to many of the same risks associated with *hyper*thyroidism—including heart attack and osteoporosis.

Other medication options that many women report benefits from and that are used by integrative and functional medicine practitioners include:

- Alternate T_4 preparations such as Tirosint, a gel that contains only T_4, glycerine, and gelatin
- Desiccated thyroid preparations (Armour Thyroid, Nature-Throid, Westhroid, Thyroid USP) that contain T_4 and T_3
- Liothyronine (Cytomel), a synthetic T_3 that is used to supplement a T_4 medication
- Liotrix (Thyrolar), a synthetic T_4/T_3 combination
- Compounded T_4/T_3, popular because they can be customized to your needs and be made free of fillers, gluten, and lactose, which are triggers for some women, and can be compounded to be sustained-released

Some women do very well on products with T_3; however, it can cause overstimulation with symptoms of agitation, insomnia, and irritability, and it carries the risks of causing hyperthyroidism. My recommendation is to stay at the lowest possible dose to relieve symptoms, and discontinue if it

Thyroid Health in Pregnancy and After Baby Is Born

Thyroid hormone plays a major role in fertility, pregnancy, birth, and our health as new mommas—including sleep, mood, energy, weight loss, and the ability to produce enough breast milk. My recommendation is that all women who are thinking about having babies get tested for thyroid function, and if you have had a known thyroid problem in the past, or test positive now even if just for thyroid antibodies, you work to optimize your thyroid health with the right nutrients, lifestyle, and the overall SOS Solution.

A history of hormonal problems, including PCOS—the leading cause of infertility—infertility itself, miscarriage, postpartum depression, trouble producing breast milk, and more, can all be related to hypothyroidism.

Thyroid disease in pregnancy represents big risks for babies, so if you're pregnant or planning to be soon, definitely have your thyroid labs done. Even if you test positive only for TPO antibody (see page 268), you could have subclinical hypothyroidism that needs treatment, and your risk of developing hypothyroidism during and after pregnancy is significantly increased, so have your labs followed. If you test positive for Hashimoto's, or just elevated TPO antibody in pregnancy, take *selenium* (see page 282) until your baby is at least six months old; it has been shown to reduce TPO antibody and development of Hashimoto's. If you're starting thyroid medication for the first time in pregnancy, I recommend starting with levothyroxine (Synthroid), because it is the standard that OBs will know how to manage for you (they often don't know how to properly dose many of the other medications, and proper dosing is critical for pregnancy health), and then changing to other medications only if you are not getting an appropriate response.

Tens of thousands of new moms in their first year after giving birth struggle with undiagnosed thyroid problems, their symptoms mistakenly chalked up to the normal challenges of motherhood. But exhaustion, depression, difficulty losing weight, and difficulty producing enough breast milk aren't just a "normal part of having a baby." They can also be telltale signs of hypothyroidism—and struggling with hypothyroidism as a new mom makes the job exponentially more exhausting and can lead to anxiety, stress, guilt, and depression.

New moms are vulnerable to autoimmune thyroid problems due to naturally occurring immune and hormonal changes that occur during pregnancy and after birth. Rates are as high as 17 percent, and at least 2.5 times higher in women who already have an autoimmune disease, a thyroid problem after a previous pregnancy, hypothyroidism going into pregnancy, or elevated TPO antibodies. While you might go straight into hypothyroidism, many moms pass through a phase of hyperthyroidism first, further confounding the diagnosis—which is often missed, and making you feel crazy because you're swinging from one extreme to the other.

Symptoms of *hyperthyroidism* include:

- Insomnia, agitation, and anxiety
- Fatigue
- Heart palpitations
- Weight loss
- Heat intolerance
- Irritability
- Tremor

Symptoms of *hypothyroidism*, for a refresher, are listed on page 42.

Testing is no different than that done at any other time, and treatment is the same, though many doctors suggest waiting a few months to treat hypothyroidism. In my experience, this practice leaves new moms feeling awful, when treatment could transform their lives and their relationships with their babies.

If, after your baby is born, you have no symptoms but

abnormal labs, repeat the thyroid labs every four to eight weeks until they return to normal. If you have hyperthyroidism, symptoms can be safely treated while breast-feeding with 40 to 120 mg of propranolol. Atenolol may be recommended instead of propranolol, but is not the best choice for breast-feeding moms. My first choice, however, before turning to medication for symptom support, is to use herbs for controlling symptoms, especially irritability, agitation, anxiety, and heart racing, whenever possible. The two most helpful herbs are motherwort® (*Leonurus cardiaca*) and lemon balm (*Melissa officinalis*), thirty to sixty drops of the liquid extract of each, two to six times a day, which is safe while breast-feeding. Radioiodine treatment and antithyroid drugs are not useful in hypothyroidism and can lead to numerous serious pregnancy complications as well as impact the growth, development, and intellectual abilities of the baby, and in new mothers, are leading causes of postpartum depression, affecting an estimated one in twelve new mothers, as well as low breast milk production, so are not advised.

If you have symptomatic hypothyroidism, thyroid hormone supplementation is the optimal treatment to get you feeling back to normal quickly, is safe while breast-feeding, and can make a huge difference in breast milk production. Levothyroxine (T_4) at a dose of 50 to 100 mcg a day is usually recommended regardless of the level of TSH, though individual dosing adjustments may need to be made. Other medications, including Armour Thyroid, can be considered.

is not working within a couple of weeks of maximizing the dose. If you are experiencing agitation, go to the lowest dose; if you still experience symptoms, discontinue. There is debate over the superiority of bioidentical hormones (naturally derived products) versus synthetic; I find this completely a matter of personal preference.

I generally start patients on Armour; however, if you're not comfortable with it because it's less conventional, your doctor refuses to prescribe it, or you don't want to take a pork-based product, you can start with levothyroxine—or consider finding another prescriber. It's best to start at a low dose, and titrate up over a few weeks until you get symptom resolution. When you start to feel really good, stay on that dose for six weeks, then retest. If your labs are normal, or heading that way, you've found your medication and dose.

Timing is important when taking a thyroid hormone supplement. It should be taken at least thirty minutes before eating, at approximately the same time each day, and four hours apart from other supplements and medications. Iron, calcium, and soy protein supplements may particularly interfere with absorption. If you're taking a bedtime dose, it should be two hours after your last meal of the day.

I'm Taking Thyroid Hormone Supplementation, but I Still Don't Feel Better

Sometimes taking thyroid hormone doesn't do the trick. If you're taking thyroid hormone supplementation and you aren't feeling better, it could be a matter of timing, as I just mentioned. Here are some of the additional reasons you might not be getting adequate benefits from your thyroid hormone supplementation:

You are taking the wrong dose or the wrong medication: Work with your primary provider to optimize your dose. If that doesn't work, you might need to try another medication. You might need T_4, or a combination of T_4 and T_3.

You could be taking a medication that blocks thyroid hormone: The most common are PPIs (Prilosec) and other antacids, oral contraceptives, antifungal medications, cholesterol-lowering drugs, antiarrhythmics, lithium, and hormone replacement.

You may have problems with thyroid hormone conversion: If you're not converting T_4 to T_3 in your tissues, especially your liver, where this mostly occurs, then T_4 isn't going to help. You may need T_3, along with working to improve T_4 to T_3 conversion. The causes of poor conversion include stress, depression, chronic pain, excessive dieting, diabetes, insulin resistance, or metabolic syndrome, leptin resistance, excessive exercise, iron deficiency, chronic inflammation, environmental toxins, and some hormone imbalances—all also associated with SOS!

You may have cellular resistance to thyroid hormone: Your body has been
making enough, but your cells haven't been taking it in due to depression, inadequate nutrition, obesity, leptin insulin resistance, diabetes,
chronic fatigue syndrome, fibromyalgia, inflammation, autoimmune
disease, or systemic illness. Because the SOS Solution has been
reversing these underlying causes, your cellular receptivity can be
completely restored as a result.

You haven't fully eliminated a Root Cause: Remember that this four-week
plan is the *start* of a lifelong plan and that you might need more time
to heal one or more of your Root Causes.

How and When Do I Go Off of Thyroid Hormone Supplementation?

If you're feeling incredible improvement and would like to know whether
you can go off of your thyroid medication, it's best to work with your primary
provider to create a plan for slowly reducing the medication dose while periodically retesting (no more than every six weeks, the amount of time it takes
thyroid changes to be reflected in your labs) to trend your TSH, FT_4, and FT_3
levels, which should stay steady. If they shift back into a hypothyroid pattern,
or if symptoms return, you need to stay on thyroid hormone supplementation longer, or indefinitely, though you might find that your testing holds
steady at a lower dose than you'd been on. If you are able to go off of your
medication, retest again six and twelve weeks after discontinuing to make
sure you're staying steady, and then again if *any* symptoms recur. Note that
thyroid antibodies can stay elevated for months or even over a year, so are not
an indication that you need to remain on thyroid medication if these other
labs are normal and you have no symptoms. However, elevated antibodies do
indicate that you want to continue to heal your Root Causes.

If you've had hypothyroidism in the past and become pregnant, it's imperative that you have your levels checked and go onto medication if needed.

Healing Thyroid Function . . . Naturally

Is There a Special Diet for Hashimoto's?

Yes, there is—and you are already on it! The Reboot (and Replenish Plan,
soon to follow) provides what you need: a low-inflammatory, nutrient- and

antioxidant-rich, high-in-fiber, gut-healthy, toxin-free plan that keeps your blood sugar steady, provides the amino acids your body needs to transport hormones and support optimal detoxification, and more.

There are a few special considerations:

- Individuals with autoimmune thyroiditis have an almost fivefold increased risk of developing celiac disease, and this can happen at any time, so I recommend all patients who have Hashimoto's remain gluten-free.

- Do not overeat raw forms of the *Brassicaceae* veggies (page 150) (don't exceed more than twice weekly); and generally avoid juicing vegetables in this family.

- Limit soy. A review of the literature demonstrates that women with normal thyroid function and normal dietary iodine intakes are not at risk for developing thyroid problems; even when consumed up to three times a week, soy does not affect thyroid function in otherwise healthy women. However, since soy can interfere with the activity of the thyroid in women on thyroid hormone supplementation, I recommend limiting soy products to a maximum of once weekly if you have Hashimoto's, or preferably, avoid them.

- Keep your blood sugar steady. Healthy, slow-burning whole grains and energy vegetables (page 149) can benefit you. If you're following a Paleo diet, then this is considered modified Paleo, which many Paleo proponents recommend in your situation.

What Herbs and Supplements Can I Take to Help?

Unless Hashimoto's labs or symptoms are severe, I start with herbs and supplements for six weeks, trend symptoms, recheck labs, and *then*, if needed, start on thyroid hormone supplementation. While there are numerous nutrients that support thyroid function, the ones in the table on pages 280-82 are those I most commonly recommend. They address the most common nutritional insufficiencies and the inflammation that can be at the root of Hashimoto's and can be taken if you are on thyroid medication. In addition to a wide variety of colorful vegetables giving you ample

SOS Rx: Thyroid Support		
Herb/ Supplement	**Uses and Cautions**	**Dose**
Curcumin⊘	When there are elevated TPO antibodies, I always begin by reducing inflammation in the system and removing any triggers. NAC and Pycnogenol can be taken alternatively, or along with curcumin. (See pages 222 and 228 for these other supplements.)	1,200 to 2,400 mg/day
Guggul⊘	An herbal medicine, guggul has been shown to improve thyroid function, increasing conversion of T_4, the inactive form of thyroid hormone, to T_3, the active form. This herb should not be taken in pregnancy, but can be taken while breast-feeding. Discontinue if baby gets a tummy upset when you take the herb, and discontinue when thyroid levels normalize.	750 mg/day

vitamins A, C, and E, and your core supplements (pages 166–67), consider the supplements on the table above in combination (don't duplicate any supplements you're already taking, such as vitamin D).

The Hashimoto's-Iodine Dilemma

Iodine is essential for the production of thyroid hormones, and low iodine is the leading cause of hypothyroidism in countries where iodine deficiency is prevalent. However, excess iodine can also equally lead to Hashimoto's, and many women report a worsening of Hashimoto's symptoms when they supplement even with small amounts of iodine. This appears to be a problem when there is a concurrent selenium insufficiency.

I recommend dulse seaweed as a great source of iodine in my practice— you can get dulse flakes at major health food stores (also see "Resources" on page 393), and add these to salads or soups, or sprinkle them on grains. They're an acquired taste, but if you like sushi, you'll like this. A dose is about 2 teaspoons a day for a small amount of dietary iodine. Many natural

Herb/ Supplement	Uses and Cautions	Dose
Iron	Iron deficiency tells your thyroid to conserve energy, leading to decreased production of thyroid hormone.	30 to 60 mg iron amino chelate/ day
	Dietary sources of iron: red meat and dark-meat poultry have a highly absorbable form, and eaten several times weekly can quickly boost your iron; also helpful are leafy greens, red beans, and dried apricots and raisins (though these are high in sugar).	
	If you test low, you might also want to supplement with iron chelate, a form of iron that is non-constipating, taken along with 500 mg of vitamin C to increase absorption.	
	PPIs should not be taken with iron because they block absorption, and iron should not be taken with your thyroid medication because it blocks it; take iron and your thyroid medication four hours apart.	

thyroid support products on the market contain iodine, so read labels before taking to make sure you're not getting too much. If you do supplement with iodine and feel worse, discontinue taking it. Also be mindful not to use iodized salt if you don't tolerate it.

Unlike selenium, iodine supplementation has *not* been found to be helpful in preventing postpartum thyroid disease; however, all pregnant women should receive 200 to 300 mcg of iodine in pregnancy for the development and health of the baby; don't rely on the amount routinely found in prenatal vitamins and seaweed to get the required amount.

Healing Hashimoto's Hair Loss

The beauty of the SOS Solution is that in the process of healing your Root Causes and healing SOS, you're automatically addressing the most common

SOS Rx: Thyroid Support		
Herb/ Supplement	**Uses and Cautions**	**Dose**
Selenium	The body turns selenium into the powerful antioxidant glutathione. Selenium protects the thyroid from the inflammation and oxidative stress that is suppressing function and damaging thyroid tissue, and several studies have shown that it can reduce TPO antibodies. It is also critical in the conversion of T_4 to T_3. It decreases the risk of developing postpartum thyroiditis in women who are positive for TPO antibodies, and can be started during pregnancy and continued into the postpartum period to reduce risk. While some suggest that enough can be obtained from one or two Brazil nuts daily, I recommend other selenium-rich foods, including mushrooms, lamb, turkey, chicken, eggs, cod, and halibut, with the inclusion of Brazil nuts if you enjoy them, but not as a replacement for a supplement.	Up to 200 mcg/day (do not exceed)
Vitamin D	Circulating levels of vitamin D_3 have been found to be low in those with Hashimoto's and other autoimmune conditions. Supplementing with D_3 at 4,000 IU daily (2,000 IU daily in pregnancy) may help prevent or reverse autoimmune thyroid disease. Levels can be rechecked every six weeks to measure levels and indicate when to stay at a steady dose or decrease the dose. (I don't recommend exceeding serum levels of 70 nM.)	2,000 to 4,000 IU/day (2,000 IU/day in pregnancy)
Zinc	Involved in the conversion of T_4 to T_3; important if you appear to be having problems with thyroid hormone conversion.	30 mg/day; take with your meals to prevent nausea

Key: ⊘ = Not safe for use in pregnancy.

symptoms of Hashimoto's. One of the symptoms that women find most disturbing is hair thinning, so I want to give this some attention. Little is known for certain about nutritional factors and hair thinning in women. However, iron deficiency, even without anemia but with low ferritin (see page 383), appears to play a role; in fact, hair loss probably won't stop unless the serum ferritin level (see page 382) is at least 70 mcg/L. The role of the essential amino acid L-lysine in hair loss also appears to be important.

One study found that a significant proportion of women responded to L-lysine and iron therapy. See iron on page 281; the dose for L-lysine is 1,000 mg daily. I recommend trying this combination for six weeks, and observe for improvement.

Congratulations! Making big changes isn't easy—but you're doing it! You've spent twenty-one days giving your body a much-needed Reboot while adding the elements your body needs to heal your SOS Root Causes. You've been busily eliminating toxins, boosting detoxification, healing your digestive system, balancing blood sugar, and bridging your phytonutrient gap. You've been recharging your batteries, restoring your gut flora, and resetting your metabolism and hormones. You've been getting rid of body and mind triggers that have been sapping your energy, and adding practices that have been replenishing resources that got depleted from living in chronic overdrive. You took out the triggers that were causing inflammation and putting you into SOS, making you tired, keeping your brain foggy, and making you feel fat and frumpy. The 21-Day Reboot gave you a chance to start over with a clean slate.

I hope you're in love with how you feel and that your friends are asking you what you've been doing because they want some, too. Even if you're just beginning to notice changes, which may be the case if you started out with a bigger mountain to climb, that's okay. Everyone benefits at her own pace. Some women need a little extra time on the Reboot. Feel free to take that; you do not have to jump into the Replenish Plan yet. Healing takes time, and you've only been at it for a few weeks. You're likely still in the process of healing some of your Root Causes. When your cells start to get the nourishment they need, your self-repair mechanisms get going again and it's almost impossible for your body *not* to respond and perform its best.

Oral Contraceptive Pills (OCPs) and Your Thyroid

While you've probably heard of the more common risks associated with the Pill, such as blood clots, what is less common knowledge is that OCPs increase sex hormone–binding globulin, which binds to active thyroid hormones in your blood, rendering them unable to get to your cells and do their work. OCPs also cause insulin resistance and inflammation, identifiable by high levels of C-reactive protein in studies of OCP users. They also can affect mood, primarily causing depression in users, as well as a chronic state of estrogen dominance. If you're struggling with these problems and are ready to switch, OCP alternatives include natural family planning along with condoms (97 percent effective with no side effects) or the IUD, which, contrary to what many of us think because of the widely publicized problems with a much earlier version, the Dalkon Shield, are very safe and effective, even if you've not had a baby yet.

WHAT'S NEXT?

Transitioning from the Reboot to the full-on Replenish Lifestyle means reintroducing a few foods into your diet and learning how to take this plan forward so you can eat healthily for life. During this week you'll mindfully reintroduce some of the foods you removed and pay attention to how you respond. What you'll discover will become the basis of your personal Replenish Lifestyle. It's a fun week of discovering what works for you—and I think you'll be pleasantly surprised at just how relaxed the lifestyle is.

Now is a great time to go back and fill out those questionnaires from chapter 3. You'll be surprised to learn what has changed, and what symptoms you've already left behind. Don't worry if you haven't seen big results just yet—there is still a lot of program ahead, and I promise this experience will be life-changing.

WEEK 3: RECHARGE, DAY BY DAY

You are the one that possesses the keys to your being.
You carry the passport to your own happiness.

—DIANE VON FURSTENBERG

Week 3 Sample Daily Meal Plan

Breakfast Example

8–12-oz. Smoothie (Shake)
or
Breakfast protein + good-quality fat (+ optional veggie)

Lunch Example

Protein entrée + green veggie + rainbow veggie + energy veggie + good-quality fat

Dinner Example

Protein entrée + green veggie + rainbow veggie + energy veggie + good-quality fat + small amount of fermented veggie (if tolerated)

Week 3
Sample Daily Menus and Lifestyle

	Day 15	Day 16	Day 17
Morning practice	The Quickie meditation (page 199)	Dry brush (page 232) in morning shower	5 minutes of deep breathing (page 191) and stretch
Fresh Start	Drink a glass of room-temperature or warm water with a squeeze of lemon.		
Breakfast + Daily Dose Supplements	Smoothie Bar	Frittata + mixed greens with Olive Oil Lemon Dressing	Smoothie Bar
Mid-morning	Rise and Shine Muffin or Power Balls	Jump Start Detox Nutrient Broth	Coconut yogurt with raw cacao nibs and berries or Olive Oil Granola
Mindful lunch + SOS Solution Supplements (if you've personalized your plan ahead)	Salmon Caper Board or other board option	Fresh Turkey "Russian" Wrap or Vegan Nori Wrap	Make Your Own Salad + soup leftovers
Mid-afternoon	½ apple sliced with 1 tbsp. almond butter	Handful dry-roasted almonds with cayenne dash	Coconut yogurt with raw cacao nibs and berries or Olive Oil Granola

Day 18	Day 19	Day 20	Day 21
The Quickie meditation	Dry brush in morning shower	5 minutes of deep breathing and stretch	Day off
Breakfast Scramble or Omelet + optional mixed greens with Olive Oil Lemon Dressing	Smoothie Bar	Breakfast Scramble or Omelet + optional mixed greens with Olive Oil Lemon Dressing	Power Parfait with optional Olive Oil Granola
Smoothie Bar	½ size any It's a Wrap	Jump Start Detox Nutrient Broth	Snack Stash option
Mediterranean Board	The Art of the Buddha Bowl leftovers)	Thai Lettuce Wrap	Make Your Own Salad + Butternut Squash Curry Coconut Soup leftovers
Snack Stash option	Handful dry-roasted almonds with cayenne dash	½ size any It's a Wrap	Snack Stash option

Week 3
Sample Daily Menus and Lifestyle

	Day 15	Day 16	Day 17
Cortisol Reset	Reset your cortisol for the evening with 15 minutes of any Replenish Repair Kit practice		
Dinner + SOS Solution Supplements (if you've personalized your plan ahead)	Baked Walnut-Crusted Chicken + Sautéed Spinach with Pine Nuts	Make Your Own Salad + a soup	Basil Coconut Curry Tagine + Sautéed Spinach (or Dandelion Greens) and Pine Nuts or Curried "Popcorn" Cauliflower + ½ cup cooked grain (brown basmati rice)
Replenish Self-Care	Replenish Bath	Gratitude or Worry Journal	Digital Detox and read

Day 18	Day 19	Day 20	Day 21
Miso-Glazed Salmon with Scallions and Sesame Seeds + Roasted Maple Winter Squash or Sautéed Orange Ginger Carrots + Roasted Broccoli	The Art of the Buddha Bowl	Rosemary Bean Soup + mixed greens salad or Roasted Brussels Sprouts	Tuscan Pasta Salad + Mediterranean Cilantro Chicken + mixed greens with Olive Oil Lemon Dressing or Sautéed Spinach with Pine Nuts
Gratitude or Worry Journal	Digital Detox and read	Replenish Bath	Gratitude or Worry Journal

REPLENISH

Eat for Life

Reboot: Remove Food Triggers • Reframe: Chronic Emotional and Mental Stress • Repair: Root Causes and SOS Damage • Recharge: Your Adrenals and Thyroid • **Replenish: No More Running on Empty**

One cannot think well, love well, sleep well, if one has not dined well.

—Virginia Woolf

THE REPLENISH LIFESTYLE

The beauty of this book and plan is that you're already living the Replenish Lifestyle. You got here without even knowing it. And notice I'm still not calling it a diet, because it's not. There's no "restricting" for a few weeks in which you drop weight, only to put it back on when you go back to your usual diet because you can't stand the restriction anymore.

This is different. It's a lifestyle.

Frankly, it's also a diet rebellion. It's a rebellion against the food industry that feeds you junk that is stealing your health and with it your life by saying, "Heck, no—I'm not buying into that anymore." It's also a rebellion against the constant exhausting pursuit of trying to be perfect, skinnier, and "cleaner." Overrestriction just makes you crave more sweets. It increases your cortisol. And it sets you up for failure.

The goal of the Replenish Lifestyle is very simple: to keep you feeling physically, mentally, and emotionally restored, nourished, energetic, and at ease in your body—so you're never running on empty. You do this by eating fresh, vital foods, at the right times of day to keep your natural rhythms in balance, give your body vital information, bring your life satisfaction, keep inflammation down, keep blood sugar and insulin normal, and keep your cortisol in healthy circadian rhythm. I promised that this plan is not about food deprivation. It's absolutely not. You'll see exactly that when I discuss the 95/5 rule.

But there's more to the Replenish Lifestyle than just the foods it includes. It's about empowered eating: learning to recognize which foods feel good in your body and eating that way because you want to—and because you know that healthy is the new sexy—and that's how you want to feel. It's about thinking of food as something that helps you create your best self, not about food control, which creates *more* stress.

And it's about giving yourself Permission to Pause in life—including with your food choices—so you enjoy the choices you're making, understand why you're making them, and feel good about yourself as you do make them, even if that's indulging once in a while. This is what it takes to make this plan successful not just for a few weeks or months, but as a new way of living that keeps you healthy for the rest of your life.

THE FOOD REINTRODUCTION PROCESS

Reintroducing foods into your diet is straightforward and easy. You simply add foods back in systematically, each for two to three days at a time, observing how you tolerate them based on symptom responses. One caveat here is that you'll only be reintroducing *real foods*. Refined carbohydrates, refined sugars, processed foods, artificial ingredients, additives, preservatives, and poor-quality oils are absolutely not a part of the Replenish

Lifestyle. They are energy sappers, not builders. So let's make them a thing of the past.

Here's what to keep out permanently:

- High-fructose corn syrup, "added sugar" in foods, sugar substitutes, and artificial sweeteners
- White flour and refined (fast-burning) carbohydrates
- Hydrogenated or partially hydrogenated fats/oils—avoid all fats and oils except for those listed as healthy in chapter 4 and on your Replenish Shopping List
- Sodas, including diet and "natural" sodas
- Sweetened beverages (including sweetened coffee and tea) and bottled fruit juice
- "Junk" foods of all kinds
- All artificial colors, preservatives, and additives
- Monosodium glutamate (MSG) and other artificial flavors

Should You Reintroduce?

I'll be honest. My daily diet is pretty darn close to the Reboot plus the 95/5 rule. Gluten-containing foods and dairy, both of which I tolerate well, are actually not part of my daily fare. They are on my 95/5 list. I feel better when they're an occasional thing, not a regular part of what I eat. It all comes down to paying attention to how your food makes you feel, and if it is giving you the energy, focus, vitality, and good feeling in your skin that you want, and then making personal choices.

If you're feeling incredible on the Reboot, if you've noticed dramatic changes in your symptoms by removing gluten and dairy, or other items you discovered were a trigger, you do not have to reintroduce any of the Reboot NO foods into your diet. In fact, once my patients discover that a specific food or food group was a contributor to how awful they felt, they never want to reintroduce it!

If that's the case for you, too, that's totally cool. If you have just started to get awesome results, or even baby ones but you're really noticing the shift start to happen, then I strongly urge you to keep going on the Reboot for another three weeks, then decide whether and what to reintroduce.

The most common foods women are generally curious about reintroducing are gluten-containing products, dairy, coffee, and something sweet now and then. Here are some guidelines for helping you decide whether to introduce gluten and dairy, after which I'll show you how. Then we'll chat about coffee and sugar. Note that if you're still *craving* sugar, refined carbs, alcohol, or other food triggers, this means that you haven't fully gotten to the Root Cause driving the craving, so please revisit page 142 and don't reintroduce these foods as long as the craving is the driver. Pleasure and desire feel different than craving—there's a sense of wanting rather than an uncontrollable *having to have.*

Should You Stay Gluten-Free?

If you did not notice any improvement after having gluten out of your diet for three weeks, then it's reasonable to *try* to reintroduce it in small amounts as an occasional part of the diet, as long as you stick to whole-grain forms. This is not license to eat a high-carb, processed-flour diet, which is one of the Root Causes of suffering for millions of people. Further, gluten intolerance masquerades as numerous illnesses that most Americans, and even the medical community, just take for granted as facts of life or natural consequences of aging. If you reintroduce gluten and experience any recurrence of the symptoms that got you to read this book in the first place, then do yourself a favor and keep gluten out of your diet.

Need Milk?

Dairy products (milk, yogurt, and cheese) aren't a problem for everyone. In the book *Blue Zones* Dan Buettner explores the diets and lifestyles of groups of people around the world with the highest numbers of centenarians—people who live to be over one hundred. Among several of these groups dairy is a regular part of the diet. Among the Sardinians, for example, who boast a shockingly large number of centenarians, the daily diet consists largely of bread, cheese, bean soup, and veggies, with meat about once a week. It's not just that many people live into their eighties, nineties, and some into their early hundreds, but they are doing it medication-free, and often living independently, working on their farms well into their nineties. Good-quality fats, which can be found in whole-milk dairy products, give us long-lasting, sustainable energy, reduce insulin spikes, keep us feeling full longer, and enhance carbohydrate metabolism, actually *enhancing* weight loss!

For a substantial number of people, however, dairy is an inflammatory trigger. Unlike in Sardinia, our milk isn't coming from the cows, goats, and sheep we're raising; it's coming from antibiotic-laden, hormone-filled cows. And unlike Sardinians, who grow up close to the land, where they are eating foods from their gardens, naturally inoculated with microbes from the soil, and are themselves raised largely antibiotic-free, there are numerous factors that impair our guts that may make dairy less tolerable.

In case you're wondering about the safety of remaining dairy-free, in contrast to the government recommendation of three glasses of low-fat milk per day for women, leading nutrition scientists David Ludwig and Walter Willett (one of my personal heroes) reported in *JAMA Pediatrics* what many in the natural wellness world have been pointing out for decades, that:

- Humans have no nutritional requirement for animal milk, which is a modern addition to the diet on an evolutionary scale.

- Low-fat and fat-free milk don't keep the fat off of us—and may, in fact, increase obesity. The emphasis on *low-fat* milk stems from misconceptions about the risks of fat in the diet, namely that fat makes you fat and that all fat is bad and causes heart disease, which, when it comes to healthy fat, just isn't true.

- Countries with higher rates of milk consumption also have higher rates of osteoporosis, and in addition, other scientists have shown a possible connection between high dairy consumption in some women and ovarian cancer, breast cancer, and heart disease.

- There is no evidence of the safety of lifelong exposure to the growth hormones naturally found in milk. They are, in all likelihood, triggers for some of our own hormonal problems. (I've had more women tell me their acne cleared up after going off of dairy than almost any other single dietary change.)

Instead, focus on plant-based sources of calcium such as green leafy vegetables, sesame seeds, beans and legumes, almonds, good-quality fats, and plant-based and nonvegetarian protein sources including beans, legumes, fish, poultry, and meat.

How to Reintroduce Foods

Reintroducing foods is simply a matter of paying attention to your symptoms as you add foods back in, noticing if symptoms return. This can happen after eating it once, or symptoms may creep back over several weeks, so you do have to pay close attention, even if the initial reintroduction doesn't trigger a recurrence.

Here's how the reintroduction works:

1. You'll reintroduce only a single food or food category (for example, gluten, dairy, fruit, beans) every three days.

2. Pick a food (for example, corn) or category (for example, nightshades) to reintroduce. Foods that you might try reintroducing include dairy, gluten (and cross-reactive grains such as corn or oats), and nuts if you've removed them. Then see how you do with various grains and beans if you've kept these out of your personal plan.

3. Include a typical-size portion of that food (for example, a slice of bread, ¼ to ½ cup of yogurt, etc.) at two meals each day, for three consecutive days.

4. Pay close attention to how you feel in the couple of hours after eating the food, and also pay close attention to how you feel over those few days, and record your findings (see the table on page 298).

5. If you experience any of the symptoms on the list below (or any recurrence of others you may have had before), then that food is either not right for you at all, or at least not yet.

   - Fatigue
   - "Brain fog"
   - Sleep disruption
   - Anxiety, depression, mood changes
   - Diarrhea, constipation, or severe digestive symptoms
   - Joint pain and swelling
   - Runny nose, watery eyes, dark circles under your eyes, allergy symptoms
   - Skin rash, itching, hives, canker sores, eczema

- Autoimmune symptoms / flares of Hashimoto's thyroiditis, inflammatory bowel disease (ulcerative colitis, Crohn's), rheumatoid arthritis, psoriasis, or vitiligo
- Cravings that come back with a vengeance
- Water retention—for example, rings get tight or there are lines on the ankles after removing your socks

In that case, remove the food, keep it out of your diet for another six to twelve weeks, and follow the 4R Program for Gut Health for another six weeks. Then try reintroducing the food again. If you're still not tolerating it, keep it out indefinitely, or seek an integrative or functional medicine practitioner for additional support.

6. If you have a food reaction, wait at least one day, and until any symptoms that reappeared clear up, before reintroducing the next food.

7. Pick the next food or food group to reintroduce, and repeat the process until you have trialed any of the foods you'd like to reintroduce.

Recommended Food Reintroduction Order

Here's the basic order I recommend for reintroducing foods that you've been avoiding. Remember to leave at least one day between each new food you trial, and discontinue any foods that cause any symptoms:

- Gluten
- Corn (and other gluten cross-reactives, page 139)
- Dairy
- Beans and legumes
- Nuts (unless you are truly allergic)
- Nightshades
- Yeast and vinegars
- Fruits

If you tolerate the reintroduction of gluten, dairy, or other food categories, it's still important to continue paying close attention to how you feel in ensuing weeks and months. If symptoms do begin to creep back in, repeat Reboot week one. Whichever foods you easily tolerate, plus the core Replenish Foods, form your personalized Replenish Lifestyle.

Seven-Day Food Reintroduction Journal (Covers Reintroducing Two Foods)			
Day 1			
Food Reintroduced			
After this meal I felt:	Breakfast:	Lunch:	Dinner:
Digestion			
Energy			
Mood			
Inflammation/ Allergy			
Sleep			
Other			
Day 2			
Food Reintroduced			
After this meal I felt:	Breakfast:	Lunch:	Dinner:
Digestion			
Energy			
Mood			
Inflammation/ Allergy			
Sleep			
Other			

Seven-Day Food Reintroduction Journal			
Day 3			
Food Reintroduced			
After this meal I felt:	Breakfast:	Lunch:	Dinner:
Digestion			
Energy			
Mood			
Inflammation/ Allergy			
Sleep			
Other			
Day 4			
Food Reintroduced			
After this meal I felt:	Breakfast:	Lunch:	Dinner:
Digestion			
Energy			
Mood			
Inflammation/ Allergy			
Sleep			
Other			

Seven-Day Food Reintroduction Journal		
Day 5		
Food Reintroduced		
After this meal I felt:	Breakfast:	Lunch:	Dinner:
Digestion		
Energy		
Mood		
Inflammation/ Allergy		
Sleep		
Other		
Day 6		
Food Reintroduced		
After this meal I felt:	Breakfast:	Lunch:	Dinner:
Digestion		
Energy		
Mood		
Inflammation/ Allergy		
Sleep		
Other		

Seven-Day Food Reintroduction Journal			
Day 7			
Food Reintroduced			
After this meal I felt:	Breakfast:	Lunch:	Dinner:
Digestion			
Energy			
Mood			
Inflammation/ Allergy			
Sleep			
Other			

Can I Have Coffee Now?

You might be surprised to find that you don't miss coffee at all once you've been off of it for a few weeks. You may even notice that you're less tired during the day, are sleeping better at night, and have fewer sugar cravings, and that long-standing hormonal problems such as PMS and breast tenderness improve or disappear. Some women do miss the ritual, in which case green, chai, or noncaffeinated herbal tea makes a lovely substitute for a hot (or cold) beverage. Yet others really do miss their coffee.

If you're missing your coffee because you're feeling tired without it, or you feel an addiction-like craving for it, you still have Root Causes that need attention. Coffee craving usually happens when you're not getting enough sleep or you're still having trouble with adrenal depletion. In your case, I'd keep the coffee out and work on healing issues by continuing to work on your Root Causes and supporting your adrenal health. If, how-ever, coffee is just a ritual and beverage you love, and you're able to func-tion and sleep without it, you're not craving it, but you just love and want some, then by all means add it in. But keep it to decaf if possible, no more than one cup per day, have it with a meal, not instead of one, and don't have it past midday. Some of my patients are thrilled to enjoy it on weekends only—a great option. Keep it unsweetened, and use whole cow's milk if you tolerate dairy, or an alternative to milk, such as coconut milk or almond milk.

What About Sugar? The 95/5 Rule

The next question is how *often* one can safely indulge in food simply for the pleasure of it.

People talk about the 80/20 rule—if you do the best thing 80 percent of the time, you can get away with anything. But 20 percent is a big amount. Twenty percent junk food in a diet is a whole lotta junk, and you can't stay healthy on that.

I personally follow the 95/5 rule in my life—I don't deprive myself of a piece of our local organic goat's milk caramel that melts like butter in my mouth and tastes heavenly (my favorite thing in the world) once every couple of months when I go to the store that sells it, and I have some dark chocolate most days of the week. I have only two rules: I only indulge in things that are real food, and I don't beat myself up after. I enjoy it with no guilt, shame, or blame.

So yes, I am saying that some sugar is okay now and then. A little more fruit in season, if you don't get gas, bloating, or dysbiosis symptoms (page 79) is reasonable, up to two servings per day; a little honey in your chai tea once in a while, a homemade dessert, a piece of your grandmother's pie that you've been enjoying since you were a kid. Yes. Sugar is a flavor that signals nourishment. It all depends on context, amount, quality, and frequency. But this only works if you can make it the exception, not the rule, and stay completely honest with yourself. If you have a history of sugar addiction, or if you have prediabetes, metabolic syndrome, or PCOS, it might not be as easy for you to safely indulge without tracking and monitoring how often it's happening. If you think about 95/5—well, that's a very small percentage of your overall food intake.

EAT FOR HOW YOU WANT TO FEEL: THE REPLENISH MANIFESTO

The key questions to come back to are *How do I want to feel?* and *How is this going to make me feel?*

Food is one of the most important forms of medicine we have—as I said before, it can truly heal your life. If eating a food is going to make you physically sick, for example, if you're highly gluten-sensitive and eating some pasta or a croissant is going to send you into an inflammatory flare, this is not a good idea. But if you really want a chocolate chip cookie, you're not gluten-intolerant or can get your hands on a really delicious gluten-free one, and you don't have diabetes—in other words, if it's not going to actually make you physically sick, then by all means have one—or several—but the trick there is to feel *really* good about it. ENJOY THE INDULGENCE. In my opinion, guilt can make you just as sick as sugar.

There's really only one *cardinal* rule to the Replenish Lifestyle—and that's *Eat to stay replenished.* Who doesn't want that? With each food choice comes the question "Is this going to help me to feel replenished?" How we feel replenished will vary with the time of day, what's going on in your life, and the demands you have on your energy. But if you can ask yourself this question, and take those thirty golden seconds with Permission to Pause to hear the answer your body is giving you, you'll be living the plan.

The Replenish Lifestyle is about making friends with food again—having a healthy food relationship, not a conflicted one. It's about learning to love eating healthily, while also sometimes simply eating what you love, without guilt or regret. A strange thing can happen when you start to experience success—strangely, many women self-sabotage. It gets back to what we talked about in chapter 5, "Reframe"—if your pattern is that feeling good feels unusual, and feeling bad is the normal default, your inner world might start to freak out a little and try to cling to feeling bad just because it's more familiar. This is where you get to remind yourself how you really want to feel, and reframe those automatic negative thoughts and feelings into a bold new one: I'm a mature woman and I get to choose how I want to feel, and I love feeling great. Shout that out to the universe! Really—go ahead, shout it out right now.

Eating to stay replenished eventually becomes second nature, but we live in a sea of junk foods and advertising that is meant to keep pulling us back down, meant to keep us hostage to the food industry's constant hawking of sugar, diabetes, and death, so you do have to stay committed and remind yourself *why* you're doing this—why you're choosing to break the mold and live outside of the box, making healthy your choice. It's a rebel stand in this day and time—and I invite you to take it.

Always choose real food. The fewer ingredients, the better. The closer it looks to how it is in nature, the healthier. Make 99 percent of your diet—or 100 percent if you can—nutrient-dense foods rather than empty calorie bombs of sugar, processed carbs, toxic fats, and inflammation. A really awesome practice is to stock your pantry and fridge with foods that have only one ingredient on the label. Remember to ask yourself, "What kind of information is this food going to give to my body?" It's a powerful question, and you now have enough food knowledge to answer that. You know that eating a perfect plate of gorgeous fresh veggies with an organic quinoa salad and chickpeas is going to give your body energy balance messages, eating dark, juicy berries is going to give your body optimal detox messages, and eating some energy veg or grain in the evening is going to give your body calming, cortisol-resetting messages. On the other hand, what's a Big Gulp or a bag of Oreos going to tell you?

SELF-LOVE IS THE
MOST IMPORTANT INGREDIENT

Self-love is the ingredient I see missing from most diets. And it's probably why most diets fail. Self-love is the main ingredient in the Replenish Lifestyle. It's the secret sauce to success, to feeling better, to reaching the moon and stars of your goals. And it's neuroscience, baby. So keep a jar of it in every room. Have some in your handbag. Stash some in your desk drawer. Sprinkle some into every pot you stir, salad you mix, smoothie you drink. Indulge in it like the finest dark chocolate.

It's time for women to get off the guilt wagon. All of us. We spend so much time body bashing, and beating ourselves up for not being "enough." Ironically, when we beat ourselves, we create mental SOS, and that statistically makes us more, not less, likely to binge again. I hope by now that you're well on your way to telling yourself a different story. But old thought patterns sometimes die hard. So this is a reminder:

How do you want to feel? I know you want to feel energetic, vibrant, and in charge of your body and life, so say, "Heck, yeah" out loud to this new way of eating—and being. Declare your intention to the universe. Eat empowered, eat for pleasure, eat to stay. Sprinkle self-love on everything. Stay replenished. You deserve it.

WEEK 4: REPLENISH, DAY BY DAY

Week 4 Sample Daily Meal Plan

Breakfast Example

8–12-oz. Smoothie (Shake)
or
Breakfast protein + good-quality fat (+ optional veggie)

Lunch Example

Protein entrée + green veggie + rainbow veggie + energy veggie + good-quality fat

Dinner Example

Protein entrée + green veggie + rainbow veggie + energy veggie + good-quality fat + small amount of fermented veggie (if tolerated)

Week 4
Sample Daily Menus and Lifestyle

	Day 22	Day 23	Day 24
Morning practice	The Quickie meditation (page 199)	Dry brush (page 232) in morning shower	5 minutes of deep breathing (page 191) and stretch
Fresh Start	Drink a glass of room-temperature or warm water with a squeeze of lemon.		
Breakfast + Daily Dose Supplements	Smoothie Bar	Frittata + mixed greens with Olive Oil Lemon Dressing	Smoothie Bar
Mid-morning	Hippie Mix	Coconut yogurt with raw cacao nibs and berries or Olive Oil Granola	½ apple sliced with 1 tbsp. almond butter
Mindful lunch + SOS Solution Supplements (if you've personalized your plan ahead)	Mediterranean Board (dinner leftovers)	It's a Wrap option	Leftover frittata + Make Your Own Salad choice
Mid-afternoon	Hardboiled egg with Himalayan sea salt sprinkle	Guacamole with veggies	Hippie Mix

Day 25	Day 26	Day 27	Day 28
The Quickie meditation	Dry brush in morning shower	5 minutes of deep breathing and stretch	Day off
Breakfast Scramble or Omelet + optional mixed greens with Olive Oil Lemon Dressing	Smoothie Bar	Breakfast Scramble or Omelet + optional mixed greens with Olive Oil Lemon Dressing	Power Parfait with optional Olive Oil Granola
Handful dry-roasted almonds with cayenne dash	Coconut kefir or Power Parfait	Rise and Shine Muffin or Power Balls	Hard-boiled egg with Himalayan sea salt sprinkle
The Art of the Buddha Bowl (possibly with salmon leftovers)	Parisian Salmon Salad leftovers + mixed green salad with Olive Oil Lemon Dressing	Hearty Beef Stew + steamed kale or green leafy salad	It's a Wrap option
2 squares dark chocolate + handful almonds	Hummus with veggies	Handful dry-roasted almonds with toasted nori shreds	Hippie Mix

Week 4
Sample Daily Menus and Lifestyle

	Day 22	Day 23	Day 24
Cortisol Reset	Reset your cortisol for the evening with 15 minutes of any Replenish Repair Kit practice		
Dinner + SOS Solution Supplements (if you've personalized your plan ahead)	Baked Walnut-Crusted Chicken + Sautéed Spinach with Pine Nuts	Miso-Glazed Salmon with Scallions and Sesame Seeds + Garlicky Green Beans	Big Fat Greek Salad with Grilled Tangy Chicken + optional Mediterranean Quinoa Salad or Garlic-Rosemary Fingerling Potatoes
Replenish Self-Care	Replenish Bath	Gratitude or Worry Journal	Digital Detox and read

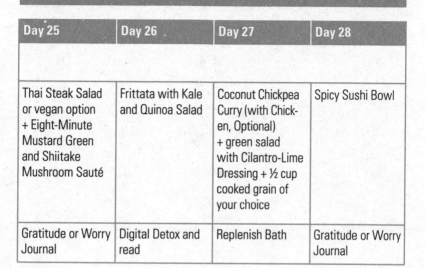

Day 25	Day 26	Day 27	Day 28
Thai Steak Salad or vegan option + Eight-Minute Mustard Green and Shiitake Mushroom Sauté	Frittata with Kale and Quinoa Salad	Coconut Chickpea Curry (with Chicken, Optional) + green salad with Cilantro-Lime Dressing + ½ cup cooked grain of your choice	Spicy Sushi Bowl
Gratitude or Worry Journal	Digital Detox and read	Replenish Bath	Gratitude or Worry Journal

CLOSING THOUGHTS
Staying Replenished Cell to Soul

You're as beautiful, as beautiful, you're as beautiful . . . as you feel.
—CAROLE KING

I F THERE'S ANYTHING I hope you take away from this book, it's this: You deserve to live your life in a way that keeps you replenished. No more running on empty, and with it running your adrenals and thyroid into overtime.

Self-care is not an indulgence or a luxury. It's essential to your health. It's a radical reclamation of your right to hit a pause button when you need to take care of yourself, and it's essential to supporting your self-repair mechanisms on every level. And you deserve it. You don't have to lean in, try to have everything, be everything, do everything for everyone all the time, and you can still be excellent at all you do. You deserve to live in a way that prevents you from ever getting into SOS again—even as a super-high-achieving woman. You deserve to create enough time to listen to your body, recognize your old stories, and create new ones. You deserve time to eat well, to take stock of what you're being exposed to environmentally and change it, and to sleep enough. And when you live this way, you restore healthy cortisol rhythms, keep inflammation in check, and keep your cravings and appetite healthy, your hormones in balance, and your mind clear.

You've got a whole set of power tools now. And I think women should have power tools. You have the tools to Reboot and Reframe, to Repair and

Recharge. You know how to find your You Zone and get your relaxation response on. You have the tools to stay Replenished. Now it's a matter of taking those tools forward into a sustainable lifestyle that keeps you out of SOS. How does it work?

It all starts with the question I asked you a few weeks ago: *How do you want to feel?* You must check in with yourself often enough to recognize how you are truly feeling. And when you're not feeling how you want to, you recalibrate. Remember, there's no perfect spot of balance that we stay in permanently. We keep recalibrating. You've actually learned all of the tools you need over the past few weeks to do this.

Remember, too, staying connected can help to counterbalance the normal stresses of everyday life, and the bigger ones should they happen. How can you stay connected? Through friends, relatives you love being with, church, synagogue, community action groups, yoga class, meditation groups, and, of course, my online community at avivaromm.com/adrenal-thyroid -revolution, where women can gather virtually to connect, share, learn, support each other, and stay inspired.

You've made an incredibly important choice in reading this book—it was a statement of hope and belief that you can turn your health around. And you are doing it. You've got this amazing and precious life that deserves to be lived well and celebrated. These Replenished Living skills aren't yours just for a day, a minute, or while you have this book in your hands. These are yours for a lifetime. They are what we, as women, didn't learn in school, might not have learned from our mothers, aunts, or older sisters, because they didn't know, and probably didn't learn from our doctors, who didn't know either. As Maya Angelou said, "Do the best you can until you know better. Then when you know better, do better." You've now become the one who knows. And you get to pass on the example and legacy of self-care, self-love, and Replenished Living to those women (and men) in your life who you love, reach, and teach. You might just change more lives than your own.

Wishing you a Replenished Life.

With love,

Dr. Aviva

RECIPES
The Replenish Kitchen

You don't need a silver fork to eat good food.
—PAUL PRUDHOMME

THIS CHAPTER will guide you to easily create the meals provided for your 21-Day Reboot, and will take you into the Replenish Lifestyle and well beyond. These recipes, from my own kitchen, are SUPER SIMPLE and really work. All of the recipes are gluten-free and dairy-free (though I do sometimes suggest adding feta or goat cheese to accent a recipe if you do include dairy occasionally *after* the Reboot), and with the exception of the fruit in the smoothies and natural sugar in the desserts, all the recipes are sugar-free.

The recipes are arranged by menu category (smoothies, wraps, salads, etc.). Most sections start with an example of how to prepare a recipe in that category. You then simply substitute the ingredients in the tables, in the amounts provided, following the same instructions as for the given recipe.

You can use any of the recipes in that section as a substitute for any in the weekly menus, too.

Even if you've never cooked before, you'll know how to after three weeks, and if you're an experienced cook, you'll have fun with the elegance and simplicity of the suggestions I've made. If you're totally new to cooking, or at least to cooking natural foods, no worries—visit the Natural MD Kitchen at my website, avivaromm.com, for a video and recipe library that will teach you all the basics and more. I also add new recipes regularly to keep you inspired and nourished. I promise you that becoming a great chef is easy, and so rewarding! Once your energy begins to climb, your waistline to shrink, and other unwanted symptoms begin to melt away, you'll be a lifelong convert to the cooking-at-home lifestyle that is one of the pillars of health.

THE REPLENISH SHOPPING LIST

This is a comprehensive list for stocking your pantry and includes more than the ingredients required for the recipes to show you what's possible beyond this book. You do not need to purchase everything on this list at once. Rather, print a copy out at avivaromm.com for each week, check off any ingredients you'll need to create your menus for the week you're on, and take the shopping list with you to the grocery store. You can also jot in the amounts next to the item.

Red Meat, Poultry, and Fish
(organic, grass-fed and -finished preferred)

- ☐ Atlantic mussels, farmed blue
- ☐ Beef
- ☐ Chicken, skinless white breast
- ☐ Farmed bay shrimp
- ☐ Mackerel
- ☐ Salmon
- ☐ Scallops
- ☐ Tilapia, U.S. farmed
- ☐ Turkey, skinless white breast
- ☐ Wild Alaskan sardines

Beans

- ☐ Black beans
- ☐ Chickpeas (garbanzo beans)
- ☐ Great Northern beans
- ☐ Kidney beans (red and white)
- ☐ Lentils
- ☐ Lima beans
- ☐ Navy beans
- ☐ Pinto beans
- ☐ Pure Pea protein powder (for smoothies)
- ☐ Refried beans, vegetarian
- ☐ Split peas
- ☐ Sprouted organic rice powder (for smoothies)
- ☐ Tofu (organic)
- ☐ White beans (cannellini or Northern)

Grains (gluten-free)

- ☐ Brown rice
- ☐ Buckwheat groats (kasha)
- ☐ Corn tortillas (sprouted)
- ☐ Millet
- ☐ Oats (rolled)
- ☐ Quinoa
- ☐ Rice noodles (Asian), rice pasta
- ☐ Wild rice (or pink, black, or other varieties)

Nuts and Seeds

- ☐ Almonds, almond butter
- ☐ Brazil nuts
- ☐ Cashews
- ☐ Chia seeds
- ☐ Flaxseeds
- ☐ Natural nut and seed butters
- ☐ Pecans
- ☐ Pine nuts
- ☐ Pumpkin seeds
- ☐ Sesame seeds
- ☐ Sunflower seeds, sunflower butter
- ☐ Tahini (sesame seed paste)
- ☐ Walnuts

Energy Vegetables

- ☐ Beets
- ☐ Carrots
- ☐ Mushrooms (all varieties)
- ☐ Parsnips
- ☐ Potatoes (NS)
- ☐ Pumpkins
- ☐ Spinach
- ☐ Squash (all varieties of "winter" squash)
- ☐ Sweet potatoes

Green Vegetables

- ☐ Arugula
- ☐ Bok choy
- ☐ Broccoli (fresh or frozen)
- ☐ Broccoli rabe (rapini)
- ☐ Brussels sprouts
- ☐ Cabbage (all varieties)
- ☐ Cauliflower (fresh or frozen)
- ☐ Chard (all colors)
- ☐ Collard greens
- ☐ Corn (frozen, organic)
- ☐ Dandelion greens
- ☐ Endives
- ☐ Escarole
- ☐ Kale
- ☐ Lettuce (all varieties)
- ☐ Mustard greens
- ☐ Snow peas
- ☐ Spinach (fresh or frozen)
- ☐ Sprouts

Rainbow Vegetables

- ☐ Artichokes
- ☐ Asparagus
- ☐ Bell peppers (all colors) (NS)
- ☐ Carrots
- ☐ Celery
- ☐ Chili peppers
- ☐ Cucumber
- ☐ Daikon radish and leaves
- ☐ Eggplant
- ☐ Green beans (fresh or frozen)
- ☐ Leeks
- ☐ Mushrooms (shiitake, portobello, others)
- ☐ Onions
- ☐ Peas
- ☐ Peppers (red and green bell) (NS)
- ☐ Peppers (jalapeño, serrano, etc.) (NS)
- ☐ Radishes
- ☐ Sea vegetables (all varieties)
- ☐ Shallots
- ☐ Snow peas (fresh or frozen)
- ☐ Sprouts
- ☐ Summer squash
- ☐ Tomatoes (NS)
- ☐ Zucchini

Fruit

- ☐ Apple (all varieties)
- ☐ Apricots
- ☐ Avocados
- ☐ Bananas (fresh or frozen)
- ☐ Blackberries (fresh or frozen)
- ☐ Blueberries (fresh or frozen)
- ☐ Cherries (fresh or frozen)
- ☐ Coconut
- ☐ Cranberries
- ☐ Figs (fresh)
- ☐ Grapefruit
- ☐ Grapes
- ☐ Kiwis
- ☐ Lemons
- ☐ Limes
- ☐ Mangoes (fresh or frozen)
- ☐ Nectarines
- ☐ Oranges
- ☐ Peaches (fresh or frozen)
- ☐ Pears
- ☐ Plums
- ☐ Pomegranates
- ☐ Raisins
- ☐ Raspberries (fresh or frozen)
- ☐ Strawberries (fresh or frozen)
- ☐ Tangerines

Fats and Oils

- ☐ Almond oil
- ☐ Avocado oil
- ☐ Coconut butter and oil
- ☐ Ghee (or organic butter)
- ☐ Olives (green, black)
- ☐ Olive oil (extra-virgin)
- ☐ Sesame seed oil (plain and toasted)
- ☐ Walnut oil

Beverages

- ☐ Green tea
- ☐ Herbal teas

Dairy Alternatives (and optional dairy)

- ☐ Almond milk (unsweetened or make your own)
- ☐ Coconut yogurt
- ☐ Feta cheese (organic, sheep's milk)
- ☐ Coconut kefir
- ☐ Coconut milk

Fresh and Dried Whole or Ground Herbs and Spices

- ☐ Basil
- ☐ Bay leaves
- ☐ Black pepper
- ☐ Cardamom
- ☐ Cayenne (NS)
- ☐ Chili powder (NS)
- ☐ Cilantro (fresh)
- ☐ Cinnamon
- ☐ Cumin
- ☐ Curry powder
- ☐ Dill
- ☐ Garlic (fresh or powdered)
- ☐ Ginger
- ☐ Mint
- ☐ Oregano
- ☐ Paprika (NS)
- ☐ Parsley
- ☐ Red chili flakes (NS)
- ☐ Rosemary
- ☐ Salt (sea salt, Himalayan salt)
- ☐ Thyme
- ☐ Turmeric

Condiments and Extras

- ☐ 72 percent dark chocolate if desired
- ☐ Apple cider vinegar
- ☐ Balsamic vinegar
- ☐ Champagne vinegar
- ☐ Chicken, beef, or vegetable stock (or make from scratch)
- ☐ Crushed canned tomatoes (NS)
- ☐ Dijon mustard
- ☐ Gluten-free tamari (or Bragg's Aminos if you don't eat soy)
- ☐ Maple syrup
- ☐ Raw cacao powder and nibs
- ☐ Red and white miso
- ☐ Rice vinegar

Fermented Foods

- ☐ Kimchi
- ☐ Sauerkraut

THE RECIPES

The Smoothie Bar

Smoothies are perfect for an on-the-go but complete breakfast or afternoon pick-me-up. Making up your own smoothies is ridiculously easy once you know the basics. All smoothies contain a protein source, a healthy liquid that usually adds additional protein and/or fat; healthy fat, fruits, or vegetables; and health "extras."

How to Make a Smoothie

Place the following ingredients into your blender:

   1 scoop plant protein powder

   1–2 tbsp. of a healthy fat, often a nut butter, which adds protein

   ½ cup total mixed fruit (frozen makes the smoothies so much creamier and more delicious, but you can use fresh)

   ¾–1 cup liquid (depending on the thickness you prefer) of choice (usually chilled almond milk, coconut milk, coconut kefir, goat's milk if you eat dairy)

   Optional nutrient boosts

Blend all ingredients in a blender until smooth.

Serves: 1
Prep and cook time: 3 minutes

Make Your Own Smoothie

Chai-liscious Detox

Anti-inflammatory and detox support

Protein:	1 serving plant-based protein powder
Healthy Fat:	1 tbsp. almond butter

Fruit/Vegetable:	1 frozen banana Optional 1 cup spinach
Liquid:	Coconut milk
Nutrient Boost:	1 tsp. turmeric powder (or 1 inch fresh turmeric) ½ tsp. grated fresh gingerroot ¼ tsp. crushed cardamom seeds

Hot Mama Super Smoothie

Hormone-supporting, adrenal-boosting power

Protein:	1 serving plant-based protein powder 1 tbsp. hemp seeds
Healthy Fat:	1 tbsp. coconut oil
Fruit/Vegetable:	½ to 1 frozen banana ½ cup frozen black cherries 1 pitted Medjool date (optional for some sweetness)
Liquid:	Unsweetened almond milk
Nutrient Boost:	1 to 2 tsp. maca powder 1 tbsp. raw cacao powder Optional: ½ tsp. bee pollen

Omega Brain Power

Super antioxidant brain and inflammation support

Protein:	1 serving plant-based protein powder
Healthy Fat:	1 tbsp. coconut oil Optional brain boost: MCT oil (order from Bulletproof Coffee, for example)
Fruit/Vegetable:	1 cup berries (strawberries, blueberries, raspberries)
Liquid:	Unsweetened almond milk
Nutrient Boost:	1 tbsp. pre-soaked chia seeds 1 tsp. hemp seeds 1 tsp. freshly ground flaxseeds Optional 1 tsp. omega-3 fish oil

Make Your Own Smoothie

Green Dream

Green-powered, antioxidant, anti-inflammatory

Protein:	1 serving plant-based protein powder 1 tbsp. ground flaxseeds
Healthy Fat:	½ ripe avocado
Fruit/Vegetable:	1 frozen banana 1 cup baby spinach
Liquid:	Coconut water
Nutrient Boost:	1 tbsp. fresh lemon juice 1 tsp. finely grated gingerroot

Berry Bliss

Protein:	2 tbsp. ground flaxseeds
Healthy Fat:	2 tbsp. walnuts
Fruit/Vegetable:	1 frozen banana 1 cup blueberries or mixed berries
Liquid:	Almond milk
Nutrient Boost:	Optional 1 tsp. finely grated gingerroot

Almond Butter Cup Shake

Antioxidant, energy-boosting, delicious

Protein:	1 tbsp. pre-soaked chia seeds
Healthy Fat:	2 tbsp. almond butter
Fruit/Vegetable:	½ avocado
Liquid:	Almond milk
Nutrient Boost:	1 tbsp. raw cacao powder

Tropical Refresh

Protein:	½ cup coconut yogurt or unsweetened organic yogurt (after Reboot) or 1 scoop sprouted rice protein powder
Healthy Fat:	1 tbsp. coconut oil

Fruit/Vegetable:	1 cup mixed frozen pineapple and mango chunks, kiwi if available
Liquid:	1 cup coconut or almond milk
Nutrient Boost:	1 tbsp. freshly ground flaxseed, 1 tsp. turmeric powder, or ½-inch section fresh turmeric root ½-inch section fresh grated gingerroot

Choco-Cherry Greenie

From Alexandra Jamieson
Functional nutrition coach, certified in applied positive psychology
Author, *Women, Food, and Desire*

Protein:	1 scoop protein powder
Healthy Fat:	1 tbsp. coconut oil or ½ avocado
Fruit/Vegetable:	1 cup fresh spinach 1 cup frozen cherries ½ banana
Liquid:	Almond or coconut milk
Nutrient Boost:	½ tsp. cinnamon 1 tbsp. raw cacao powder

Power Parfait

A nice change of pace—just scoop the yogurt into the cup and add toppings for this one. Eat with a spoon, not a straw!

Protein:	½ cup coconut yogurt or unsweetened organic yogurt (if past the Reboot and you tolerate dairy)
Healthy Fat:	2 tbsp. almond butter
Fruit/Vegetable:	Summer: 1 cup blueberries, blackberries, and/or raspberries Winter: ½ chopped apple
Liquid:	None
Nutrient Boost:	Topping options: ¼ cup chopped toasted almonds or walnuts 2 tsp. toasted ground flax-seeds 2 tsp. cacao nibs 1 tsp. maple syrup or raw honey

The Breakfast Scramble or Omelet Option

How to Make a Breakfast Scramble

Place 1 tbsp. of your oil of choice into a cast iron or stainless steel skillet.

Bring to medium heat so the oil melts.

Sauté ½ cup mixed vegetables; if you use onions, sauté those first for 2 minutes until translucent, then add the remaining veggies, which should be sautéed for about 3 to 5 minutes until they are bright in color and coated in the oil.

Season the veggies with the recommended herbs and flavorings.

If you're using eggs, beat them and then add a dash of salt and black pepper, or other seasonings of your choice.

Either add in your tofu, or remove the veggies and scramble 2 eggs in the skillet, adding the veggies back when the eggs are finished.

This makes a complete breakfast meal. If having for lunch or dinner, serve over a bed of rice noodles, quinoa or other grain, or a sprouted rice tortilla.

How to Make an Omelet or "Fried Egg"

Prepare your skillet, eggs, and veggies as above, but instead of scrambling, let the eggs set and after a few minutes flip the whole thing to cook on the other side. Should be golden yellow and firm on both sides. Slide onto a plate and top with your veggies.

Serves: Each scramble or omelet below serves 1 person.
Prep and cook time: 12 minutes

Make Your Own Break Scramble or Omelet

Asian

Protein: ¼ brick tofu or 2 eggs

Veggies: ½ cup mixed sautéed scallions or sliced yellow onion, shiitake mushrooms, finely chopped napa cabbage, and broccoli; if you tolerate nightshades, add in red bell pepper (NS)

Fat (Cooking Oil): 1 tbsp. coconut or sesame oil, lightly heated

Seasoning and Finishing Touches:
1 tbsp. gluten-free tamari or Bragg's Liquid Aminos, sesame seeds

Optional: Serve with Slow Starch:
½ small sweet potato or ¼ cup wild or brown rice

Hippie Tofu

Protein: ¼ brick tofu

Veggies: 2 cups baby spinach, ¼ cup roasted or fresh red bell pepper (NS), ¼ cup sweet corn, and green onion

Fat (Cooking Oil): 1 tbsp. olive oil or coconut oil, lightly heated

Seasoning and Finishing Touches:
1 tsp. powdered turmeric, ½ tsp. ground cumin seed, salt and pepper to taste

Optional: Serve with Slow Starch:
¼ cup quinoa tabouli, sweet potato fries, or roasted potatoes with rosemary (NS)

Mexican Egg

Protein: 2 eggs

Veggies: ¼ cup red bell pepper (NS), 1 cup baby spinach, ¼ cup finely chopped red onion, 2 tbsp. black olives (optional)

Fat (Cooking Oil): 1 tbsp. olive oil, lightly heated

Seasoning and Finishing Touches:
Minced cilantro, ¼ to ½ avocado, fresh salsa

Optional: Serve with Slow Starch:
½ small sweet potato or ¼ cup sweet potato fries/nuggets

Make Your Own Break Scramble or Omelet

Asparagus and Onions

Protein:	2 eggs
Veggies:	½ diced yellow onion, 8 stalks asparagus—just the upper two-thirds
Fat (Cooking Oil):	1 tbsp. olive oil, lightly heated

Seasoning and Finishing Touches:
Chopped fresh chives, dollop of coconut yogurt (optional), and a sprinkle of fresh or dried dill

Optional: Serve with Slow Starch:
Roasted potatoes with rosemary (NS)

Fast, Filling Frittatas

How to Make a Frittata

Ingredients:

10 free-range eggs

4 cups mixed veggies of your choice—see recipes below for ideas

1 tbsp. olive oil for sautéing

Seasonings/spices of your choice

½ tsp. salt and few dashes pepper or red pepper flakes (NS)

Optional additional savory ingredients:

¼ cup chopped smoked salmon

6 slices bacon, baked then crumbled

½ cup feta cheese or ¼ cup Parmesan if you eat dairy *and only after the Reboot*

To prepare:

Preheat the oven to 400 degrees.

Sauté all the vegetables and fresh seasonings (garlic, ginger) in olive oil for 3 to 5 minutes, until glistening and just on the edge of tender, and turn off the heat. I sauté mine in a large cast iron skillet and bake the whole thing in the same skillet. If you don't have a cast iron pan, sauté in your usual sauté pan, then bake the whole thing in a casserole dish.

In a bowl crack the eggs and mix in your seasonings. Beat lightly for 30 seconds.

If you are making this dish in a cast iron skillet, crumble your feta over the vegetables if you are including it. Then, feta or not, simply pour the egg mix over the vegetables. If you are using a casserole pan, mix the veggies, eggs, and feta (optional) in a bowl and pour into a lightly oiled casserole dish.

Pop the skillet or casserole dish into the oven and bake 25 minutes, until very lightly brown on top and firm to the touch.

Serve plain or with some of your favorite hot sauce.

Serves: 6 to 10 people
Prep and cook time: 35 minutes

Make Your Own Frittata

Paleo Skillet Frittata

Protein:	10 eggs
Veggies (choose 2 or 3):	½ bunch chopped kale ½ cup zucchini, quartered and sliced small 1 diced red onion
Fat (choose 1 + cooking oil):	Olive oil (I have also used some of the bacon fat as an alternative)
Herbs/Spices:	2 cloves garlic Salt and pepper
Optional Protein Additions:	6 slices bacon, cooked by baking, crumbled into "batter," or leftover hamburger or pieces of grilled chicken ¼ cup fresh feta (after the Reboot only)
Serve with/on:	Serve on bed of arugula or mixed greens

Make Your Own Frittata

Frittato Italiano

Protein: 10 eggs

Veggies (choose 2 or 3):

1 yellow onion, diced
2 cups frozen spinach or 1 bunch asparagus, cut into bite-size pieces
1 red bell pepper, chopped (NS)

Fat (choose 1 + cooking oil):
Olive oil

Herbs/Spices: 1 cup chopped basil or 1 tsp. dried
½ tsp. dried oregano
¼ tsp. red pepper flakes (NS)
¼ tsp. black pepper
½ tsp. salt

Optional Protein Additions:
¼ cup fresh Parmesan cheese (after the Reboot only)

Serve with/on: Serve on bed of arugula or mixed greens

Latin Vibe Frittata

Protein: 10 eggs
½ cup cooked black beans

Veggies (choose 2 or 3):

½ cup roasted sweet potato nuggets (optional if you have time or leftovers—incredibly delicious)
½ bunch chopped cilantro
1 diced yellow onion
1 diced green bell pepper (NS)
½ cup frozen corn (if past the Reboot)

Fat (choose 1 + cooking oil):
Olive Oil

Herbs/Spices: ½ tsp. chipotle pepper (NS)
½ tsp. cumin
Sea salt
Black pepper

Optional Protein Additions:
    None

Serve with/on: Top with avocado or guacamole and extra cilantro, optional salsa

East Meets West Frittata

Protein: 10 eggs

Veggies (choose 2 or 3):
    2 cups small broccoli florets
    ¾ cup chopped shiitake mushrooms
    1 small bunch scallions, chopped
    1 diced red bell pepper (NS)

Fat (choose 1 + cooking oil):
    Coconut or sesame oil or ghee

Herbs/Spices: 2 tsp. fresh grated ginger
    2 cloves minced garlic
    ¼ tsp. black pepper
    2 tbsp. gluten-free tamari or 1 tsp. sea salt

Serve with/on: Top with extra scallions and, if you like it, Sriracha; serve on bed of mixed salad greens or sautéed veggies

The Lunch (or Dinner) Board

I sometimes serve my lunch—or a late afternoon snack—on a beautiful locally handcrafted wooden cutting board when I'm home lunching alone. I know that may sound funny, but I believe that the aesthetic—the presentation of food, how it appeals to all of our senses, not just aroma and taste—is part of the healthy digestion process. In fact, your brain starts to stimulate your digestive powers even when you just think about food. When you see appealing food, the effect can be amplified. Eating a lovely spread also creates a feeling of spaciousness, elegance, and time—it slows me down, makes me more present and conscious of my food, and as you've learned, this also improves your health. It's also a cognitive break from eating off of a plate, though I also recommend making a small investment in yourself and your kitchen now and then by collecting beautiful and fun dishes, utensils, and cups. I now treat myself along these lines for my birthdays and holidays—preferring lovely kitchen things over other gifts.

Below are some of my favorite lunch boards. I've done them with breakfast sandwiches. They work well for summer dinners, and even winter dinners accompanied by a soup, stew, or chili. I also put out larger but similar spreads for casual company visits and as appetizers when I have guests. Use these as springboards for your own ideas.

Serves: 2

Prep and cook time: 20 minutes to prepare board and ingredients

Make Your Own "Board"

The Middle East Board

Mains:	Scoop of hummus 2 falafel patties ¼ to ½ cup quinoa tabouli
Scoopers:	Boston lettuce leaves Gluten-free crackers (Mary's Gone Crackers are a big fave in my house) Crudités
Sides:	Olives in a small bowl
Dips:	Olive oil with a pinch of salt or Tahini Sauce
Extra Goodness:	Small bowl of dry-roasted, unsalted pistachio nuts or toasted almonds

The Mediterranean Board

Mains:	Amie Valpone's Sun-Dried Tomato Oregano Hummus (NS) Tuscan Kale Salad Tuscan Pasta Salad
Scoopers:	Gluten-free crackers

Sides:	Roasted cherry tomatoes (NS)
	Olives in a small bowl
	Artichoke hearts
	Roasted fingerling potatoes (NS), blanched green beans, and/or asparagus
Dips:	Fresh pesto
Extra Goodness:	Small bowl of dry-roasted, unsalted pistachio nuts or toasted almonds
	Goat cheese (if you eat dairy and are past the Reboot)

The Mex Board

Mains:	Sweet Potato and Kale Salad
	Mexican Black Beans
Scoopers:	Gluten-free crackers, veggie sticks (celery, carrot, and jicama are faves)
Sides:	Fresh salsa
Dips:	Guacamole
Extra Goodness:	Curried "Popcorn" Cauliflower

Salmon Caper Board

Mains:	Smoked salmon (or trout)
	Amie Valpone's Sun-Dried Tomato Oregano Hummus (NS)
	Rosemary roasted potatoes (NS)
Scoopers:	Sliced tomatoes (NS)
	Sliced red onion
	Gluten-free crackers
Sides:	Capers
	Pickled veggies
	Kimchi
Dips:	Dollop of coconut yogurt with a dash of salt and fresh or dried dill
Extra Goodness:	Bed of mixed greens with splash of Champagne vinegar or squeeze of lemon

The Art of the Buddha Bowl

How to Make a Buddha Bowl

A Buddha bowl typically contains:

A prepared grain—for example, rice, wild rice, quinoa, millet, or rice noodles, onto which you layer . . .

A portion of a sautéed or grilled protein (beef, chicken, tofu, or red lentil or chickpea dahl, for example), onto which you layer . . .

Lots of veggies—usually about 2 cups cooked per bowl—either steamed, sautéed, or baked (or a combo).

Then you top with:

A few tablespoons of sauce and . . .

A few tablespoons of chopped raw veggies—for example, mung bean sprouts or chopped cilantro

Plus:

A few tablespoons of a pickled vegetable if it mixes with the meal— for example, sauerkraut or kimchi—on the side (not as appropriate with Indian bowls, for example, dahl).

To prepare:

Cook 1 cup grain or 2 servings Asian rice noodles ahead of time (takes 30 minutes for grains, 10 for rice noodles). Sauté your meat of choice or tofu, or have your lentil or other dahl prepared ahead of time (takes 10 minutes for meat or tofu, 20 to 30 minutes for dahl). Steam, bake, or sauté your veggies. Mix your sauce. Chop your raw veggies as needed. Layer as above. Serve with the pickled veggies.

Serves: 2
Prep and cook time: 35 minutes

You're a Dahl Buddha Bowl

For the lentils:

Sauté 1 small chopped onion in 1 heaping tbsp. coconut oil.

Add 2 tsp. curry powder and sauté for 30 seconds.

Add 1 cup red lentils and sauté for another 30 seconds.

Add 3 cups water, cover, and simmer for 25 minutes.

Check and stir periodically to keep from sticking.

Add ½ tsp. salt at the end and stir.

For the veggies:

Cube 2 sweet potatoes, place in a baking tray, and drizzle with olive oil. Bake in a 400-degree oven for 25 minutes.

Cut 1 small head broccoli into florets (save the stems for another dish) and add to the sweet potatoes in the oven for the last 10 minutes of cooking.

Steam 3 cups washed, chopped kale for 6 to 8 minutes in a steamer basket.

To serve:

When all the ingredients are done cooking, place ½ cup of the cooked rice into a bowl, add a healthy scoop of the red lentils, then layer on the kale, then the roasted sweet potatoes and broccoli. Sprinkle on salt and black pepper to taste, and enjoy! Optionally top with a small handful of mung bean sprouts or 1 tbsp. chopped fresh cilantro.

Serves: 2 as a main dish or 4 as a complement
Prep and cook time: 40 minutes

Make Your Own Buddha Bowl

Broccoli Sesame Noodle Bowl

Slow Starch (Cook your grain or starch and put into the individual serving bowl first):
> Rice or soba noodles

Protein (Then layer on):
> Select from a chicken recipe below

Veggies (And on top of that layer):
> 4 cups combined broccoli, bell pepper (NS), bean sprouts, snow peas

For sautéing with or layered on . . . :
> 1 to 2 tbsp. coconut oil

Top off with seasoning and finishing touches:
> Ginger, tamari, garlic, sesame seeds

Spicy Sushi Bowl

Slow Starch (Cook your grain or starch and put into the individual serving bowl first):
> Quinoa, brown rice, pink rice, or rice noodles

Protein (Then layer on):
> Miso-Glazed Salmon

Veggies (And on top of that layer):
> Kale, shiitake mushrooms

For sautéing with or layered on . . . :
> Sesame oil

Top off with seasoning and finishing touches:
> Scallions, fresh avocado to garnish

Teriyaki Steak Bowl

Slow Starch (Cook your grain or starch and put into the individual serving bowl first):
> Jasmine rice or rice noodles

Protein (Then layer on):
> Teriyaki steak, chicken, or tofu, or use Tahini Sauce as your protein

Veggies (And on top of that layer):
> Bok choy, shiitake mushrooms, broccoli, chili peppers (NS)

For sautéing with or layered on . . . :
> Coconut oil

Top off with seasoning and finishing touches:
> Basil, scallions, garlic, tamari, side of sauerkraut or kimchi

Eastern Wisdom Bowl

Slow Starch (Cook your grain or starch and put into the individual serving bowl first):
> Quinoa, rice noodles, roasted sweet potatoes, or millet

Protein (Then layer on):
> Tofu (baked with miso/tamari marinade)

Veggies (And on top of that layer):
> Baked broccoli, finely sliced napa cabbage salad

For sautéing with or layered on . . . :
> Coconut oil

Top off with seasoning and finishing touches:
> Miso, tamari, toasted pumpkin, and/or sunflower seeds, side of sauerkraut or kimchi

Black Bean and Sweet Potato Bowl

Slow Starch (Cook your grain or starch and put into the individual serving bowl first):
> Quinoa, roasted sweet potatoes, roasted butternut squash, or an organic gluten-free tortilla (corn-free while on the Reboot)

Protein (Then layer on):
> 1 cup cooked Mexican Black Beans (or Pinto Beans), seasoned with ¼ cup cumin, chili powder (NS), and salt and black pepper to taste

Veggies (And on top of that layer):
> 1 cup chopped romaine lettuce
> 1 chopped tomato (NS)
> ¼ finely minced red onion

For sautéing with or layered on . . . :
> 1 ripe avocado, sliced thinly, or guacamole

Make Your Own Buddha Bowl

Top off with seasoning and finishing touches:
Toasted pumpkin seeds (1 tbsp. per bowl), ¼ cup chopped cilantro per bowl
Squeeze juice from ¼ lime per bowl over the top
Optional: ¼ tsp. freshly chopped jalapeño (NS) or habanero pepper sprinkled on top (NS)

Green Tara Lentil Bowl

Slow Starch (Cook your grain or starch and put into the individual serving bowl first):
1 cup cooked brown basmati rice

Protein (Then layer on):
1 cup green or red lentil dahl or Coconut Chickpea Curry (with Chicken, Optional)

Veggies (And on top of that layer):
Roasted Broccoli
Roasted Cauliflower

For sautéing with or layered on . . . :
Coconut oil or ghee for cooking

Top off with seasoning and finishing touches:
Fresh cilantro
Fresh chopped cucumber
Fresh chopped red onion
½ tsp. fresh ginger
Dollop of coconut yogurt (or organic dairy yogurt if past Reboot)

Spreads, Dips, and Pesto

Serves: 2 to 4
Prep and cook time: 10 minutes

Make Your Own Dip or Spread

Classic Hummus

(goes with Middle Eastern and Mediterranean meals)
To prepare, blend all ingredients in a food processor on high speed until smooth.

Base:	1 cup cooked garbanzo beans
Oil:	¼ cup tahini 2 tbsp. olive oil
Liquid:	2 tbsp. water or to the consistency you prefer (thick or thinner)
Savory:	¼ cup fresh lemon juice
Seasoning:	¼ tsp. roasted paprika powder (NS) Optional dash of cumin powder Serve with a drizzle of olive oil and dash of the paprika (NS)

Guacamole

(goes with Mexican/Latin meals)
To prepare, mash avocado in a bowl until creamy and then blend in the other ingredients with a fork until well mixed.

Base:	1 ripe avocado
Oil:	The avocado
Liquid:	The lemon juice
Savory:	1 to 2 tbsp. fresh lemon juice
Seasoning:	1 clove minced garlic 2 tbsp. chopped fresh cilantro 2 tbsp. chopped fresh tomato (NS) 2 tsp. finely minced red onion Salt to taste

Walnut Basil Pesto

(goes with Italian and Mediterranean meals)
To prepare, blend all ingredients in a food processor on high speed until smooth.

Base:	1 cup walnuts
Oil:	½ cup olive oil

Make Your Own Dip or Spread

Liquid:	None
Savory:	None
Seasoning:	1 cup fresh basil leaves
	2 cloves garlic
	½ tsp. salt, or to taste
	Optional ¼ cup grated Parmesan (if you eat cheese and only after the Reboot)

Amie Valpone's Sun-Dried Tomato Oregano Hummus (NS)

Amie Valpone is the founder of TheHealthyApple.com and the author of Eating Clean: The 21-Day Plan to Detox, Fight Inflammation, and Reset Your Body.

Ingredients:

1 cup white cannellini beans

4 tsp. salt

½ tsp. dried oregano

1 tbsp. freshly squeezed lemon juice

½ tbsp. minced garlic

2 tbsp. organic sun-dried tomatoes in oil (NS)

To prepare:

Combine all ingredients in a food processor and puree until smooth. Transfer to a serving bowl and serve with gluten-free whole-grain crackers or avocado toast, or add to a Buddha bowl. Store leftovers in a sealed container in the refrigerator for up to 3 days.

Serves: 2
Prep and cook time: 15 minutes

Eat-a-Rainbow Salads

Serves: 2
Prep and cook time: 10 to 35 minutes (longer if preparing grains or certain protein dishes such as Thai beef or chicken ahead of time)

Make Your Own Salad

Nappy Raw Citrus Salad

Green:	1 small napa cabbage, sliced very finely crosswise
Vegetable:	2 grated carrots 4 chopped scallions 1 finely chopped red pepper (NS) 1 cup chopped fresh basil ¼ cup chopped fresh cilantro ¼ cup bean sprouts
Protein:	Satay beef, chicken, or tofu
Fat:	Coconut oil for cooking
Dressing:	Grapefruity Ginger-Lime-Cilantro or Spicy Thai Dressing

Not Your Mother's Slaw

Green:	½ red and ½ green cabbage, chopped finely or minced in the food processor
Vegetable:	2 carrots, grated or minced in the food processor 2 tbsp. finely minced red onion ½ jalapeño, finely minced (NS) 1 bunch finely chopped cilantro
Protein:	Serve with Fiesta Fish
Fat:	Serve with avocado
Dressing:	Juice of ½ to 1 lime or Cilantro Lime-Dressing

Make Your Own Salad

Mexicali Black Bean Salad

Green:	1 head romaine lettuce
Vegetable:	¼ small red onion, chopped ¼ cup chopped tomatoes (NS) Fresh cilantro If you have them on hand, add ¼ to ½ cup roasted sweet potato nuggets
Protein:	½ cup Mexican Black Beans ½ cup shredded chicken (optional)
Fat:	1 avocado, sliced
Dressing:	Cilantro Lime-Dressing

Big Fat Greek Salad

Green:	3 cups mixed greens or large head of romaine, torn or chopped into large pieces
Vegetable:	2 cucumbers, chopped ½ cup cherry tomatoes (NS) 1 red bell pepper, chopped (NS) ¼ to ½ small red onion, finely chopped
Protein:	1 can chickpeas
Fat:	Olives (optional) ¼ cup feta cheese (optional after Reboot) or ½ avocado, sliced
Dressing:	Olive Oil Lemon Dressing (with oregano)

Tuscan Kale Salad

Green:	1 bunch lacinata kale, chopped into small pieces and massaged for 2 minutes with olive oil, salt, and lemon
Vegetable:	1 cup cherry tomatoes (optional) (NS)
Protein:	1 cup chickpeas and/or grilled chicken
Fat:	¼ cup pine nuts
Dressing:	Olive Oil Lemon Dressing A couple "twists" fresh black pepper 1 clove crushed garlic

Thai Steak Salad

Green:	1 large head butter lettuce or 1 small napa cabbage, sliced very finely crosswise
Vegetable:	1 cup bean sprouts 1 cucumber, chopped 1 red bell pepper, chopped (NS) Handful of cilantro or basil
Protein:	½ pound grilled sirloin tips or satay steak (chicken or tofu okay too)
Fat:	¼ cup toasted cashews (or peanuts if after the Reboot and no allergy)
Dressing:	Spicy Thai Dressing

Kale and Quinoa Salad

Green:	1 bunch de-stemmed and chopped kale (any variety), massaged for 2 minutes with squeeze of lemon, a few pinches of salt, and 1 tbsp. olive oil
Vegetable:	1 cup roasted sweet potatoes or delicata squash
Protein:	1 cup cooked quinoa
Fat:	⅓ cup toasted walnuts
Dressing:	Olive Oil Lemon Dressing

Marti Wolfson's Parisian Salmon Salad

Marti Wolfson, M.S.N.

Ingredients:

2 3.75-oz. cans sockeye salmon

2 tsp. Dijon mustard

4 tsp. olive oil

2 tsp. white wine vinegar

Salt

Pepper

2 cups cooked gluten-free pasta (I recommend Tinkiyada)

2 cups arugula

To prepare:

In a medium bowl mix the salmon, mustard, olive oil, and vinegar together with a fork until well combined. Add salt and pepper to taste. Fold in the cooked pasta and arugula.

Serves: 2

Prep and cook time: 10 minutes

Vegan Quinoa Tabouli

For a light meal, serve the tabouli salad and falafel (see page 364) over a bed of lettuce with some fresh olives on the side. For a heartier meal, accompany with hummus and pita bread or gluten-free crackers, grilled summer vegetables, and even a salmon dish.

There's about 30 minutes of prep involved—but the dish is simple to make, and the results are impressive!

Ingredients:

1 cup dry quinoa

¼ cup fresh lemon or lime juice

1 to 2 cloves fresh crushed garlic

¼ cup extra-virgin olive oil

1 tbsp. chopped fresh or 1 tsp. dried peppermint leaf

3 tbsp. finely minced red onion

2 medium tomatoes, diced (NS)

1 cucumber, diced

1 ½ tsp. salt

Fresh black pepper

1 cup freshly chopped parsley

To prepare:

Rinse quinoa for 2 minutes and combine in a pot with 2 cups water. Bring to a boil, then turn heat down to lowest setting and cook covered for 15 minutes. Turn off heat and let stand, covered, for 5 more minutes. Fluff with a fork and set aside. Combine lemon juice, garlic, oil, and peppermint, and mix thoroughly. Add onion, tomato, and cucumber. After the quinoa has cooled a bit, add seasonings/veggies. You can put the bowl in the fridge if you want it to cool thoroughly while you make the falafel.

Serves: 4
Prep and cook time: 25 minutes

Most Incredible Mediterranean Quinoa Salad—EVER!

Ingredients and prep:

Rinse and cook 2 cups quinoa.

Grill or oven-roast 2 large or 3 small bunches asparagus. To oven-roast, cut the asparagus into thirds and toss onto a baking tray, drizzle with olive oil, and salt, and bake at 400 degrees for about 15 minutes.

Toast ½ cup pine nuts.

Cut 1 pint cherry tomatoes in half (NS).

When the quinoa and asparagus are done, put into a large serving bowl. Add in pine nuts and tomatoes. Then add ⅓ cup golden raisins, and, optionally, ⅓ cup cubed feta cheese. (Or go vegan by skipping the feta.)

Add in plenty of olive oil—even ¼ cup works for me—a few splashes of red wine vinegar, and salt and pepper to taste.

Serve warm, at room temperature, or cool. Enjoy.

Serves: 4 to 6
Prep and cook time: 30 minutes

Tuscan Pasta Salad

Ingredients:

- ½ package cooked rice pasta (I prefer rotini, which is in the spiral shape, or penne; you can make this recipe with rice spaghetti as well.)
- 4 cups roasted broccoli
- ½ cup chopped red pepper (NS)
- ½ cup halved cherry tomatoes (NS)
- 1 ½ cups cooked garbanzo beans
- 1 ½ cups cooked red kidney beans
- ½ cup toasted pine nuts
- 1 clove garlic, crushed
- 1 cup fresh chopped basil leaves
- ¼ tsp. red pepper flakes (NS)
- ¼ tsp. black pepper (ideally, freshly ground)
- ⅓ cup Balsamic Shallot Vinaigrette (page 344)
- Optional: ⅓ cup chopped pitted green or black olives

To prepare:

Mix all ingredients in a large serving bowl. Serve warm, at room temperature, or cool. Add salt to taste if needed.

Serves: 4
Prep and cook time: 25 minutes

Salad Dressings and Sauces

How to Make a Salad Dressing

Combine all ingredients in your blender or food processor. Blend on high speed until smooth, about 1 minute. Dressings typically store well in a glass jar for 3 days in the fridge. Separation of the oil and other ingredients is normal—just whiz back in your blender or give the dressing a whisk or shake before using. Here are my favorite recipes. Use them as alternatives on any of the Replenish salads, and also as dips on your lunch boards. You'll also find some of these appearing in the Buddha bowls and wraps.

Serves: 2 to 4
Prep and cook time: 5 minutes

Make Your Own Salad Dressing

Green Goddess Dressing

Oil:	⅓ cup olive oil or ½ ripe avocado 2 tbsp. water for a creamy dressing
Herbs/Spices:	½ cup cilantro leaves 1 clove garlic, minced
Savory:	3 tbsp. fresh lime juice
Other:	¼ tsp. salt, or to taste

Olive Oil Lemon Dressing

Oil:	⅓ cup olive oil
Herbs/Spices:	Optional for variety also add: 1 tbsp. fresh or 1 tsp. dried rosemary leaves 1 tbsp. fresh or 1 tsp. dried oregano leaf Dash of black pepper
Savory:	3 tbsp. fresh lemon juice (you can use Champagne vinegar for a slightly different flavor)
Other:	¼ tsp. salt, or to taste

Cilantro-Lime Dressing

Oil:	⅓ cup olive oil
Herbs/Spices:	1 whole bunch of cilantro, stems mostly removed
Savory:	Juice of 2 fresh limes
Other:	¼ tsp. salt, or to taste 1 tsp. minced jalapeño (NS) or ¼ tsp. red pepper flakes (NS)

Make Your Own Salad Dressing

Honey Dijon Dressing

Oil:	⅓ cup olive oil
Herbs/Spices:	None
Savory:	1 tbsp. red wine vinegar 1 tbsp. Dijon mustard
Other:	¼ tsp. salt, or to taste 1 to 2 tbsp. raw honey

Balsamic or Champagne Shallot Vinaigrette Dressing

Oil:	⅓ cup olive oil
Herbs/Spices:	1 shallot, finely minced
Savory:	3 tbsp. balsamic vinegar or Champagne vinegar (the latter for a lighter taste)
Other:	¼ tsp. salt, or to taste

Spicy Thai Dressing

Oil:	⅓ cup toasted sesame oil
Herbs/Spices:	½ to 1 serrano pepper, seeded and minced, depending on how spicy you like it (NS) ½ cup fresh basil leaves
Savory:	3 tbsp. lime juice 2 tbsp. tamari (or 1 tbsp. Bragg's Aminos if you don't use soy)
Other:	¼ tsp. salt, or to taste 1 tsp. honey (optional)

Tahini Sauce

Oil:	½ cup tahini
Herbs/Spices:	1 clove garlic, crushed
Savory:	¼ cup fresh lemon juice 2 tbsp. water
Other:	¼ tsp. salt, or to taste

Spicy Tahini Sauce

Oil:	½ cup tahini
Herbs/Spices:	2 cloves garlic, crushed
Savory:	¼ cup fresh lemon juice 2 tbsp. water ¼ tsp. cayenne pepper (NS)
Other:	¼ tsp. salt, or to taste

Grapefruity Ginger-Lime Cilantro Dressing

Oil:	⅓ cup olive oil
Herbs/Spices:	¼ cup fresh cilantro leaves ½ inch fresh gingerroot, grated Dash of cayenne pepper (NS)
Savory:	¼ cup fresh pink grapefruit juice
Other:	¼ tsp. salt, or to taste

Fresh Basil Vinaigrette

Oil:	⅓ cup olive oil
Herbs/Spices:	¼ bunch of fresh basil leaves 1 clove garlic, minced
Savory:	⅓ cup water ¼ cup lemon juice 1 tsp. Dijon mustard
Other:	None

Creamy Cashew Dressing

Oil:	⅓ cup olive oil ⅓ cup raw cashews
Herbs/Spices:	1 clove garlic, crushed
Savory:	⅓ cup water ¼ cup lemon juice 1 tsp. Dijon mustard
Other:	None

It's a Wrap

Serves: Each recipe serves 1
Prep and cook time: 5 to 35 minutes, depending on whether your protein and grain are cooked ahead of time

Make Your Own Wrap

Cajun Lime Fish "Taco"

Wrapper:	Boston lettuce leaves, or if you eat corn after the Reboot, sprouted corn tortilla
Protein:	Fiesta Fish (can do with tofu, seasoned as for Fiesta Fish, or Mexican Black Beans if you are vegan)
Vegetable:	Not Your Mother's Slaw

Healthy Fat and Secret Sauce:
2 tbsp. guacamole per taco
Lime juice to taste
Salsa is terrific, too

Chicken Fajita "Taco"

Wrapper:	Boston lettuce leaves, gluten-free wrap, or 100 percent sprouted corn tortilla
Protein:	Fajita chicken or Mexican Black Beans
Vegetable:	Bell pepper (NS), red onion, romaine lettuce

Healthy Fat and Secret Sauce:
Avocado, cilantro, cumin, jalapeño pepper (NS)

Thai Lettuce Wraps (beef, chicken, or tofu wrap)

Wrapper:	Boston lettuce leaves or napa cabbage leaves; separate the leaves from the head and keep whole
Protein:	Teriyaki Steak Buddha Bowl
Vegetable:	¼ cup sautéed shiitake mushrooms ½ cup mixed raw mung bean sprouts, fresh cilantro, matchstick carrots, and scallions for layering on

Healthy Fat and Secret Sauce:
Sesame oil for sautéing
Spicy Thai Dressing

Hummus Wrap

Wrapper: Gluten-free wrap, romaine or Boston lettuce, or steamed collard
                greens

Protein: Hummus
                Optional scoop of Cauliflower or Vegan Quinoa Tabouli
                Optional falafel patty

Vegetable: Cucumber, tomato (NS), sprouts, red onion, chopped Kalamata
                olives

Healthy Fat and Secret Sauce:
                Tahini or Spicy Tahini Sauce

Nori Rice Wrap

Wrapper: Roasted nori sheets

Protein: Brown rice or cooked quinoa with Nappy Raw Citrus Salad
                using tofu

Vegetable: Mung bean sprouts, kimchi

Healthy Fat and Secret Sauce:
                Cilantro-Lime, Grapefruity Ginger-Lime-Cilantro, or Spicy Thai
                Dressing

Vegan Nori Wrap

Wrapper: Roasted nori sheets

Protein: Hummus

Vegetable: Carrot, avocado, red onion

Healthy Fat and Secret Sauce:
                Spicy Tahini Sauce

Fresh Turkey "Russian" Wrap

Wrapper: Romaine or Boston lettuce leaves

Protein: Sliced organic deli turkey

Vegetable: Sauerkraut

Healthy Fat and Secret Sauce:
                Avocado and/or Green Goddess Dressing

The Art of Greens and Rainbow Veggie Sides

Sautéed Kale and Toasted Walnuts

This recipe is a great intro to kale for greens newbies. Everyone loves it. It works whether your guests are vegan, Paleo, macrobiotic, or following a Mediterranean diet, because we all agree on one thing: greens are good for you!

There are only five ingredients. It's *easy*. And *quick* (15 to 20 minutes). And satisfying.

Ingredients:

> 2 tbsp. extra-virgin olive oil
>
> 2 bunches prewashed and cut kale (If you cut and wash your own kale—I do—add 5 minutes to the prep time.)
>
> 2 cloves garlic, minced
>
> ⅓ cup toasted walnuts, finely chopped
>
> 1 tbsp. tamari, aminos, or other similar salt seasoning

To prepare:

Heat oil in a large skillet or wok. Sauté the kale for about 5 to 7 minutes until glistening, bright green, and tender. Add the fresh garlic and sauté for another 1 to 2 minutes. Add the walnuts and tamari (or alternative) and sauté for another minute.

Serves: 2
Prep and cook time: 15 minutes

Roasted Broccoli

Ingredients:

3 cups of broccoli crowns, cut into florets

1 tbsp. olive oil

½ tsp. salt

Optional dash of garlic powder

To prepare:

Preheat the oven to 425 degrees. Toss with the olive oil and salt. Roast for 10 minutes. Toss and roast for an additional 5 to 10 minutes or until slightly crunchy. Sprinkle on garlic powder (optional) and stir. Serve hot.

Serves: 2
Prep and cook time: 25 minutes

Roasted Brussels Sprouts

Ingredients:

4 cups Brussels sprouts

2 tbsp. olive oil

½ tsp. salt

Pinch of red pepper flakes (NS)

2 tsp. balsamic vinegar

To prepare:

Preheat the oven to 425 degrees. Wash Brussels sprouts in a large colander. Trim the ends off and slice in half. Place Brussels sprouts on a baking sheet or in a large cast iron skillet. Add any leaves that may have fallen off when you trimmed them. Toss with olive oil and salt. Roast for 15 minutes and then stir. Roast for another 5 minutes and then remove from oven. Toss on remaining seasonings and stir. Serve hot or at room temperature.

Serves: 2
Prep and cook time: 30 minutes

Ginger-Lime Kale

Ingredients:

1 tbsp. coconut oil

1 clove garlic, finely minced

1 tbsp. fresh ginger, minced

¼ tsp. fresh chopped jalapeño pepper (NS) or dash of red pepper flakes (NS)

1 bunch of kale (any kind); remove the stems and chop into bite-size pieces

¼ cup coconut milk (full-fat)

¼ tsp. salt

2 tbsp. fresh lime juice

To prepare:

Melt oil in a skillet. Sauté the garlic, ginger, and, if using, fresh jalapeño for 1 minute. Add the kale and sauté for 3 minutes. Add coconut milk and sauté for another 5 minutes. Add salt, lime juice, and red pepper flakes (if not using jalapeño). Serve hot.

Serves: 2
Prep and cook time: 20 minutes

Sautéed Spinach (or Dandelion Greens) with Pine Nuts

Ingredients:

1 tbsp. olive oil

1 small red onion, sliced thinly

8 cups raw spinach, washed (or the same amount of fresh dandelion greens, washed and chopped into 1-inch sections, for a more bitter flavor and liver detox boost)

¼ cup pine nuts, toasted for 1 minute

½ tsp. salt (or tamari)

To prepare:

Lightly heat olive oil in a large skillet. Sauté the onion until slightly translucent, add the greens, and sauté until soft, about 3 minutes. Add the toasted pine nuts and salt (or tamari). Serve hot.

Serves: 2
Prep and cook time: 10 minutes

Sweet Potato and Kale Salad

Ingredients:

   4 sweet potatoes, peeled and chopped into bite-size chunks

   Extra-virgin olive oil

   1 tsp. smoked paprika (NS)

   Salt and pepper

   1 bunch of curly kale

   Juice of ½ lime

   ½ cup frozen organic corn (omit if you don't tolerate corn or aren't past the Reboot)

   1 tsp. honey (optional)

To prepare:

Preheat the oven to 400 degrees. Put sweet potatoes onto a baking tray, drizzle with olive oil, and toss in the paprika, salt, and pepper. Roast for 35 to 40 minutes, or until potatoes are soft on the inside and just a little crisp on the outside. Remove the stems from the kale and chop the leaves into bite-size pieces. Put into a bowl, add lime juice and a pinch of salt, and then "massage" the kale with your hands for 3 minutes to soften. Heat a skillet until hot and add the corn, stirring frequently until slightly brown. Then add it to the kale. Add the sweet potatoes to the kale and corn when done. Toss it all together, drizzle with honey if using, and serve. Leftovers are delicious at room temperature. I serve this dish with vegetarian chili and sliced avocado on the side.

Serves: 4 to 6
Prep and cook time: 50 minutes

Against the Grain Cauliflower Tabouli

Ingredients:

- 1 cauliflower (about 1 1/2 pounds)
- 1 chopped medium organic tomato (NS), or 1/2 cup halved cherry tomatoes (NS)
- 1/2 organic cucumber, peeled and diced
- 2 tbsp. minced red onion
- 1/2 to 1 cup finely chopped Italian parsley
- 1 to 2 tbsp. finely chopped fresh mint
- 1/4 cup olive oil
- 1/4 cup lemon juice
- 2 tbsp. sesame tahini
- 1 clove garlic, crushed (optional)
- Salt to taste

To prepare:

Cut the cauliflower into florets and place in a steamer basket. Steam for 5 to 8 minutes, then let cool in the pot. Place half of the florets into a food processor and pulse about 10 to 15 times to a crumbly consistency. Transfer to a bowl. Repeat with the other half of the florets, and then add to the same bowl. Allow to cool for another 10 minutes. Add the remaining ingredients. Mix well, cool, and serve.

Serves: 4 to 6
Prep and cook time: 20 minutes

Eight-Minute Mustard Green and Shiitake Mushroom Sauté

Ingredients:

- 3 cups shiitake mushrooms, sliced in half or quarters, depending on their size
- 2 tbsp. olive oil

1 bunch of fresh mustard greens, chopped (not too small)

4 cloves fresh garlic, chopped

Tamari or salt

Rice wine vinegar

To prepare:

Sauté shiitake mushrooms in olive oil for 2 minutes, stirring often. Add the mustard greens and garlic. Sauté for about 5 minutes. Add a light drizzle of tamari (or a few pinches of salt if you don't use soy) and a very light splash of rice wine or other light vinegar. Serve hot.

Serves: 2
Prep and cook time: 10 minutes

Curried "Popcorn" Cauliflower

Stefanie Sacks, M.S., C.N.S., C.D.N., culinary nutritionist, author of
What the Fork Are You Eating?, stefaniesacks.com

Ingredients:

2 tbsp. coconut oil

4 cloves garlic, minced

½ small red onion, finely diced

2 tbsp. curry powder

1 tsp. ground cumin

1 head cauliflower, chopped into small, popcorn-like pieces

¼ cup roughly chopped cilantro

Juice of 1 lime

Salt to taste

To prepare:

In large sauté pan, heat oil on medium, then add garlic, onion, curry, and cumin. Cook until slightly browned (about 2 minutes). Add cauliflower and mix to coat cauliflower; toss regularly until cauliflower is golden and tender. Finish with cilantro, lime juice, and salt.

Serves: 2
Prep and cook time: 10 minutes

Garlicky Green Beans and Roasted Almonds

Ingredients:

- 1 lb. green beans, with ends cut off
- 1 tbsp. olive oil
- 2 cloves garlic, finely minced
- Salt
- ¼ cup chopped roasted almonds (see page 371 in "Snack Stash and Sweet Treats")

To prepare:

Steam the green beans for 5 minutes. Drizzle with olive oil and crushed garlic. Sprinkle with a pinch of salt. Toss with the almonds. Alternatively, you can sauté the green beans in the oil.

Serves: 2
Prep and cook time: 10 minutes

Energy Veggie Sides

Sautéed Orange Ginger Carrots

Ingredients:

- 1 tbsp. coconut oil
- 1 tbsp. grated fresh ginger
- 4 carrots, peeled and grated
- 2 tbsp. freshly squeezed orange juice
- Pinch of salt

To prepare:

Heat oil in a skillet until melted. Sauté the ginger for 1 minute. Add the carrots and sauté for 3 minutes. Add the orange juice and cover the skillet. Simmer for 2 minutes. Turn off the heat. Add a pinch of salt. Serve hot.

Serves: 2
Prep and cook time: 10 minutes

You Can't Beat These Roasted Beets

Ingredients:

4 medium red beets

4 medium heirloom tomatoes (NS)

1 bunch of fresh cilantro

2 to 4 tbsp. extra-virgin olive oil

Salt and black pepper to taste

4 tbsp. chèvre (plain or garlic/chive; omit if you're not past the Reboot or don't tolerate dairy)

Several tbsp. fresh dill (if available) or 1 tsp. dried dill weed

To prepare:

Preheat the oven to 400 degrees. Wash the beets, trim off the very top and bottom, wrap in foil, place on a baking tray, and bake for 75 minutes. Meanwhile, wash and slice the tomatoes and lay them on a serving platter. Chop the cilantro. When the beets are done cooking, open the foil and run the beets under cool water. Then gently rub off the skin. It should peel off super easily. Slice the beets thinly and lay over the tomatoes. Drizzle the olive oil and sprinkle the cilantro over the tomatoes and beets, sprinkle on salt and pepper to taste, and sprinkle the chèvre and dill over the whole thing. Serve immediately or chilled. Amazingly delicious!

Serves: 4
Prep and cook time: 85 minutes

How to Make Roasted Veggies

Ingredients:

4 cups veggies—for the root veggies, cut into cubes (with the exception of sweet potato fries); for the rainbow veggies, cut into quarters or eighths—so big chunks, basically.

Olive or coconut oil

Salt and black pepper

Additional herbs as recommended in the table

To prepare:

Cut the veggies into 1- to 2-inch cubes. For the winter squash, cut into "rings" or halve. Toss in a bowl with the olive oil, salt, and seasonings. Place the veggies on a baking tray (lay out the squash rings or place the squash halves facedown) and bake at 400 degrees for 40 minutes. For all but the sweet potato fries and the rosemary roasted potatoes, I start by covering the tray for 30 minutes, then bake uncovered for the remaining time. The veggies should be tender but not mushy. For slightly drier veggies, spread the mixture over two baking trays rather than one.

Serves: 4
Prep and cook time: 50 minutes

Make Your Own Roasted Veggies

Oven-Roasted Sweet Potato Fries

Root Veggies:	4 sweet potatoes, cut into "French fry" shapes or 1-inch bite-size pieces
Rainbow Veggies:	None
Oil:	2 tbsp. olive oil drizzled over
Seasonings:	Salt + Optional additional varieties: Roasted paprika (NS) Rosemary Garlic Cayenne (NS)

Rosemary Roasted Root Veggies

Root Veggies:	4 cups of a variety of root vegetables—choose from sweet potatoes, parsnip, carrots, small potatoes (NS), beets cut into 2-inch chunks
Rainbow Veggies:	1 red and 1 yellow onion cut into 4 wedges
Oil:	2 tbsp. olive oil drizzled over
Seasonings:	¼ tsp. salt, to taste ½ tsp. dried rosemary (or, if you have fresh rosemary, cook 2 to 3 sprigs in with the veggies)

Garlic-Rosemary Fingerling Potatoes (NS)

Root Veggies:	1 lb. fingerling potatoes, whole or sliced in half (NS)
Rainbow Veggies:	1 bulb garlic, separated into cloves and peeled
Oil:	2 tbsp. olive oil drizzled over
Seasonings:	¼ tsp. salt, to taste ½ tsp. dried rosemary (or, if you have fresh rosemary, cook 2 to 3 sprigs in with the veggies)

Roasted Maple Winter Squash

Root Veggies:	2 medium delicata squash (scoop out pulp and seeds, and cut crosswise into 1-inch rings) or 1 medium butternut squash (scoop out pulp and seeds, and cut lengthwise)
Rainbow Veggies:	None
Oil:	Delicata squash: drizzle rings with olive oil and optionally 2 tsp. maple syrup and dash of cinnamon; butternut squash: rub the outside with olive oil and, when done, turn over, sprinkle with maple syrup and cinnamon, and bake 5 more minutes
Seasonings:	Salt Cinnamon Maple syrup (only after Reboot)

Soup's On

My grandma, a classic (i.e., stereotypical) Jewish grandma and cook, would almost always have a pot of vegetable soup, barley soup, split pea soup, or, dare I say, the classic chicken soup waiting for us upon our arrival. Soups go so far back into my personal comfort memories that they are practically a part of my lizard brain! So I REALLY LOVE SOUPS because they are ALL ABOUT THE LOVE to me! During the cooler months, I usually make some kind of soup at least once a week. And I always remember my grandma.

Soups are amazing because:

- You can make a great soup from practically anything you have in your fridge and pantry.
- You can feed a lot of folks from one pot.
- You can have leftovers for several days.
- One-pot meals are easy to make and clean up from!
- They are warm, cozy, friendly, and nourishing, and fill your home with an aroma of deliciousness.
- I occasionally use soup recipes—mostly when I want to try something new or taste someone else's style of cooking—but I mostly make them up.

Vegan Detox Nutrient Broth

Potassium broth helps to alkalize your system and provides you with essential electrolytes to keep your cells happy and energized while you detox. It is easy and inexpensive to make. The addition of turmeric and rosemary adds an antioxidant boost that also lends some support to your liver. This recipe makes 6 to 8 cups. Prepare it the day before you begin your detox. It keeps in the fridge for up to five days and can even be frozen for future use! If you feel hungry, have an extra cup!

Ingredients:

- 4 medium organic white potatoes (NS) (or sweet potatoes if sensitive to nightshades or during Reboot), cleaned but not peeled
- 6 large organic carrots, cleaned but not peeled
- 2 large organic yellow onions
- 6 stalks organic celery
- 1 cup chopped fresh organic parsley
- 1 tbsp. turmeric powder
- 1 tsp. dried rosemary
- 2 tsp. good quality salt
- 12 cups filtered (or pure) water

To prepare:

Chop the veggies and place them and the parsley, turmeric, and rosemary into a large stainless steel pot. Add the salt. Cover with water. Bring to a boil, then simmer for 1 hour. Strain out and discard the vegetables, saving the broth. Drink 1 to 2 cups daily.

Serves: 6 to 8
Prep and cook time: 80 minutes

Butternut Squash Curry Coconut Soup

Ingredients:

- 1 1/2 tbsp. olive oil
- 3/4 cup sliced shallots
- 1 tbsp. minced or grated fresh ginger
- 1 garlic clove, minced
- 9 cups peeled and cubed butternut squash (about 3 lb.)
- 3 cups chicken or vegetable broth
- 1/2 tsp. salt, plus more to taste
- 1 tsp. Thai red curry paste

¾ cup light coconut milk

2 tsp. fresh lime juice

To prepare:

In a large pot over medium heat, warm the olive oil. Add the shallots and cook until softened, 2 to 3 minutes. Add the ginger and garlic and cook until fragrant but not browned, about 1 minute more. Add the squash, broth, and the ½ tsp. salt, increase the heat to high, and bring to a boil. Reduce the heat to maintain a simmer, cover, and cook until the squash is tender when pierced with a fork, about 20 minutes. Let cool slightly. Put the curry paste in a small bowl and stir in the coconut milk until well blended. In a blender or food processor, puree the soup, in batches if necessary, until smooth. Return the soup to the pot and stir in the coconut milk mixture. Heat the soup until just hot, then stir in the lime juice and adjust the seasoning with salt. Ladle the soup into warm bowls and serve immediately.

Serves: 4
Prep and cook time: 40 minutes

Rosemary Bean Soup

Ingredients:

2 tbsp. olive oil

2 yellow onions, chopped

2 carrots, chopped

3 celery stalks, chopped

½ sweet red pepper, chopped (NS)

4 cloves garlic, chopped

1 small head broccoli, cut into small florets

Some handfuls of fresh spinach leaves

16 oz. organic vegetable or chicken broth

6 cups water

1 sprig fresh rosemary or ½ tsp. dried rosemary

15.5-oz. can kidney beans

15.5-oz. can garbanzo beans

¼ tsp. red pepper flakes (NS)

Salt and pepper to taste

To prepare:

Heat the oil in a large pot over medium heat and sauté the onion until slightly translucent. Add the carrots, celery, red pepper, garlic, and broccoli and sauté for about 3 minutes. Add the broth, water, and rosemary, bring to a boil, turn down, and simmer vigorously for 30 minutes. Stir a few times here and there. Add the beans and seasonings. Cook another 10 minutes. Voilà! Done, gorgeous, and delicious.

Serves: 6 to 8
Prep and cook time: 50 minutes

Make Your Own Soup

Tortilla Soup

Liquid:	2 cups chicken stock, 1 can crushed tomatoes (NS)
Vegetable:	1 red bell pepper (NS), 1½ cups corn, 1 jalapeño pepper (NS), 1 yellow onion
Protein:	1 lb. shredded chicken, 1 can black beans
Fat:	4 tbsp. olive oil or coconut oil
Seasoning:	Cumin, garlic, chili powder to taste, minced cilantro

Hearty Beef Stew

Liquid:	4 cups beef stock or bone broth
Vegetable:	4 small Yukon potatoes (NS), 2 stalks celery, 2 carrots, 1 yellow onion, 1 cup frozen peas
Protein:	1 lb. grass-fed cubed beef
Fat:	2 tbsp. olive oil
Seasoning:	Thyme, 1 bay leaf, 2 tbsp. tomato paste (NS), black pepper and salt to taste

Beans, Beans

Moroccan Spinach, Coconut, and Chickpeas

Ingredients:

   1 tbsp. coconut oil

   1 tsp. finely grated gingerroot

   2 garlic cloves, crushed

   1 shallot, diced

   1 red bell pepper, cut into thin strips (NS)

   ½ tsp. ground turmeric

   1 tsp. ground cumin

   ¼ tsp. ground cinnamon

   2 tbsp. coconut cream

   1 cup water

   1 lb. spinach leaves

   2 cans (approx. 12 oz. each) chickpeas, drained

   Salt to taste

To prepare:

Heat the oil in a skillet over medium heat. Add the gingerroot and garlic and stir-fry for half a minute. Add the shallot and bell pepper and stir-fry for 5 to 6 minutes until slightly softened. Stir in the spices and coconut cream. Sauté for 2 to 3 minutes, then pour in the water and bring to a boil. Add the spinach and chickpeas and cook for 5 to 6 minutes, or until the spinach has just wilted. Season with salt to taste.

Serves: 4
Prep and cook time: 15 minutes

Mexican Black Beans (or Pinto or Kidney Beans)

Ingredients:

2 tbsp. olive oil

1 yellow onion, chopped

1 red bell pepper, chopped (NS)

1 bunch of fresh cilantro, stemmed and chopped

½ cup frozen corn (optional)

½ to 1 whole jalapeño, minced (optional) (NS)

2 cloves garlic, minced

1 tsp. cumin powder

1 tsp. chili powder

Salt to taste

2 cups cooked black beans (or use pinto or kidney beans for variety)

To prepare:

Heat the oil in a skillet. Sauté the onion for 1 minute. Add the remaining seasonings and veggies, sautéing for 3 minutes. Add the cooked black beans and sauté for 3 more minutes.

Serves: 4
Prep and cook time: 12 minutes

Coconut Chickpea Curry (with Chicken, Optional)

Ingredients:

2 tbsp. coconut oil

1 large onion, diced

3 cloves garlic, chopped

1 inch of gingerroot, peeled and minced

1 tsp. each of ground cumin, ground turmeric, and garam masala

15.5-oz. can chickpeas, drained and rinsed (or 1 ½ cups cooked
    chickpeas)

14.5-oz. can diced tomatoes (NS)

1 can either full-fat (my preference) or "lite" coconut milk

½ large head of cauliflower, broken into florets

Salt to taste

¼ cup chopped cilantro

To prepare:

Heat the coconut oil in a medium pot. Sauté the onion, garlic, and ginger, cooking until softened, 2 to 3 minutes. Add all of the spices, stirring for about 1 minute. Add the chickpeas, tomatoes, coconut milk, and cauliflower. Bring to a quick boil, then reduce the heat to a simmer and cook for 25 minutes. Be careful when cooking, as it can easily scorch, so stir regularly. Salt to taste. Can serve over whole-grain rice with a topping of fresh cilantro.

Serves: 4 servings as a side dish, 2 or more servings as a main protein
Prep and cook time: 35 minutes

Baked Falafel

Ingredients:

4 cups cooked chickpeas (2 BPA-free 15.5-oz. cans or 2 cups dried chickpeas soaked and then cooked)

3 cloves garlic, crushed

½ cup each of scallions and celery, finely minced

2 eggs, beaten

3 tbsp. tahini

½ tsp. ground cumin

½ tsp. turmeric

1 ½ tsp. salt

¼ tsp. cayenne pepper (NS)

Dash of black pepper

To prepare:

Mash the chickpeas well and combine with all of the other ingredients. I commonly use a food processor to get a thorough mix, but you can do this by hand. Chill well in the fridge—about 30 minutes. Preheat the oven on bake to 400 degrees. With damp hands, form the batter into 1-inch-diameter balls and place onto a well-oiled baking sheet. Bake for about 30 minutes—the balls should look well-formed and slightly brown on top. Don't worry: they will firm up more once they come out of the oven and cool. Serve with Tahini Sauce (see recipe on page 344), in a hummus wrap, or as part of a Mediterranean board.

Serves: 4

Prep and cook time: 80 minutes (including chill time in the refrigerator)

The Meat of the Matter

Fiesta Fish Tacos

Ingredients:

4 fillets of high-quality farm-raised tilapia, flounder, or other low-mercury whitefish

1 tbsp. olive oil

Cajun spice (buy from a company that includes no MSG, caking agents, or sugar)

To prepare:

Preheat the oven to 400 degrees. Rub the fillets on both sides with olive oil, then sprinkle thoroughly on both sides with the Cajun spice. Place on a parchment-paper-lined cookie sheet. Bake for 20 minutes. Serve with Not Your Mother's Slaw (page 337) and Guacamole (page 335).

Serves: 2 to 4

Prep and cook time: 25 minutes

Miso-Glazed Salmon
with Scallions and Sesame Seeds

Ingredients:

2 6-oz. fillets of salmon

2 tbsp. sweet white miso

1 tbsp. toasted sesame oil

1 tsp. honey or maple syrup

Sesame seeds

Scallions

To prepare:

Preheat the oven to 425 degrees. Lay salmon on a parchment-lined baking sheet. In a small bowl whisk together the miso, toasted sesame oil, and honey or maple syrup. Spread a thin layer over each salmon fillet and sprinkle with sesame seeds. Bake in the oven for 15 to 20 minutes. Garnish with thinly sliced scallions.

Serves: 2
Prep and cook time: 30 minutes

Chicken (or Tilapia) Basil Coconut
Curry Tagine

This dish is incredibly easy to make, beyond fantastically flavorful, and every ingredient is good for you—from the light, protein-rich poultry to the heart-healthy fish to the antioxidant, immune-boosting, cholesterol-lowering seasonings (and it is gluten-free!).

Ingredients:

1 tbsp. olive oil

1 yellow onion, chopped

½ red bell pepper, cut into medium chunks (NS)

3 cloves garlic, chopped

3 1/8-inch-thick slices of fresh ginger

1/2 fresh chili pepper, minced (NS)

4 chicken breasts (or 4 pieces tilapia or other low-mercury whitefish)

1/2 cup chopped fresh basil leaves

1/3 cup golden raisins

1 tsp. curry powder

Salt to taste (about 1/8 tsp.)

8-oz. can coconut milk

1 thin stalk of fresh lemongrass

To prepare:

Heat the olive oil in a skillet and sauté the onion for about 1 minute, then add the red pepper, garlic, ginger slices, and chili pepper. Stir for 1 to 2 minutes. Layer the chicken or fish over this, and then top with the basil and raisins. In a measuring cup, dissolve the curry powder and salt into the coconut milk and pour this over everything. Lay the lemongrass on top of it all and cover the pot. Simmer for 20 minutes. Serve hot. I accompany the fish with steamed delicata squash cut into pretty rings and sautéed spinach with garlic. It is an amazingly yum meal!

Serves: 2 to 4
Prep and cook time: 35 minutes

Baked Whole Lemon-Rosemary Chicken

Ingredients:

1 whole organic chicken

1 tsp. salt

1/2 tsp. black pepper

1 lemon

2 sprigs fresh rosemary

To prepare:

Preheat the oven to 400 degrees. Clean the cavity of the chicken, discarding giblets. Thoroughly wash the chicken and pat it dry. Place chicken breast-side up in a roasting pan, cast iron skillet, or baking tray with sides and sprinkle generously with salt and pepper inside and on all of the outside surfaces of the bird. Wash a lemon and poke small holes all around it with a fork or a chopstick. Stuff the rosemary and the lemon into the open cavity. Place the chicken into the oven. After an hour, open the oven and test the chicken for readiness with a meat thermometer. The chicken is done when it registers 165 degrees in the thickest part of the thigh. If not done yet, continue roasting the chicken and check it every 10 minutes until it is done.

Serves: 4
Prep and cook time: 85 minutes

Mediterranean Cilantro Chicken

Ingredients:

4 boneless, skinless chicken breast halves (about 1 ½ to 2 lbs.)

1 tbsp. olive oil

1 large yellow onion, thinly sliced

1 pint cherry tomatoes, halved or whole (NS)

⅓ cup pitted green olives, halved (optional)

1 cup packed fresh cilantro, chopped with any extra stem removed

Juice of 1 lime

Salt and pepper to taste

To prepare:

Season the chicken with salt and pepper on both sides, heat the oil in a large skillet over medium-low heat, and cook the chicken until lightly browned and just cooked through—turning once. It should take 10 to 15 minutes. Transfer the chicken to a plate. Raise the heat to medium and cook onion 5 to 7 minutes until softened. Add tomatoes and olives (if using), and cook until tomatoes soften and release their juices, about 1 to 2 minutes. Put the chicken back into the pan, and layer the vegetables over it. Add the cilantro and lime juice, salt, and pepper, and gently toss into the vegetables. Transfer all to a platter and serve.

Serves: 2
Prep and cook time: 30 minutes

Grilled Tangy Chicken

Ingredients:

4 tbsp. olive oil

2 tbsp. balsamic vinegar and 1 tsp. Dijon mustard, or 4 tbsp. lime juice

Salt

Black pepper

2 chicken breasts, butterflied (you can ask your butcher to do this for you)

To prepare:

In a medium bowl, mix together the olive oil, balsamic vinegar, and Dijon mustard (or lime juice), and a pinch of salt and black pepper. Place the chicken in the bowl and spoon the marinade over the top. Refrigerate for 1 hour up to overnight. Fire up your grill and cook on a medium grill temperature for about 6 minutes on each side, or bake in a 400-degree oven for 25 minutes.

Serves: 2
Prep and cook time: 20 minutes, plus 1 hour to marinate chicken

Baked Walnut-Crusted Chicken

Ingredients:

¾ cup walnuts

½ tsp. salt

⅛ tsp. black pepper

2 chicken breasts, butterflied (you can ask your butcher to do this
for you)

2 tbsp. olive oil

To prepare:

Preheat the oven to 400 degrees. Place walnuts into a food processor
along with salt and pepper. Process until mealy in texture. Transfer to a
flat plate. Lightly coat the chicken breasts with olive oil and dip them into
the walnut mixture until they are fully coated. Place on a baking sheet
and bake in the oven for 30 minutes.

Serves: 2
Prep and cook time: 45 minutes

Satay Chicken, Beef, or Tofu with Spicy Tahini Sauce

Ingredients:

1 lb. boneless, skinless chicken breasts, cut crosswise into 2-inch
pieces, or thighs

For the marinade:

¼ cup fresh lime juice

1 tbsp. gluten-free tamari or Bragg's Aminos

1 tbsp. minced fresh ginger

½ tsp. chili flakes (NS)

4 garlic cloves, minced

Optional: 1 small jalapeño pepper, minced (NS)

Optional after Reboot: 1 tsp. honey or maple syrup

Spicy Tahini Sauce (page 344)

To prepare:

Place the chicken in a shallow baking dish. Whisk together all of the
marinade ingredients and pour over the chicken, then stir to coat. Cover

and place in the fridge for 1 to 4 hours. Place the chicken breast pieces on skewers and grill for about 4 minutes on each side or sauté the chicken in 2 tbsp. coconut oil.

Serve over the Thai Napa Salad, in a Buddha bowl, or in a wrap with Spicy Tahini Sauce (or if past the Reboot and not allergic, peanut sauce).

Serves: 2
Prep and cook time: 20 minutes plus 1 to 4 hours to marinate chicken.

Snack Stash and Sweet Treats

Toasty Savory Nuts and Seeds

While you can purchase decent-quality roasted nuts and seeds, it's easy to toast your own, and they are much fresher.

Ingredients:

1 cup of one or more of the following: raw almonds, walnuts, sunflower, or pumpkin seeds

Optional ingredients:

½ tsp. of any of the following:

Garlic powder

Curry powder

Onion powder

1 sheet of toasted nori seaweed, torn into bite-size pieces, or ¼ cup toasted dulse seaweed pieces

To prepare:

Preheat the oven to 350 degrees. Place nuts or seeds in a thin layer on a cookie sheet. Bake for 10 minutes. Toss on any seasonings you like. Cool to room temperature and then store in a glass jar or container.

Serves: 4
Prep and cook time: 12 minutes

Hippie Mix

Pick several of the following. A good ratio to follow is:
    2 parts mix-and-match nuts (1/2 cup total)
    2 parts mix-and-match seeds (1/2 cup total)
    1 part mix-and-match dried fruit or chocolate (1/4 cup total)

Ingredients to chose from:

Dry-roasted or raw cashews

Dry-roasted or raw almonds

Pecans

Walnuts

Sunflower seeds

Pumpkin seeds

Goji berries

Jujube dates

Mulberries

Raisins

Dark chocolate chips or
    chopped dark chocolate
    (70 percent or darker)

Dried coconut chips

Cacao nibs

Unsweetened dried cherries

Unsweetened dried mango

An optional dash of any of the following:

Cayenne pepper (NS)

Cinnamon

Pinch of salt

To prepare:

Mix together your favorites and enjoy! Can be stored in a container at room temperature for several weeks at a time, so make a big batch to grab and go when you need it.

Serves: 4 to 6
Prep and cook time: 5 minutes

Olive Oil Granola

Ingredients:

- 3 cups rolled oats
- 1 cup raw almonds, chopped or whole
- 3 tbsp. golden flaxseeds
- ½ cup unsweetened shredded coconut
- 1 tsp. salt
- ¼ cup good-quality extra-virgin olive oil
- ¾ cup pure maple syrup
- 1 tbsp. cinnamon
- 2 heaping tbsp. raw cocoa powder

To prepare:

Preheat the oven to 350 degrees. In a large mixing bowl, combine the oats, almonds, flaxseeds, coconut, and salt. Stir together until evenly blended. In a measuring cup, whisk together the olive oil and maple syrup. Pour liquids over the dry ingredients, and stir until the mixture is evenly coated throughout. Sprinkle on the cinnamon and cocoa powder and give the mixture a final stir. Spread the granola evenly on a large baking sheet covered with parchment paper. Bake for about 10 minutes and then give it a good stir with a spatula before cooking another 10 minutes, or until it turns a nice golden-brown color. When it's ready, remove the tray from the oven and cool completely before transferring to a large glass jar.

Serves: 8
Prep and cook time: 30 minutes

Rise and Shine Muffins

Ingredients:

- 5 eggs
- ½ cup coconut, walnut, or sunflower oil
- 2 tsp. vanilla extract

2 cups rice flour

¾ cup organic brown sugar

1 cup rolled oats

1 cup unsweetened, flaked coconut

1 cup golden raisins

1 apple, grated

2 cups grated carrots

½ cup chopped walnuts

2 tsp. ground cinnamon

2 tsp. baking powder

2 tsp. baking soda

¼ tsp. salt

To prepare:

Preheat the oven to 350 degrees. Line a regular-size muffin tin with paper baking cups. Mix all ingredients until this very thick batter is evenly moistened. Fill muffin cups three-quarters of the way. Bake 25 minutes until firm and toasty-brown-colored. Cool in the tins and then on a rack.

Serves: 8 to 16 (makes 12 to 16 muffins)
Prep and cook time: 40 minutes

Berry Chocolate (Antioxidant) Heaven Bowl

Ingredients:

2 pts. mixed fresh berries (I used blackberries, blueberries, and strawberries; cut the latter in quarters)

½ bar of 72 percent or higher dark chocolate chopped into small bits (okay, you can use cacao nibs if you're hard-core Paleo)

2 tbsp. fresh mint, chopped

To prepare:

Mix in a bowl. Serve. Seriously, that's it. Well, enjoy, too!

Serves: 2 to 4
Prep and cook time: 5 minutes

Power Ball Raw "Cookies"

How to Make Power Balls

Select from the categories below, and put all ingredients into a food processor. Chop until it's a pasty, dough-like consistency that you can roll into balls, and do just that, using 2 tbsp. of the mix per ball. A serving is 2 power balls.

This makes about 12 to 16. Store in the fridge for up to a week.

Make Your Own Power Balls

Nuts:	1 or 2 options, 1 cup total: Almonds Pecans Walnuts
Dried Fruit (pitted):	1 or 2 options, ½ cup total: Dried apricots Goji berries Medjool dates Deglet dates Raisins Dried prunes
Protein/Fat:	4 tbsp.: Almond butter (or preferred nut butter) Tahini
Protein Boosts:	Ground flaxseed Chia seeds Sunflower seeds Toasted sesame seeds

Make Your Own Power Balls

Extra Goodness: 2 or 3 options, ¼ cup total:
Shredded coconut
Raw cacao powder
Cinnamon
Vanilla extract
Bee pollen
Spirulina powder

Chocolate Chip Coconut Cookies

Ingredients:

1 ½ cups unsweetened shredded coconut

¾ cup almond flour

½ tsp. baking powder

¼ tsp. salt

1 egg

⅓ cup pure maple syrup

2 heaping tbsp. unrefined coconut oil

1 tsp. pure vanilla extract

¼ cup finely chopped dark chocolate (70 percent or darker)

To prepare:

Preheat the oven to 350 degrees. In a medium mixing bowl, mix together the shredded coconut, almond flour, baking powder, and salt. In a separate small mixing bowl, whisk together the egg, maple syrup, coconut oil (at room temperature), and vanilla extract. Pour the wet ingredients into the dry ingredients and combine. Add the chocolate and stir until evenly distributed throughout. Drop 2 tablespoons per cookie onto cookie sheet, about 1 ½ inches apart. Bake for 15 minutes or until golden brown. Be careful—they go from perfect to burned really fast.

Serves: 8
Prep and cook time: 25 minutes

I Can't Believe It's Chia (Pudding)

Ingredients:

½ cup chia seeds

1 cup cashews, soaked in filtered water for 2 to 8 hours, plus 4 cups
    filtered water (you can substitute 1 cup unsweetened almond milk
    or unsweetened coconut milk for the homemade cashew milk)

7 Medjool dates, pitted

Pinch of salt

¼ teaspoon cinnamon powder

2 tbsp. coconut butter (I skipped this ingredient but I'm sure it would
    make the pudding even creamier!)

4 tsp. vanilla extract

1 vanilla bean (optional)

Fresh berries to serve

Raw honey or maple syrup to serve

To prepare:

Place chia seeds in a medium mixing bowl and set aside. Strain the
cashews and rinse well. Place in an upright blender and add the 4 cups
filtered water, dates, salt, cinnamon, coconut butter (if using), and
vanilla extract. Remove seeds from vanilla bean (if using) and add to the
blender; place pod in bowl with chia seeds. Blend on high speed for
2 minutes and pour into bowl with chia seeds and vanilla bean pod; whisk
well. Let mixture sit for 10 to 15 minutes, whisking every few minutes to
prevent chia seeds from clumping; pudding will thicken fast. Place in the
fridge and chill for 1 hour. Remove from fridge; whisk. Remove vanilla
bean pod (if using), serve chilled, topped with berries and a drizzle of raw
honey or maple syrup if you'd like and you're past the Reboot.

Serves: 2 to 4
Prep and cook time: 90 minutes, including chill time in the refrigerator

Banana-Coconut Soft Serve

Ingredients:

4 frozen bananas (peel and freeze bananas in a freezer-safe glass storage container at least 1 day before)

4 tbsp. full-fat coconut milk

Optional:

1 cup frozen fruit (I love frozen strawberries, black cherries, or mixed tropical fruit, including mango)

Cacao nibs or dark chocolate chips

1 tsp. fresh mint leaves

Vanilla extract

Coconut flakes

To prepare:

Place the bananas and coconut milk into a Vitamix for best results, or place half of these ingredients at a time in your blender, and blend/mix at high speed until creamy. Add additional optional ingredients as desired, and whiz again for 30 seconds. Return the mixture to the glass container and freeze again for about 30 minutes, then serve. If you freeze for longer, allow to soften to your liking at room temperature before serving.

Sample combos:

Banana mango coconut

Banana chocolate chip

Mint chip

Chocolate cherry nib

Serves: 2 to 4
Prep and cook time: 35 minutes

The Flexible Foodie Flourless Chocolate Cake

"I'm fairly certain that chocolate cake is good for you," says my daughter, who also created this recipe, "once in a while . . . just saying." I'm including this, even though it has some sugar, in case you have a birthday party or special event coming up while you're on the Reboot and need something to prepare that's as close to your plan as possible but lets you serve or have something that doesn't feel restrictive to you—or your guests.

This cake is gluten-free, made with coconut oil instead of butter, and contains only six simple ingredients: unsweetened cocoa powder, bittersweet (or semisweet) chocolate, eggs, coconut oil, sugar, and vanilla. It can be served warm with whipped Greek yogurt lightly sweetened with honey and flecks of vanilla bean, or with the Banana-Coconut Soft Serve (page 378). It's outrageously delicious.

Ingredients:

Unsweetened cocoa powder, for dusting

6 organic, free-range eggs

½ cup coconut oil

12 oz. bittersweet chocolate (you can use semisweet if you prefer a slightly sweeter cake)

1 tbsp. vanilla extract

¼ cup sugar

To prepare:

Preheat the oven to 375 degrees. Grease a springform cake pan and dust with unsweetened cocoa powder. Set aside. Separate yolks and whites into 2 mixing bowls. Melt the coconut oil in a medium saucepan over low heat. Add chocolate and whisk until it's fully melted and the mixture is smooth and creamy. Let cool for a few minutes. Whisk egg yolks, vanilla, and chocolate until fully combined. Using an electric mixer, beat egg whites, and slowly add the sugar until stiff peaks form. Fold half of the egg whites into the chocolate mixture, add the remainder, and gently fold in. Pour batter into cake pan and bake for 25 minutes. Let cool for 5 to 10 minutes.

To make whipped Greek yogurt, combine ¾ cup whole Greek yogurt with 1 tbsp. honey and the vanilla seeds from half of a vanilla bean pod (or use ½ tsp. fair-trade vanilla extract). Using an electric mixer, whip for 30 seconds.

Serves: 8
Prep and cook time: 45 minutes

Great Things to Drink

Hot Herbal Tea: Keep a nice supply of herbal teas on hand. Hot and with lemon, or iced, they are a healthful alternative to coffee.

Ginger Lemon Tea: Steep 1 tsp. fresh grated gingerroot in boiling water for 5 minutes. Strain and add lemon. Drink hot. Great for digestion, aches and pains, and cold symptoms, and is a natural anti-inflammatory.

Ginger Lemon Cooler: Squeeze the juice of 1 tbsp. grated fresh ginger and ¼ fresh lemon into sparkling water. Stir and serve as is or with ice.

Love Your Liver Bitters Tonic: Use the bitters support blend (page 162) or Angostura bitters in ¼ cup sparkling water, plain or on the rocks, for a liver detox tonic and after-dinner digestive.

Chai Golden Milk: See page 157. Enjoy hot or iced with almond or coconut milk.

Pomegranate Spritzer: Stir 2 oz. pomegranate concentrate into 6 oz. sparkling water. Antioxidant-boosting.

Clean Green Mojito: Muddle 1 tbsp. fresh mint leaves in 8 oz. sparkling water and add the juice of ¼ fresh lime. Serve over ice.

Lemon-Raspberry-Basil (or Cucumber-Basil) Cooler: Muddle several fresh basil leaves and 4 fresh or frozen red raspberries in sparkling water and add a squeeze of lemon. Serve over ice. If you'd like a cucumber cooler instead, blend ¼ cucumber and ¼ cup water, strain, and add the liquid to the sparkling water with basil and lemon.

Appendix 1

THE SOS SOLUTION LAB TESTS

The testing in this appendix isn't necessary for your success with the SOS Solution. For most women, following the plan thoroughly is all you need for success. However, if you were directed here because of your scores on your questionnaires, or if you are interested in additional testing for personal knowledge, these are the most common tests I use in my medical practice to further uncover the Root Causes of SOS. If after three months on the Replenish Lifestyle you're still having symptoms in any area, I do recommend that you pursue the relevant testing in this appendix, and additional testing if needed as recommended by an integrative or functional medicine doctor.

Testing for Nutritional Deficiencies

Hemoglobin and ferritin: Fatigue, other nutritional deficiencies, and suspected celiac disease (which causes nutritional deficiencies due to poor intestinal absorption) all point to getting your hemoglobin tested, usually done as part of the complete blood count (CBC), if you've not already had this checked. A hemoglobin below 12.0 g/d is suggestive of anemia (lower than this for intense athletes or higher in those who live at high altitudes can be normal). When below normal, also get checked for serum ferritin, the storage form of iron. A normal ferritin range is between 50 and 100 mcg/L. If low, this is indicative of chronically low iron. However, if it is high, this indicates chronic inflammation and is considered a marker of SOS.

Vitamin D: Americans are notoriously low in vitamin D, so I routinely test my patients. An optimal 25 (OH) vitamin D level is between 50 and 80 ng/mL. If you are low in vitamin D (<50 ng/mL), spending more time in the sunshine is certainly healthful, but it's not enough—even if you live in the Caribbean—to bring your level to an optimal range anytime soon, so supplementation is in order (see page 167). Your vitamin D level can be rechecked twelve weeks after you begin supplementing to see if you're getting enough; if not, the dose can be raised and your levels checked again in another twelve weeks, and so on, until you are optimized.

Vitamin B_{12} and folate deficiency: If you are having numbness or tingling in any of your limbs or face, if you are generally nutritionally deficient, if you've been a vegan or vegetarian for more than two years, if you've been on an anti-reflux medication for more than six months, or if you have large red blood cells on your CBC, I recommend getting tested for vitamin B_{12}. Since vitamin B_{12} and folate deficiencies often coexist and are sometimes hard to tell apart, testing for both is recommended. A healthy B_{12} result is above 450 pg/mL, which you'll find is higher than the lower limit of lab range you'll see on your lab report because that lower level is too low to support health. A normal folate concentration is >4 ng/mL. Because vitamin B_{12} blood tests are notoriously inaccurate, and may be normal in up to 5 percent of people with a vitamin B_{12} deficiency, I also check for specific metabolic products of B_{12} and folate at the same time, which can accumulate in these deficiencies, and which are more accurate tests. These are methylmalonic acid (MMA) and homocysteine (discussed opposite). The homocysteine concentration may be elevated even before B_{12} and folate tests are abnormal, giving you an early indication of these deficiencies. Of note, even if vitamin B_{12} testing is normal, if symptoms suggest a deficiency, then supplementing for a few months and seeing if symptoms improve is recommended.

Test	What It Is	Optimal Range
Ferritin	The storage form of iron	50 to 200 mcg/L
Folate	Folate, or the synthetic form, folic acid, is a B vitamin found in leafy green vegetables and other sources, and is important for forming our genetic material and cell division, among other roles in the body.	>4 ng/mL
Hemoglobin	The oxygen-carrying capacity of your red blood cells	12 to 15.5 g/dL
Methylmalonic acid	A metabolite of vitamin B_{12} used as a blood test for adequate B_{12} and folate	70 to 270 nmol/L
25-hydroxy-vitamin D	Technically a hormone, but referred to as a vitamin because we need it in the diet. Involved in thousands of biological activities and particularly important for bone, mood, and immune system health.	50 to 80 ng/mL
Vitamin B_{12}	A water-soluble vitamin in the B-complex family involved primarily in nervous system functioning	450 to 800 pg/mL

Testing for Chronic Inflammation

Test	What It Is	Optimal Range
Highly sensitive C-reactive protein (hs-CRP)	A protein produced by your liver in response to inflammation. It is tested for by checking blood levels of highly sensitive CRP (hs-CRP).	<1.0 mg/L

Test	What It Is	Optimal Range
Homocysteine	An amino acid that occurs in the body as a metabolite in protein breakdown and other metabolic processes; important for DNA methylation and detoxification. High levels are particularly concerning because they've been associated with pregnancy problems (increased risk of miscarriage, pregnancy-induced hypertension, placental abruption, gestational diabetes), autoimmune diseases, and risks of heart disease, stroke, and Alzheimer's—not necessarily because it causes these problems, but because it is a marker of low folate status (as well as vitamin B_{12} status).	< 10.0 μmol/dL
MTHFR mutation	A gene that produces an enzyme necessary for the metabolism of folate and B_{12}, for methylation, detoxification, and protection from oxidative stress damage to cells and DNA. Two mutations ("SNPs") are medically important: the C677T and A1298c variants. The SNPs are exceptionally common: as many as 30 percent of the population has at least one, and at least 10 percent has a more complex combination of both. Variations in this gene increase your risk for all of the problems I discussed with elevated homocysteine, because this gene variation leads to the elevated homocysteine.	Most people have variations in these genes.

Blood Sugar Testing

Test	What It Is	Optimal Range
Fasting glucose	A measure of your body's fasting blood sugar, a good marker of blood sugar balance, inflammation, and health risk	70 to 85 mg/dL
Fasting insulin	A measure of your body's insulin level, a good marker for insulin resistance, inflammation, and health risk	2 to 5 μIU/dL
HDL	High-density lipoprotein is a protective form of cholesterol	>60 mg/dL
Hemoglobin A1C	An average of the impact of three months of blood sugar on your red blood cells	<5.2%

Gut Imbalances Testing

Celiac disease: I usually recommend celiac disease testing only when symptoms have improved off of gluten and I can't otherwise convince someone to stay off of it. The gold standard test is an endoscopy with a biopsy, but it's invasive and usually unnecessary. The blood tests are a good alternative. Positive celiac antibody testing is practically definitive for having celiac disease. However, negative test results don't rule out celiac; they are notoriously false negative. That's where genetic testing comes in handy. Most people who have celiac have the celiac HLA DQ2 and HLA DQ8 genes. In a gluten-sensitive patient with a lot of symptoms or an autoimmune disease, I consider the presence of these genes enough of a reason to permanently remove gluten from the diet. However, not everyone who has these genes has or develops celiac, so be careful about overdiagnosing yourself! In truth, though, the proof is in the pudding—if you do better off of gluten, stay off of it! See chapter 8 for a more detailed discussion on whether and when to reintroduce gluten after the SOS Solution Reboot.

Leaky gut: Intestinal hyperpermeability ("leaky gut") does not require testing. If you have symptoms of leaky gut, the best thing to do is the SOS Solution gut repair. However, testing is available and involves a lactulose-mannitol challenge, in which you ingest a small amount of each of these two sugars and then have a urine collection analyzed for how much of each was excreted. A high lactulose ratio indicates a leaky gut.

SIBO: The SIBO breath test involves drinking a lactulose preparation, then exhaling into a device that can measure the gases produced as a result, which indicate the presence or absence, depending on the result, of the type of bacteria in your upper gut. I only recommend doing these tests if you have symptoms that haven't cleared up on the SOS Solution. If you are sensitive to dairy, ingesting lactulose can exacerbate your symptoms, so this might not be optimal for you.

Testing for Stealth Infections

Epstein-Barr virus (EBV) and cytomegalovirus (CMV): Testing includes a complete EBV acute panel and a chronic infection panel, plus a CMV panel. Positive tests for *current* infections will be indicated on your lab results with positive IgM results.

Lyme disease: Lyme disease testing is complex and controversial. I start out by testing an ELISA, Western Blot, lyme PCR, and lyme coinfections panel. If you have positive test results, review antibiotic treatment with your primary care provider.

H. pylori: This common stomach bug is asymptomatic in most people and doesn't routinely need to be treated if not causing stomach symptoms. However, if you do have Hashimoto's and a history of known *H. pylori* infection, or frequent indigestion, it can be worthwhile to get an *H. pylori* breath test, as there is a possible correlation. Breath testing is the gold standard for active, current infection.

Adrenal/SOS Testing

Serum cortisol: Depending on the severity of your symptoms, it may be advisable to test for true adrenal insufficiency, or another condition affecting the adrenal glands or pituitary. Serum cortisol testing should be done before 9:00 A.M. A healthy cortisol level drawn at that time of day is between 10 and 15 mcg/dL (slightly higher for women over fifty). An abnormal result usually requires medical care, which can be used in conjunction with the SOS Solution.

Cortisol curve: The twenty-four-hour salivary cortisol test is a specialty test commonly recommended by integrative and functional medicine practitioners. It's done at home and is based on saliva samples gathered at four different times through the day and evening. The test is highly influenced by stress, perceived stress, diet, and other circumstances at the time of testing, so it should only be considered a snapshot, not definitive or a long-term pattern. You can assess your results by comparing your graph to the normal cortisol rhythm that is plotted next to your test result.

To learn more about how to access lab testing if you have difficulty finding it in your community, visit avivaromm.com/adrenal-thyroid-revolution.

Appendix 2

WORKiNG WITH YOUR HEALTH PRACTITIONER— OR FINDING ANOTHER

Having a supportive licensed health practitioner on your side can be an invaluable asset on your wellness journey. Unfortunately, most conventional M.D.s are sorely undertrained in the recognition and treatment of the symptoms that brought you to this book, and lack comprehensive knowledge of diagnosing and properly treating hypothyroidism. Some are open to the conversation but are (reasonably) skeptical of inadequately studied tests and treatments. Here are some tips for making it work with your M.D.:

1. Schedule an appointment specifically to discuss your current concerns, ideas, health care needs, and requests (as opposed to trying to fit this into your annual visit, for example, or tagging it onto a Pap smear or sick visit for another condition).

2. Before the appointment, think through what you're asking for help with and why, and write your key points in a notebook or on index cards. Use this as a script when you go to the doctor. This will help you to keep focused and calm, as well as make you look prepared and organized, like you've given this some thought and research.

3. At your appointment, let your doctor know that you respect her training and credentials, and so appreciate her knowledge and honesty; also let her know you'd like to learn to become the CEO of your own health, and more of an active partner in your health care, that you really welcome her partnership and advice, and that you'd love to work with a doctor who sees you this way and enjoys working collaboratively.

4. Bring a few references and resources with you. For example, at avivaromm.com/adrenal-thyroid-revolution you can download a summary of important labs and a page of medical references supporting their value for women with your set of health concerns. Or bring this book to your appointment. Let your doctor know you've been doing some "homework" on your symptoms, and you think that the tests you're asking for will shed some light on what's going on in a way that will improve your health. Ultimately, that's your doctor's goal, too! We all want to see our patients thrive in health and happiness! And we do love having positive relationships with our patients.

However, if you are unable to have an honest conversation with your doctor, if you feel your doctor is not listening or is condescending, then that's another issue—and it would probably serve you best to find another provider. You should be able to have mutually respectful conversations with your care provider, to get the answers you are seeking, and to be able to explore your concerns.

Finding the Right "Alternative" Practitioner for You

You might have better luck finding a doctor who understands what you're looking for by visiting the websites of the American Board of Integrative Medicine, American Board of Integrative and Holistic Medicine, or Institute of Functional Medicine—all have a practitioner directory. Look for someone trained as an M.D. with a residency in internal medicine, family medicine, gynecology, or endocrinology to ensure that they are appropriately medically trained to address your specific concerns. Nurse practitioners (N.P.s), advance practice registered nurses (A.P.R.N.s), and certified nurse midwives

(C.N.M.s) are also excellent options, and in most states, A.P.R.N.s and N.P.s are able to test, diagnose, and prescribe.

Naturopathic doctors (N.D.s) are also a fantastic option if they are licensed in your state. In states where they aren't licensed, you'll still find practitioners using the credential, but they may have no more than distance learning or a few weekends of training—so only work with an N.D. who has trained at one of the four-year accredited naturopathic colleges and is licensed in your state.

If you are working with an integrative or functional medicine practitioner, be certain you understand the extent of their training and experience, and don't hesitate to ask questions about the evidence behind the testing and treatments they are offering. There is use of unregulated, unsubstantiated techniques, devices, and treatments—even among M.D.s. Your practitioner should be able to provide the rationale for their use of tests and therapies, and should be able to give you a realistic appraisal of effectiveness. Your practitioner should also be willing to disclose their profit margins on any tests or supplements they are providing; while it is reasonable for practitioners to set up a profit-based business model, even in health care, this should be openly acknowledged, as it can influence recommendations made to patients in many practices.

Acupuncturists, herbalists, massage therapists, nutritionists, health coaches, yoga teachers, and other integrative practitioners can also be invaluable team members in your healing process. Similarly, make sure they are appropriately trained to offer the services they are providing.

With any practitioner, if you feel disrespected, if you feel you're being sold a bill of goods, or if there is excessive polarization *against* conventional medicine that could be keeping you from getting appropriate conventional care, find another provider. Above all, trust your intuition and judgment and practice good common sense. You're probably right.

RESOURCES

For more inspiration come visit me at my website, avivaromm.com, where you can join the Adrenal Thyroid Revolution Community and find extra resources that just couldn't fit into the book. Come on over and spend more time with me and an amazing community of women at avivaromm .com/adrenal-thyroid-revolution. Can't wait to hang out with you there!

Herbs

Adrenal Thyroid Solution Supplement Store—avivaromm.com
    /adrenal-thyroid-revolution
Frontier Natural Products Co-op—frontiercoop.com
Gaia Herbs—gaiaherbs.com
Herb Pharm—herb-pharm.com
Mountain Rose Herbs—mountainroseherbs.com

Vitamin, Mineral, Probiotic, and Fish Oil Supplements

Carlson Labs (fish oil)—carlsonlabs.com
Jarrow Formulas—jarrow.com
MegaFood—megafood.com
Nordic Naturals (fish oil)—nordicnaturals.com
NOW Foods—nowfoods.com
Rainbow Light—rainbowlight.com

Practitioner-Level Supplements

Designs for Health—designsforhealth.com
Integrative Therapeutics—integrativepro.com
Klaire Labs—klaire.com
Metagenics—metagenics.com
Pure Encapsulations—pureencapsulations.com

Good Food You Can Order at Home

Maine Seaweed—theseaweedman.com
Thrive Market—thrivemarket.com
Vital Choice Seafood—vitalchoice.com

Food and Fish Safety

EWG—ewg.org/foodscores AND ewg.org/foodnews
Monterey Bay Aquarium—seafoodwatch.org
NRDC—nrdc.org/stories/smart-seafood-buying-guide

Personal Care and Cosmetics

Environmental Working Group—ewg.org/skindeep
Seventh Generation—seventhgeneration.com

Home Cleaning

Ecover—us.ecover.com
Environmental Working Group—ewg.org/skindeep
Real Simple—realsimple.com
Seventh Generation—seventhgeneration.com

Online Streaming Yoga Classes

YogaGlo—yogaglo.com

Acknowledgments

As solitary as the art of writing is, particularly a book, in truth it takes a village. I am deeply grateful for mine: Tracy Romm, my husband for thirty-two years, who didn't mind the DO NOT DISTURB sign hanging around my neck, who kept the rest of our world afloat for several months while I wrote, and who said that the sound of my typing in bed while he slept was comforting because it meant I was nearby. He also spell-checked every word.

My daughter, Mima, who gave me her beacons of insight, wisdom, encouragement, and good humor, reviewing and thoughtfully commenting on every aspect of this book, and kept me on point. Working with you was the very best part.

My dear friends Jeff Jump, M.D., and Robin Gellman, L.Ac., who said, "Yes, I'd love to"—and meant it—when I asked them to review my manuscript in the midst of their busy lives. A deep bow to Megan Liebmann and Amanda Swan for holding down the online and practice forts while I wrote nonstop.

A special shout-out to the "team behind the book": Alisa Bowman, who provided fabulous editorial coaching and reminded me to trust my instincts; my agent, Celeste Fine; her assistant, John Maas, and JJ Virgin for the Celeste introduction; my ever-encouraging editor, Gideon Weil (!), and his bright and generous assistant, Sydney Rogers, at HarperOne, for their belief that this book needed to be in the hands of women readers, and for helping to make that happen.

Gratitude to the special colleagues in my extended health and business community who share the belief that there is room and need for all of us to raise our voices and who have been especially supportive in a variety of personal and professional ways: Pilar Gerasimo, Gabrielle Bernstein, Kris Carr, Kelly Brogan, M.D., Lisa Rankin, M.D., Izaballa Wentz, Ph.D., Terri Cole, Jonathan Fields, Michael Wentz, and Michael Fishman, to name a few who really stepped up.

To my children, Iyah, Yemima, Forest, and Naomi, for being fabulous adults with whom I can discuss ideas and who challenge and inspire me. You are the bedrock of and healing sources in my life. To Sylvia and Eric, who have added more love to our family, and my grandbabies, who keep me out of SOS with laughter and deliciousness. To Michelle Collins, for being my soul sister, for always lifting me up, and for being my personal comedy hour in this life. You are the best medicine.

Finally, a deep thank-you to the women in my practice, courses, and online world who give my life meaning, my work purpose, my heart gratitude, and my mind inspiration. This book was written for you, and with you in mind every step of the way.

References

In order to maximize the amount of information in this book, in the setting of publisher-driven book length constraints, I chose to bring you more content, which required limiting the references provided herein. I've selected seventy key references. You'll find the complete, extensive medical and scientific bibliography of over 500 up-to-date references, for free, at avivaromm.com/adrenal-thyroid-revolution, should you wish to review the scientific evidence upon which the book is firmly based. *Thank you for your understanding, and for joining me in the Adrenal Thyroid Revolution!*

Adam, T. C., and E. S. Epel. 2007. "Stress, eating and the reward system." *Physiology & Behavior* 91 (4): 449–58.

Ader, R., Cohen, N., and Felten, D. 1995. "Psychoneuroimmunology: Interactions between the nervous system and the immune system." *Lancet* 345 (8942): 99–103.

Alcock, J., C. C. Maley, and C. A. Aktipis. 2014. "Is eating behavior manipulated by the gastrointestinal microbiota? Evolutionary pressures and potential mechanisms." *BioEssays* 36 (10): 940–49.

American Psychological Association. 2013. *Stress in America: Missing the Healthcare Connection.* Retrieved October 13, 2014. https://www.apa.org/news/press/releases /stress/2012/full-report.pdf.

Anderson, S., K. M. Pedersen, N. H. Bruun, and P. Laurberg. 2002. "Narrow individual variations in the serum T(4) and T(3) in normal subjects: A clue to the understanding of subclinical thyroid disease." *Journal of Clinical Endocrinology & Metabolism* 87 (3): 1068–72.

Aoki, Y., R. M. Belin, R. Clickner, R. Jeffries, L. Phillips, and K. R. Mahaffey. 2007. "Serum TSH and total T₄ in the United States population and their association with participant characteristics: National Health and Nutrition Examination Survey (NHANES 1999–2002)." *Thyroid* 17 (12): 1211–23.

Aschbacher, K., S. Kornfield, M. Picard, et al. 2014. "Chronic stress increases vulnerability to diet-related abdominal fat, oxidative stress, and metabolic risk." *Psychoneuroendocrinology* 46: 14–22. Retrieved August 16, 2016.

Aschbacher, K., A. O'Donovan, O. M. Wolkowitz, F. S. Dhabhar, Y. Su, and E. Epel. 2013. "Good stress, bad stress and oxidative stress: Insights from anticipatory cortisol reactivity." *Psychoneuroendocrinology* 38 (9): 1698-1708.

Aschbacher, K., M. Rodriguez-Fernandez, H. V. Wietmarschen, et al. 2014. "The hypothalamic-pituitary-adrenal-leptin axis and metabolic health: A systems approach to resilience, robustness and control." *Interface Focus* 4 (5): 20140020.

Astin, J. A., S. L. Shapiro, D. M. Eisenberg, and K. L. Forys. 2003. "Mind-body medicine: State of the science, implications for practice." *Journal of the American Board of Family Medicine* 16 (2): 131-47.

Backhaus, J., K. Junghanns, and F. Hohagen. 2004. "Sleep disturbances are correlated with decreased morning awakening salivary cortisol." *Psychoneuroendocrinology* 29 (9): 1184-91.

Barzilai, O., Y. Sherer, M. Ram, D. Izhaky, J. Anaya, and Y. Shoenfeld. 2007. "Epstein Barr virus and cytomegalovirus in autoimmune diseases: Are they truly notorious? A preliminary report." *Annals of the New York Academy of Sciences* 1108 (1): 567-77.

Bischoff, S. C., G. Barbara, W. Buurman, et al. 2014. "Intestinal permeability: A new target for disease prevention and therapy." *BMC Gastroenterology* 14: 189.

Black, P. H. 2006. "The inflammatory consequences of psychologic stress: Relationship to insulin resistance, obesity, atherosclerosis and diabetes mellitus, type II." *Medical Hypotheses* 67 (4): 879-91.

Camilleri, M., K. Madsen, R. Spiller, B. G. Meerveld, and G. N. Verne. 2012. "Intestinal barrier function in health and gastrointestinal disease." *Neurogastroenterology & Motility* 24 (6): 503-12.

Ch'ng, C. L., M. K. Jones, and J. G. Kingham. 2007. "Celiac disease and autoimmune thyroid disease." *Clinical Medicine & Research* 5 (3): 184-92.

Chrousos, G. 2005. "Stress and disorders of the stress system." *Nature Reviews Endocrinology* 5 (July): 374-81.

Clarke, S. F., E. F. Murphy, K. Nilaweera, et al. 2012. "The gut microbiota and its relationship to diet and obesity." *Gut Microbes* 3 (3): 186-202.

Cohen, S., D. Janicki-Deverts, and G. E. Miller. 2007. "Psychological stress and disease." *Journal of the American Medical Association* 298 (14): 1685-87.

Diamanti-Kandarakis, E., J. P. Bourguignon, L. C. Giudice, et al. 2009. "Endocrine-disrupting chemicals: An Endocrine Society scientific statement." *Endocrine Reviews* 30 (4): 293-342.

Dinan, T. G., and J. F. Cryan. 2012. "Regulation of the stress response by the gut microbiota: Implications for psychoneuroendocrinology." *Psychoneuroendocrinology* 37 (9): 1369-78.

Duntas, L. H. 2008. "Environmental factors and autoimmune thyroiditis." *Nature Clinical Practice Endocrinology & Metabolism* 4 (8): 454-60.

Dusenbery, M. 2015. "Is medicine's gender bias killing young women?" *Pacific Standard*, March 23. Retrieved August 10, 2016. https://psmag.com/is-medicine-s-gender-bias -killing-young-women-4cab6946ab5c#.tf4y6osaq.

Elks, C. M., and J. Francis. 2010. "Central adiposity, systemic inflammation, and the metabolic syndrome." *Current Hypertension Reports* 12: 99-104.

Emami, A., R. Nazem, and M. Hedayati. 2014. "Is association between thyroid hormones and gut peptides, ghrelin and obestatin, able to suggest new regulatory relation between the HPT axis and gut?" *Regulatory Peptides* 189: 17-21.

Epel, E., J. Daubenmier, J. T. Moskowitz, S. Folkman, and E. Blackburn. 2009. "Can meditation slow rate of cellular aging? Cognitive stress, mindfulness, and telomeres." *Annals of the New York Academy of Sciences* 1172 (1): 34-53.

Fasano, A. 2011. "Leaky gut and autoimmune diseases." *Clinical Reviews in Allergy & Immunology* 42 (1): 71-78.

Fujinami, R. S., M. G. Herrath, U. Christen, and J. L. Whitton. 2006. "Molecular mimicry, bystander activation, or viral persistence: Infections and autoimmune disease." *Clinical Microbiology Reviews* 19 (1): 80-94.

García-Bueno, B., J. R. Caso, and J. C. Leza. 2008. "Stress as a neuroinflammatory condition in brain: Damaging and protective mechanisms." *Neuroscience & Biobehavioral Reviews* 32 (6): 1136-51.

García-Prieto, M. D., F. J. Tébar, F. Nicolás, E. Larqué, S. Zamora, and M. Garaulet. 2007. "Cortisol secretary pattern and glucocorticoid feedback sensitivity in women from a Mediterranean area: Relationship with anthropometric characteristics, dietary intake and plasma fatty acid profile." *Clinical Endocrinology* (Oxford) 66 (2): 185-91.

Glaser, R. 2005. "Stress-associated immune dysregulation and its importance for human health: A personal history of psychoneuroimmunology." *Brain, Behavior, and Immunity* 19 (1): 3-11.

Goichot, B., and S. H. Pearce. 2012. "Subclinical thyroid disease: Time to enter the age of evidence-based medicine." *Thyroid* 22 (8): 765-68.

Hadhazy, A. 2010. "Think twice: How the gut's 'second brain' influences mood and well-being." *Scientific American*, February 12, 2010. Accessed September 6, 2016. http://www.scientificamerican.com/article/gut-second-brain.

Haentjens, P., A. Van Meerhaeghe, K. Poppe, and B. Velkeniers. 2008. "Subclinical thyroid dysfunction and mortality: An estimate of relative and absolute excess all-cause mortality based on time-to-event data from cohort studies." *European Journal of Endocrinology* 159 (3): 329-41.

Helfand, M. 2004. "Screening for subclinical thyroid dysfunction in nonpregnant adults: A summary of the evidence for the U.S. Preventive Services Task Force." *Annals of Internal Medicine* 140 (2): 128-41. doi:10.7326/0003-4819-140-2-200401200-00015.

Hennig, B., L. Ormsbee, C. J. McClain, et al. 2012. "Nutrition can modulate the toxicity of environmental pollutants: Implications in risk assessment and human health." *Environmental Health Perspectives* 120 (6): 771-74.

Iwata, M., K. T. Ota, and R. S. Duman. 2013. "The inflammasome: Pathways linking psychological stress, depression, and systemic illnesses." *Brain, Behavior, and Immunity* 31: 105-14.

Jacobs, E. J., C. C. Newton, Y. Wang, et al. 2010. "Waist circumference and all-cause mortality in a large US cohort." *Archives of Internal Medicine* 170: 1293.

Jin, C., and R. A. Flavell. 2013. "Innate sensors of pathogen and stress: Linking inflammation to obesity." *Journal of Allergy and Clinical Immunology* 132 (2): 287-94.

Kalantaridou, S., A. Makrigiannakis, E. Zoumakis, and G. Chrousos. 2004. "Stress and the female reproductive system." *Journal of Reproductive Immunology* 62 (1-2): 61-68.

Kau, A. L., P. P. Ahern, N. W. Griffin, A. L. Goodman, and J. I. Gordon. "Human nutrition, the gut microbiome and the immune system." *Nature* 474: 327-36.

Knutson, K. L., K. Spiegel, P. Penev, and E. Van Cauter. 2007. "The metabolic consequences of sleep deprivation." *Sleep Medicine Reviews* 11 (3): 163-78.

Korte, S. M., J. M. Koolhaas, J. C. Wingfield, and B. S. McEwen. 2005. "The Darwinian concept of stress: Benefits of allostasis and costs of allostatic load and the trade-offs in health and disease." *Neuroscience & Biobehavioral Reviews* 29 (1): 3-38.

Koster, A., M. F. Leitzmann, A. Schatzkin, et al. 2008. "Waist circumference and mortality." *American Journal of Epidemiology* 167: 1465.

Kris-Etherton, P., R. H. Eckel, B. V. Howard, S. S. Jeor, and T. L. Bazzarre. 2001. "Lyon Diet heart study: Benefits of a Mediterranean-style, National Cholesterol Education Program/American Heart Association Step I dietary pattern on cardiovascular disease." *Circulation* 103 (13): 1823-25.

Lustig, R. H., L. A. Schmidt, and C. D. Brindis. 2012. "Public health: The toxic truth about sugar." *Nature* 482 (7383): 27-29.

McDermott, M. T., and E. C. Ridgway. 2001. "Subclinical hypothyroidism is mild thyroid failure and should be treated." *Journal of Clinical Endocrinology & Metabolism* 86 (10): 4585-90.

McEwen, B. S., and P. J. Gianaros. 2011. "Stress- and allostasis-induced brain plasticity." *Annual Review of Medicine* 62 (1): 431-45.

Mechiel, S. M., J. M. Koolhaas, J. C. Wingfield, and B. S. McEwen. 2005. "The Darwinian concept of stress: Benefits of allostasis and costs of allostatic load and the trade-offs in health and disease." *Neuroscience & Biobehavioral Reviews* 29 (1): 3-38. doi:10.1016/j.neubiorev.2004.08.009.

Miller, G. E., S. Cohen, and A. K. Ritchey. 2002. "Chronic psychological stress and the regulation of pro-inflammatory cytokines: A glucocorticoid-resistance model." *Health Psychology* 21 (6): 531-41. doi:10.1037/0278-6133.21.6.531.

Miller, M. D., K. M. Crofton, D. C. Rice, and R. T. Zoeller. 2009. "Thyroid-disrupting chemicals: Interpreting upstream biomarkers of adverse outcomes." *Environmental Health Perspectives* 117 (7): 1033-41.

Montgomery, J. 2012. "Survival mode and evolutionary mismatch." Retrieved May 12, 2016. *Psychology Today.* https://www.psychologytoday.com/blog/the-embodied-mind/201212/survival-mode-and-evolutionary-mismatch.

Morris, Z. S., S. Wooding, and J. Grant. 2011. "The answer is 17 years, what is the question: Understanding time lags in translational research." *Journal of the Royal Society of Medicine* 104 (12): 510-20.

Nabi, H., M. Kivimaki, G. D. Batty, et al. 2013. "Increased risk of coronary heart disease among individuals reporting adverse impact of stress on their health: The Whitehall II prospective cohort study." *European Heart Journal* 34 (34): 2697-705.

Neeland, I. J., C. R. Ayers, A. K. Rohatgi, et al. 2013. "Associations of visceral and abdominal subcutaneous adipose tissue with markers of cardiac and metabolic risk in obese adults." *Obesity* (9): E439-47.

O'Connor, D., H. Hendrickx, T. Dadd, et al. 2009. "Cortisol awakening rise in middle-aged women in relation to psychological stress." *Psychoneuroendocrinology* 34 (10): 1486-94.

Raison, C. L., L. Capuron, and A. H. Miller. 2006. "Cytokines sing the blues: Inflammation and the pathogenesis of depression." *Trends in Immunology* 27 (1): 24-31.

Raison, C. L., and A. H. Miller. 2013. "Malaise, melancholia and madness: The evolutionary legacy of an inflammatory bias." *Brain, Behavior, and Immunity* 31: 1-8.

Rodondi, N., W. P. den Elzen, D. C. Bauer, et al. 2010. "Subclinical hypothyroidism and the risk of coronary heart disease and mortality." *Journal of the American Medical Association* 304 (12): 1365-74.

Ros, E., M. A. Martínez-González, R. Estruch, et al. 2014. "Mediterranean diet and cardiovascular health: Teachings of the PREDIMED study." *Advances in Nutrition* 5 (3): 330S-336S.

Rutters, F., S. L. Fleur, S. Lemmens, J. Born, M. Martens, and T. Adam. 2012. "The hypothalamic-pituitary-adrenal axis, obesity, and chronic stress exposure: Foods and HPA axis." *Current Obesity Reports* 1 (4): 199-207.

Seeman, T. E., L. F. Berkman, P. A. Charpentier, D. G. Blazer, M. S. Albert, and M. E. Tinetti. 1995. "Behavioral and psychosocial predictors of physical performance: MacArthur Studies of Successful Aging." *Journals of Gerontology Series A: Biological Sciences and Medical Sciences* 50 (4): M177-83.

Segerstrom, S., and G. Miller. 2004. "Psychological stress and the human immune system: A meta-analytic study of 30 years of inquiry." *Psychological Bulletin* 130 (4): 601-30.

Spiegel, K., E. Tasali, R. Leproult, and E. V. Cauter. 2009. "Effects of poor and short sleep on glucose metabolism and obesity risk." *Nature Reviews Endocrinology* 5 (5): 253-61.

Taylor, S., L. C. Klein, B. P. Lewis, T. L. Gruenewald, R. A. Gurung, and J. A. Updegraff. 2000. "Biobehavioral responses to stress in females: Tend-and-befriend, not fight-or-flight." *Psychological Review* 107 (3): 411-29.

Valls-Pedret, C., A. Sala-Vila, M. Serra-Mir, et al. 2015. "Mediterranean diet and age-related cognitive decline." *JAMA Internal Medicine* 175 (7): 1094-103.

Walsh, S., and L. Rau. 2000. "Autoimmune diseases: A leading cause of death among young and middle-aged women in the United States." *American Journal of Public Health* 90 (9): 1463-66.

Wartofsky, L., and R. A. Dickey. 2005. "The evidence for a narrower thyrotropin reference range is compelling." *Journal of Clinical Endocrinology & Metabolism* 90 (9): 5483-88.

Weiss, G., L. T. Goldsmith, R. N. Taylor, D. Bellet, and H. S. Taylor. 2009. "Inflammation in reproductive disorders." *Reproductive Sciences* 16 (2): 216-29.

Zellner, D. A., S. Loaiza, Z. Gonzalez, et al. 2006. "Food selection changes under stress." *Physiology & Behavior* 87 (4): 789-93.

Index